The Great Stink of Paris
and the Nineteenth-Century Struggle
against Filth and Germs

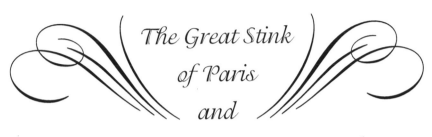

The Great Stink of Paris and the Nineteenth-Century Struggle against Filth and Germs

DAVID S. BARNES

Johns Hopkins University Press
Baltimore

Johns Hopkins Paperback edition, 2018
2 4 6 8 9 7 5 3 1

Johns Hopkins University Press
2715 North Charles Street
Baltimore, Maryland 21218-4363
www.press.jhu.edu

The Library of Congress has cataloged the hardcover edition of this book as follows:
Barnes, David S.
The great stink of Paris and the nineteenth-century struggle against filth
and germs / David S. Barnes.
p. cm.
Includes bibliographical references and index.
ISBN 0-8018-8349-0 (hardcover : alk. paper)
1. Social medicine—Europe—History. 2. Social medicine—France—History.
3. Diseases—Europe—History. 4. Diseases—France—History. I. Title.
[DNLM: 1. Public Health—history—France. 2. Health Knowledge, Attitudes,
Practice—France. 3. Communicable Disease Control—history—France.
4. Sanitation—history—France. 5. Bacteriology—history—France.
WA 11 GF7 2006]
RA418.3.E85B37 2006
306.4′61—dc22   2005023385

A catalog record for this book is available from the British Library.

ISBN-13: 978-1-4214-2565-8
ISBN-10: 1-4214-2565-3

Special discounts are available for bulk purchases of this book.
For more information, please contact Special Sales at 410-516-6936 or
specialsales@press.jhu.edu.

To Joan

Contents

Acknowledgments

I am grateful to the editors of *Historical Reflections / Réflexions historiques* and to the University of Minnesota Press for permission to reprint material previously published in "Scents and Sensibilities: Disgust and the Meanings of Odors in Late Nineteenth-Century Paris," *Historical Reflections / Réflexions historiques* 28 (2002): 21–49, and in "Confronting Sensory Crisis in the Great Stinks of London and Paris," in William A. Cohen and Ryan Johnson, eds., *Filth: Dirt, Disgust, and Modern Life* (Minneapolis: University of Minnesota Press, 2005). Research for this project was generously funded by the National Endowment for the Humanities; the National Institutes of Health (Publication Grant #7G13LM007212-02); the Georges Lurcy Educational and Charitable Trust; the William F. Milton Fund, the Joseph H. Clark Fund, and the Faculty of Arts and Sciences of Harvard University; and by the School of Arts and Sciences of the University of Pennsylvania.

The intellectual and personal debts I have incurred in the course of the research and writing of this book seem to be proportional to the length of its gestation. In France, Joël Surcouf and Pascal Mory helped guide me through various archival thickets, as did the archivists and librarians at the Bibliothèque administrative de la ville de Paris, the Archives de la Préfecture de Police in Paris, the Archives départementales de la Côte-d'Or in Dijon, and the Archives municipales du Havre. Lion Murard and Patrick Zylberman encouraged and challenged me and gave freely of both their expertise and their advice. The faculty of the Medicine, Health, and Society Research Center (CERMES) in Paris extended a warm welcome to me and gave my work a supportive and critical reception. Alain Corbin not only inspired much of this project with his pathbreaking work on the history of senses, sensibilities, and *mentalités* but also encouraged and advised me in the early stages of my research on the intersection of disgust and bacteriology in the late nineteenth century.

David Nickles, Lynda Yast, Theresa Levitt, and Elly Truitt provided research assistance at critical stages. Judith Lajoie, Stephanie Nasson, Stacey DiCicco, Yuri Hospodar, and Patricia Johnson contributed invaluable administrative help. Michael Drake rescued me on several occasions with his technological and typographical acumen. The staffs of Countway and Widener Libraries at Harvard, the Library of the College of Physicians of Philadelphia, and Van Pelt Library at the University of Pennsylvania managed to put many old and obscure works in my hands. Charles Fineman of Widener Library, Ed Morman of the College of Physicians, and Martin von Wyss and Patrick Florance of the Harvard Map Collection deserve special thanks. Audiences at the University of Wisconsin, MIT, the University of Toronto, Yale, UCLA, Johns Hopkins, the University of Pennsylvania, and the annual meetings of the American Association for the History of Medicine, the History of Science Society, and the Society for French Historical Studies offered insightful critical feedback that was essential at every stage of this book's development. Members of the H-France and H-Sci-Med-Tech listservs likewise helped with key tips and leads along the way. (Although we historians bemoan the Internet's effect on our students' research habits, the advent of such online communities, which continuously join far-flung scholars together for discussion and advice, can only be considered a boon.)

A select group of French historians and historians of medicine thought enough of this project to give guidance and support to it from the very beginning. I am deeply indebted to Robert Nye, Ann La Berge, Matthew Ramsey, George Weisz, Cherilyn Lacy, Roger Hahn, Jeffrey Ravel, Harold Cook, Judy Leavitt, Ron Numbers, Walt Shalick, John Harley Warner, and the late Larry Holmes.

Both at Harvard and at Penn, I have been extremely lucky to be able to work with students and colleagues in an atmosphere of creative exchange and cross-fertilization. I owe special thanks to Mary Terrall, Robert Brain, Stephanie Kenen, Barbara Gutmann Rosenkrantz, Charis Thompson, David Jones, Conevery Bolton Valencius, Eric Kupferberg, and Alisha Rankin for helping nurture this project in its early stages at Harvard. Janet Tighe, Steven Feierman, Henrika Kuklick, Rosemary Stevens, Ruth Schwartz Cowan, Nathan Sivin, Susan Lindee, Sarah Igo, Ben Nathans, Andria Johnson, Gerald Prince, Michèle Richman, Maurice Samuels, and Cary Hollinshead-Strick helped coax it through its latter phases at Penn.

Allan Brandt provided both logistical and intellectual encouragement to this project. He also served as a role model of the most understated and inspiring kind. While others might be tempted to cultivate media attention or negotiate for additional time off, he remains deeply dedicated to both undergraduate and graduate teaching as well as research that is engaged in the contemporary world of health policy and disease prevention. One can find the highest standards of ethical scholarship, I learned from his example, not only in publications, but also in everyday interactions in the classroom and in the hallway.

Jennifer Malat, Nicholas King, Robert Aronowitz, and Charles Rosenberg read the entire manuscript in draft form, as did an anonymous reviewer for the Johns Hopkins University Press. Their time, good will, and acute critical faculties have greatly improved the book. It has been my great good fortune to work alongside Robert Aronowitz and Charles Rosenberg. Their warm and unpretentious manner is as rare as the wisdom and experience behind their advice, which has been invaluable to me. Rare are those who can persuasively play the roles of both good cop and bad cop, as the situation warrants. As one of these talented few, Jacqueline Wehmueller of the Johns Hopkins University Press is the consummate editor, alternating with an artist's touch between patient, supportive friend and firm, demanding taskmaster in the pursuit of a mutually desired end. Every author should be so lucky.

It is tempting, after having benefited from the help of such stellar collaborators, to blame the remaining flaws in this book on them. In the interests of honesty, I must resist that temptation.

My parents, Richard and Helena Barnes, have stayed true to their history as the earliest and staunchest supporters of my research. If not for their loving encouragement, none of this would have been possible. My sons, Daniel and Nicholas, served (especially during their toilet training) as human subjects in an ad hoc observational study on the learned nature of disgust. (I'm sure I have their consent forms around here somewhere.) With great resiliency and good humor, they have put up with periodic dislocation and a paternal fixation with bodily substances. When this project began, they were the reason I got up in the middle of the night; now, as the saying goes, they are the reason I get up in the morning. Finally, I owe the greatest debt of all to Joan Batista, my partner in everything. For her constructive skepticism, her creativity in embracing upheaval, and her tough-minded idealism, this book is dedicated to her, with love.

The Great Stink of Paris
and the Nineteenth-Century Struggle
against Filth and Germs

Introduction

This story begins and ends with a wave of foul odors in Paris. In 1880, a pervasive and disgusting stench afflicted the city for most of the summer, provoking a popular outcry and a minor political crisis. According to the consensus of medical experts and ordinary Parisians, the odors either could cause or did cause disease. In 1895, a similar stink arose in the city, again sparking anger and indignation among the population. This time, however, scarcely anyone claimed that the odors spread disease. This book tells the story of how public health knowledge and practice changed—and didn't change—during the fifteen years separating the two unpleasant episodes. The germ theory of disease was a critical ingredient in the shift but cannot alone explain it.

The years at the heart of this story coincide with the apex of Louis Pasteur's career. In 1880, Pasteur was already well known for his work on silkworms, wine, and beer, but he had only recently begun to turn his attention to the role of microorganisms in human disease. Because of his reputation for scientific innovation and problem solving, Pasteur was appointed to the national commission formed to study the Great Stink of 1880. The commission concluded that foul odors could indeed spread disease—not as generalized miasmas but as vehicles of specific pathogenic microbes. Pasteur cited a recent study at a farm north of Paris in which he claimed to have found sheep that became infected with anthrax simply by sniffing the ground beneath which sheep that had died of anthrax years earlier were buried. In effect, the centuries-old doctrine of miasmatism seemed to have gained validation from the new science of germs.[1]

In 1895, less than two months after the end of the second Great Stink, Louis Pasteur died in St. Cloud outside Paris. So great was his fame that his elaborate state funeral drew thousands of mourners into the streets of the capital as the mile-long procession led by the Republican Guard carried the coffin from the Pasteur Institute to Notre Dame Cathedral.[2] The scientist had become a symbol not just of the power of laboratory science in the modern world but also of French glory and achievement in an era marked by widespread fear of national decline. The landscape of health and disease that Pasteur left behind in 1895 would have been almost unrecognizable to a visitor from 1880: thanks in part to his development of vaccines for anthrax and rabies—and to the unprecedented publicity that work received—germs and disease had become all but synonymous by the mid-1890s, and the future of treatment and prevention clearly lay in the bacteriological laboratory. The odors of 1895 and Pasteur's state funeral did not mark the end of an era; rather, they brought further confirmation (if any was needed) that a new era of health and disease was already well under way.

The germ theory of disease changed everything and nothing at all. Seen from a bird's-eye view, the landscape of disease causation in France was reshaped dramatically—as if by an earthquake—in the span of less than twenty years. In the late 1870s, nearly all medical observers agreed on the fundamental causes of disease: heredity, climate, miasmas, immoderate lifestyles. Some diseases were considered to be contagious in some circumstances—smallpox and syphilis, for example—but even those could usually be traced to these fundamental causes. By the mid-1890s, all but a few holdouts considered living microorganisms the only true cause of infectious disease. The causal microbes for some diseases had not yet been uncovered, but that was only a matter of time. The practical strategies recommended for preventing disease, however, had changed little. Moderation, conformity with behavioral norms, avoidance of overcrowded living conditions, public and domestic cleanliness, containment and disposal of bodily excretions, and even the neutralization of contaminating odors with disinfectants figured as prominently among precautionary injunctions in 1900 as they did in 1875, or in 1840 for that matter.

The connection between filth and microbes that seems obvious today—disgusting things spread germs, germs are found in disgusting places and substances—came to be obvious through a series of developments that in a relatively short period of time left its mark indelibly on medicine and society. The chapters that follow trace the response to infectious disease at the local level in France, paying special attention to shifting etiologies and to the enactment of social, political, and cultural agendas through public health reform. From the fashionable boulevards of Paris to the most isolated rural hamlet, physicians and government officials pursued an ambitious campaign throughout the 1880s and 1890s targeting germs and filth. In their eyes, it was a battle of civilization against backwardness, and of the secular republic against its intractable reactionary enemies. The guiding light of their campaign (and the key to understanding the blend of old and new in the rise of germ theory) is what I call the "sanitary-bacteriological synthesis" (or SBS, for the sake of brevity). A flexible framework for addressing health threats rather than a strict medical doctrine, the sanitary-bacteriological synthesis brought the commonsense cultural appeal and broad applicability of the old knowledge (for example, that foul-smelling substances are bad for one's health) into harmony with the specificity and scientific mastery inherent in the new knowledge of microbes.

The SBS made possible a new way of understanding, explaining, and combating disease in society by integrating the old concerns of the sanitary movement (filth and contamination, cleanliness and morality) with a new germ-centered focus on the danger of contact with potentially sick bodies and bodily substances, tests for the presence of microbes, and the promise of their control through laboratory science. This integration took place through the language of bacteriology, with a persistent overlay of moralizing disgust, and gave rise to a new set of meanings and practices that have shaped the understanding of disease to this day. Although it is now put to use for different diseases and in different settings, the SBS governs responses to infectious disease in the early twenty-first century even more powerfully than it did in 1900. The passage of a hundred years has only made its truth more self-evident, its straightforward applicability to most diseases more obvious.

Threats to human health, we are able to see, arise from filth, behavioral transgression, and contact with sick or suspect bodies. On an instinctual level, danger can be identified with these violations of civilization's rules, but they must be verified, evaluated, and measured by the authoritative science of the laboratory. After the threat is assessed, an appropriate mix of remedies can be prescribed to keep it at bay: behavioral and environmental controls help avoid future exposure, while technical and medical intervention (ranging from gloves and masks to vaccines and therapeutic drugs) snuff out the already established spark before it becomes a full-fledged fire. The contentious and uneven transition from the sanitary to the bacteriological era is erased in the seamless blend of disgust and clinical mastery. In the age of the sanitary-bacteriological synthesis, filth still causes disease (as it always did), but only science can identify it, explain it, and cure it; and together, science and clean living can prevent it. Much remained the same after the Bacteriological Revolution, but both professional and popular understandings of health and disease changed forever in critical ways. It is impossible to fully appreciate the vagaries of health knowledge and behavior today without understanding their roots in the early SBS a century ago.

Why France? What makes this country—now seemingly consigned to the second tier of nations in international biomedicine as well as in global cultural and political influence—worth a closer look where the cultural and political roots of modern medical science and public health are concerned? A strong case could be made that both the scientific study of public health and the germ theory of disease were born in nineteenth-century France. Britain, Germany, and other countries could also lay claim to early milestones in these areas, but no nation figured as centrally in both histories as France did. When Edwin Chadwick sought guidance for sanitary reform in Britain, he looked to the French hygienists; when Joseph Lister was developing his antiseptic system of surgery, he looked to France and Pasteur for scientific inspiration.[3] Nowhere else in the world did demographic alarm, social conflict, and medical innovation mix in such a highly charged manner. In such a combustible atmosphere, the political stakes of public health before and during the Bacteriological Revolution stand out in stark relief, and otherwise hidden connections occasionally emerge into visibility.

Many other countries followed, in broad outline, the same overall trajectory described in this book. Local chronologies and manifestations varied, but viewed from a distance in retrospect, the fundamental transition from sanitary to bacteriological explanations of disease took place throughout the industrialized world.[4] Roughly similar versions of the SBS supplanted miasmatic, geographic, and moralistic etiologies in many countries in the decades immediately preceding and following 1900. What made the French experience unique was the confluence of several key elements—a proud medical and hygienic tradition, pathbreaking scientific advances, and social and political turmoil—in the same place within a relatively short period of time.

France was a large and culturally diverse country in the late nineteenth century, and generalizations must be very carefully made. This book begins and ends with Parisians' stories of foul odors and germs, but between these two episodes it pays considerable attention to provincial epidemics and their consequences. The evidence that sustains this portion of the argument was gathered from a variety of departments (the rough equivalent of counties) throughout France. The research was initially undertaken in the expectation of finding regional variations in responses to infectious disease.[5] From Lille to Montpellier, from Rennes to Dijon, and in countless towns and villages in between, local public health policies and attitudes toward disease prevention turned out to show surprising nationwide uniformity. The archival preservation of local public health records varied considerably from year to year and from department to department, but the content of those records (when and where they survive) reproduced the same local concerns and the same set of changes throughout the nation in the 1880s and 1890s. Even at the local level in the remotest corners of France, the public health agenda was being driven by officials appointed by and dedicated to a centralized republican political regime, which was determined to lead the country forward along a road paved by secularism and science.

Readers expecting to find a profession of theoretical allegiance at this point will be disappointed. In its attempt to make sense of public health and popular attitudes toward disease in the nineteenth century, this book relies less on a single grand theory than on a workaday, pragmatic bricolage of methods and analytical perspectives. The surviving record speaks in irregular and allusive bursts. To weave a coherent narrative and analysis out of it requires a creative and flexible approach, borrowing from other scholars or theorists as necessary to shed light on a particular text, belief, or practice. No single authority fits all interpretive needs. Medical knowledge represents a special challenge for historians, inasmuch as it tends to claim universal validity regardless of place and time. To assess health-related discoveries and innovations historically requires a careful touch; the social contexts out of which they emerged often explain such developments better than do retrospective evaluations of correctness or efficacy.[6]

The general orientation of this project is inspired by a motley assortment of theoretical perspectives, including Michel Foucault's exposure of the disciplinary imperatives of surveillance, measurement, and internalized norms as "grids" structuring the definition and perception of reality;[7] Pierre Bourdieu's grasp of the extent to which social hierarchies and relationships come to express themselves in everyday behaviors and bodily practices;[8] Norbert Elias's identification of long-term behavioral changes as part of a generalized movement toward the harnessing of emotions and impulses;[9] and Mary Douglas's cultural anthropology of conformity and transgression.[10]

More directly, this book's approach has been inspired by what some have called a "history of meaning," within the tradition of what used to be called history of *mentalités* and now stands at the heart of the practice of cultural history. According to this approach, ideas and values gain meaning not by being articulated in the abstract but by being grounded and enacted in specific local practices and social relations.[11] Practitioners of "microhistory" and ethnographic "thick description" have demonstrated that exploration of a single well-chosen incident, person, or place in meticulous detail can illuminate an entire culture or era.[12] Following a different path to a similar destination, historian Alain Corbin has shown such seemingly timeless and taken-for-granted realities as the smell of city streets, the sound of small-town church bells, and the visual appeal of the seacoast to have rich and profound histories.[13] The equally self-evident connection between filth and germs deserves similar treatment.

Examining local practices in detail not only preserves some of the texture of everyday experience as lived by working-class and peasant families. It also causes otherwise hidden patterns and structures of meaning to emerge into visibility. Local microhistories, as one historian recently put it, "begin with the premise that local 'phenomena of circulation, negotiation, appropriation' constitute an essential facet of a broader social reality." Historians choose the local scale of analysis "not to test national or global theses, but to retrieve the strategies and interpretations of rational actors who mobilized the resources at their disposal to construct their social world."[14] The danger of excessive localism lies in the tendency to find generalizable patterns in the idiosyncratic experiences of unrepresentative individuals or groups. Hence the need to stitch together a patchwork of detailed local stories, and wherever possible to discern in them common configurations, relationships, and conflicts.

The last quarter of the nineteenth century saw significant changes both in medical knowledge and in bodily practices and mores. Meanwhile, the fitful development of urban infrastructures and an apparent decline in rates of infectious disease may have made exposure to filth and the experience of disease seem less inevitable.[15] In retrospect, some changes appear sudden, and others gradual. In the final analysis, what changed most durably were the *meanings* of bodily substances and infectious diseases—that is, where knowledge, policy, and behavior intersected. The same old excrement; the same old "croup" and diarrheal diseases; the same old stairway odor of urine, unwashed sweaty bodies, and *renfermé* (stale air) all acquired qualitatively new meanings at century's end. The same material realities, reshaped into new configurations, combined to forge a new reality. Nothing had changed, and everything had changed.

Borrowing the dictum Steven Shapin contrived for the Scientific Revolution, it is even possible to say, "There is no such thing as the Bacteriological Revolution, and this is a book about it." A conventional history credits a hardy band of inspired researchers with vanquishing the resistance of hidebound traditionalists and bringing the light of science at long last to the study of disease. "After millennia of wishful thinking and groping in the dark," one historian has written, "medical science at last got it right."[16] The stubborn determination of these pioneers, so this story goes, finally succeeded in overcoming the resistance of their benighted, tradition-bound opponents.[17] Such a simplified and heroic history is no longer tenable. Recent scholarship has cast doubt on the revolutionary nature of changes in late nineteenth-century medical science, and even on the very notion of a single "germ theory" of disease. Whatever changes there were took place in a gradual, piecemeal fashion, historians have argued, and it is more accurate to speak of multiple germ theories, each developed under unique local circumstances and devised to meet particular (often disease-specific) professional needs.[18] Most importantly, as Charles Rosenberg and others have repeatedly reminded us, changes in medical knowledge and practice were not dictated by "the facts" or by the discovery of transcendent truths, but rather negotiated through an elaborate web of interests and relationships involving physicians as well as patients, government officials, civic leaders, educational institutions, the press, and the general public.[19]

In the realm of public health, the question of paramount interest is not how medical knowledge changed, but rather how that knowledge was translated into unprecedented authority in society as a whole, and in specific organs of government. What became known as the "new public health" turned the new science of germs into new prestige, new institutions, new laws, and new social norms. Historians have debated whether the reorientation of public health represented a narrowing or a broadening of the field.[20] Ultimately, this debate misses the point: clearly the new public health narrowed the range of factors identified as potential causes of disease. Just as clearly, it broadened the range of official interventions that could be brought to bear on the prevention of infectious disease, as well as the laws, regulations, and institutions that could facilitate those interventions.

France has figured in this historiography primarily as a land of missed opportunities. Historians have scorned France as the slow pupil in the class of advanced nations fighting the battle against infectious disease. Especially compared to Britain and Germany, France has been singled out as having failed to enact aggressive health-related legislation and to devote significant resources to existing programs.[21] A comprehensive recent study of French public health and politics in the early Third Republic laments a "thwarted utopia" in which good intentions fell victim to craven political opportunism and the inertia of entrenched local authorities. In this account, the loud and sustained outcry for public health reform in France sounds like nothing more than empty rhetoric, if not outright hypocrisy.[22]

Valuable as they are, these pictures leave many important details out and many questions unanswered. Equating public health reform with legislation or with funds appropriated at the national level is a mistake—an understandable one, but one that ignores entire dimensions of health-related knowledge, policy, and behavior. This book attempts to fill in the blanks by retelling the story of public health in France not as what it was not—a German-style expansion of legislation and bureaucracy—but as what it was: a loud, contentious, and remarkably unproductive political debate accompanied by a halting and ambivalent, but ultimately thoroughgoing, reorientation of attitudes and mores concerning bodies and health. More importantly, the chapters that follow refocus attention on local rather than national stories. Grand narratives of medical progress tend to dissolve into unpredictable idiosyncrasy when examined in local detail. Aggregated local narratives, on the other hand, can form a sometimes puzzling patchwork that nevertheless assumes a recognizable shape when fully assembled.

One of the aims of this book is to help readjust the focus of the historiography of public health. Medical debates, legislation, and policy initiatives will continue to demand our attention, as will stories of victimization and resistance told from the bottom up. And well they should. Empirical demographic assessments of various measures' effects on the health of populations should continue to challenge our assumptions regarding medical efficacy. But accounts of success and failure, hegemony and resistance, efficacy and futility encourage us to think one- or two-dimensionally about health in the past—unless, that is, they are deepened by *cultural* histories of health-related knowledge and practices. The history of public health as a subdiscipline should be about education and public outreach as well as about laws, regulations, and infrastructures; but it should also be a history of *meaning*. Local stories have more than merely anecdotal value. The early nineteenth-century families who refused hygienists' injunctions to ventilate their hovels and wash their bodies and the late nineteenth-century peasant families who accepted disinfection but resisted isolation of contagious children were manifesting much more than ignorance, or even resistance to authority.[23] They were expressing—and enacting—their own local knowledge, their own mores about bodily well-being and cultural integrity.

Historians can and should judge them (or at least assess their significance), but only after hearing them out.

Any attempt to show how filth and germs came to be conjoined cannot help but run up against a straightforward objection: it's just a fact that disgusting substances contain and spread germs—period. No amount of textual analysis or interpretive sleight of hand can change that simple truth. Excrement spreads germs. The crowding together of dirty bodies spreads germs. This much is certainly true, but the exact nature of its truth is worth emphasizing. The Bacteriological Revolution established a new kind of truth in which the existence of a particular microbe in a tested sample was enough to identify a person, place, or thing as a health hazard, regardless of whether actual cases of disease were associated with that person, place, or thing.[24]

But germs lurk everywhere—not just in disgusting or marginal contexts. Farms, handshakes, facial hair, pets, kisses—all kinds of places, behaviors, and substances can contain or spread microbes. Yet those that are culturally appropriate in context—that is, not disgusting or otherwise unacceptable— are rarely singled out as threats to public health. We continue, as ever, to associate disease with society's stigmatized zones. We do so now, however, using the precisely calibrated science of microbes. The laboratory produces the undeniable fact that yes, excrement spreads germs.

This book examines perceptions of infectious disease in nineteenth-century France, and yet the three best-known infectious diseases of nineteenth-century France are almost entirely absent from its pages. Tuberculosis, smallpox, and cholera occupied the first ranks of microbial killers, but the fundamentally exceptional way in which health authorities approached the fight against them places them outside the scope of a historical study of infectious disease *in general* in the late nineteenth century. For one thing, their story has already been told—and at some length. Each of these three diseases has already been the object of ample and sustained attention from historians of nineteenth-century France; for the most part, the diseases discussed in this book have not.[25]

Even though it was widely understood to be contagious after Robert Koch's 1882 identification of its causal bacterium, tuberculosis was not officially declared a "contagious disease" in France until well into the twentieth century, and it was not subject to the routinized rules, investigations, and reports of the public health authorities during the period covered by this book.[26] In contrast, smallpox was widely considered to be contagious, but as early as 1800, preventive policy was reduced to a single intervention not applicable to any other disease: vaccination. For better or for worse, every smallpox-related development, proposal, intervention, or opinion was immediately reduced to or translated into a commentary of some sort on vaccination policy. The fight against smallpox traveled a singular path not followed for any other disease in the nineteenth century.[27] Asiatic cholera was an exotic, imported disease rather than a homegrown domestic problem. As such, its prevention consisted almost entirely of barring its entry into France. All of the anxiety and concern about cholera were channeled into case detection, quarantine policies, and the monitoring of port cities and international commerce. As far as public health policy was concerned, like tuberculosis and smallpox, cholera was sui generis.[28] Although all three were clearly infectious and preventible, these diseases were fought with separate weapons on separate battlefields. The story of domestic French infectious disease control in the early bacteriological era lies in the histories of more prosaic, homegrown epidemic diseases such as typhoid fever, diphtheria, influenza, measles, scarlet fever, dysentery, and whooping cough.

This book retells the triumph of germ theory and the emergence of the sanitary-bacteriological synthesis not through the pronouncements of scientists or the deliberations of official medical institutions, but through the negotiation of public health knowledge and policy at ground level. The two traumatic episodes of foul odors in Paris in 1880 and 1895 serve as bookends here (chapters 1 and 6), showing how disgusting emanations first did, then did not spread disease. In chapter 1, the Great Stink of 1880 became a full-fledged public health crisis, and scientific luminaries such as Pasteur warned of their potential to spread disease. Chapter 2 recounts the backstory of this drama, in which "public hygiene" claimed for itself the status of a scientific discipline and—decades before germs arrived on the scene—first enunciated some of the core elements that would continue to define disease control in France into the twentieth century. Chapters 3 through 5 shift attention away from Paris, investigating the details of responses to infectious disease in provincial towns and villages during the 1880s and 1890s. These chapters examine in turn the shifting etiological taxonomy of infectious disease (chapter 3); hygienists' efforts to preach the "gospel of germs" through educational programs and specific disease control policies such as isolation and disinfection (chapter 4); and the obsession of local health authorities with a cultural agenda of cleanliness, which operated in concert with a social agenda promoting the integration of the peasantry into national life and a political agenda of anticlerical republicanism (chapter 5). Chapter 6 revisits the notorious odors of Paris, which themselves revisited the capital in 1895. This time, they were a nuisance, intolerable to civilized sensibilities but largely harmless to human health. Disgusting substances still carried germs, but they no longer did so through malodorous emanations. In this subtle shift lies the key to understanding the power of a cultural history of public health: what reshaped perceptions and behaviors was not the germ theory of disease per se, but rather the extensive series of accommodations through which scientific and cultural demands were reconciled: in short, the sanitary-bacteriological synthesis.

The SBS is still very much with us today. Product marketing, news media, popular books, and museum exhibits continually tell us what we already know intuitively: germs are "gross," and disgusting substances are dangerous because they can spread germs. The public eats it up, figuratively speaking. We are fascinated and terrified in equal parts by this alliance, it seems, and we will spend our money on both the books, movies, and museum exhibits that scare us and the soaps, sprays, and toothpastes that promise to protect us. These celebrations of fear and progress may pay homage to the founding fathers of bacteriology, but they do not generally depict the connection between filth and germs itself as historically produced. Louis Pasteur's legacy lives on, not only in pasteurization and in the Pasteur Institute and in the name of multinational pharmaceutical giants (Aventis Pasteur, Sanofi Pasteur), but also in the lessons of Rosières and the Great Stink commission. Whether we realize it or not, when we buy a particular brand of toothpaste or deodorizing spray or hand soap because it kills germs, we are reenacting the SBS in our own lives, and we are choosing to validate a certain set of potential health threats while ignoring others. The historical roots and ramifications of that impulse deserve deeper examination.

1

"Not Everything That Stinks Kills"

Odors and Germs in the Streets of Paris, 1880

*I*n the late summer of 1880 in Paris, death was in the air, and it smelled like excrement. That, at least, was the prevailing opinion at the time, shared and vociferously proclaimed by scientists, medical doctors, elected representatives, and ordinary Parisians. For more than two months, oppressive and insufferable odors pervaded the air of the capital, occasionally disappearing and then reappearing with even greater intensity according to the indecipherable rhythm of mysterious forces. More than a mere annoyance, the stench that gripped the city between late July and early October of 1880 represented a genuine public menace, a clear and present danger to the health of the population that needed to be met with a correspondingly drastic public response: "Complaints came from all sides. . . . The press protested violently against the government's negligence. . . . People approached one another with but one greeting: 'Do you smell that? What a stench!' It was a real public calamity. Parisians were panic-stricken; public officials were anguished; cabinet ministers were troubled."[1]

Parisians high and low, powerful and plebeian exercised themselves into a frenzied mixture of terror and outrage during the Great Stink of 1880.[2] The chorus of popular protest—"The odors are truly unbearable"; "We've never seen anything like this!"; "This can't go on!"[3]—was seconded by the official sanction of scientific authority. A government commission composed of the nation's leading medical scientists (including the great Louis Pasteur himself) concluded, "These odors that have spread over Paris . . . *can* pose a threat to the public health."[4]

For two months, predictions of impending plagues vied for headlines with political recriminations and vivid descriptions of the sickening stench.

Ten years after the Prussians laid siege to the city in 1870–71, Parisians once again described themselves as besieged by a ruthless and implacable force. Even allowing for the hyperbole characteristic of French public discourse (especially in the popular press), the intensity of the complaints is striking. "Our great and beautiful city . . . [is being] turned into an immense cesspool, which soon . . . will be uninhabitable," one newspaper claimed.[5] "The foul stench sweeping down on Paris has provoked a general outcry . . . [and] public lamentations," another reported.[6] Disgust, anger, and fear combined in a volatile mix, which, although it seemed to dissipate with the odors when autumn fell, testifies to the depth of the anxieties that beset a society in the throes of dramatic historical change.

There are times when one must take such animated public complaints and dramatic lamentations with a grain of salt. After all, to take one obvious example, the weather can cause widespread death and destruction—and provoke considerable, spirited discussion among the population—without signifying any important historical developments. What makes the Great Stink of 1880 (that is, the public reaction as well as the odors themselves) different from any of a number of extreme or unpleasant meteorological phenomena?

The answer lies in the widespread, almost reflexive assumptions of Parisians in 1880 regarding the spread of disease and the nature of government responsibility. Although officials and ordinary citizens debated the cause of the odors as well as appropriate public and private remedies, there was a remarkable degree of consensus on two central issues: first, that the smells represented an urgent danger to the public health, and second, that the authorities—that is, the government, in consultation with scientific and technical experts—bore a correspondingly urgent responsibility to do something about them. The deep-rooted familiarity and persistence of the first thesis and the novelty of the second in 1880, among other things, mark the Great Stink as a historical watershed.

Eighteen eighty, in fact, was a pivotal year in several respects. In what can be seen as a crucible of modernity, fundamental changes were reshaping French politics, science, and culture to an extent that only became clear much later. A durably republican, democratic political regime came to power for the first time; a nation humiliated by military defeat grappled with demographic decline and a perceived loss of national vitality; the memory of revolutionary upheaval and the threat of social conflict continued to haunt the wealthy, while intractable poverty and injustice nurtured bitter resentment among the poor; a rural exodus put a tremendous strain on urban housing and infrastructure, while in the capital a new standard of state-sponsored reshaping of the built environment was emerging; new imperatives of civilized behavior subverted old mores and lowered thresholds of tolerance for previously accepted practices and substances; and a radically new science identified tiny living organisms invisible to the unaided eye as the causes of everything from the fermentation of beer and wine to deadly diseases.

In the midst of these changes, the collective response to disgusting smells in 1880 was fundamentally different from anything seen previously in Paris and from anything yet to come. In particular, the combination of a persistent, quasi-miasmatic belief in pathogenic smells and the demand for progressive, technocratic governmental intervention signaled both the dawn of a new age and the impossibility of leaving behind the old one. Beneath the straightforward expressions of sheer disgust and inchoate apprehension that characterized the Great Stink lies a welter of intersecting anxieties and agendas, which can only be untangled through a careful mapping of the political, scientific, and cultural landscape of Paris in the early Third Republic.

It was Alain Corbin who in 1982 first called scholarly attention to the secret history of the sense of smell. It is significant that this pioneering work, blending social history, cultural history, and medical history, focused on eighteenth- and nineteenth-century France, a place and time in which malodorous conditions of material life clashed with new standards of civilized living. To Corbin, the determined efforts of Frenchmen to cultivate pleasurable odors and banish disgusting ones opened up the heart of a society actively engaged in the project of reshaping and reinventing itself. In his view, the odors of 1880 signaled the end of the old regime of smell, the demise of the previously intimate connection between foul odors and disease that had figured prominently in early nineteenth-century medicine and public health. According to Corbin, the characteristic "pre-Pasteurian" anxiety surrounding foul-smelling emanations from bodies and decaying organic matter had been definitively replaced in the years around 1880 by new bacteriological etiologies in which odors were absent.[7] Although the broad outlines of this story still hold true, a detailed analysis of the situation in 1880 shows that the chronology and details of this account need clarification and adjustment. In particular, the extent to which the odors-disease nexus had been severed by 1880 must be reexamined; the same is true of the decisiveness with which the new germ theory of disease banished disgusting phenomena from the etiological landscape.

Other historians have considered the odors of 1880 as a noisy intrusion into the debate over waste disposal in Paris, a noteworthy development in the inexorable (if slow) move toward a modern sewage system.[8] It certainly was this, but it was much more as well. Arising at a critical historical moment, the Great Stink of 1880 simultaneously ratified age-old beliefs and provoked new needs and new demands. This particular microhistory was shaped by a variety of divergent and contingent macrohistories—the rise of germ theory, the development of the French political system, the shifting boundary between the tolerable and the disgusting in civilized society, among others—while in turn it played a role (even if in some cases only an imperceptibly small one) in shaping these disparate long-term historical trajectories.

Historians such as Robert Darnton and Edward Berenson have shown how apparently isolated and bizarre events—a cruel yet light-hearted massacre of cats in a printer's shop in the late 1730s, the assassination of a newspaper editor by the wife of a government official in 1914—can crystallize and encapsulate the values and meaning systems of a distant world. In a sense, it is precisely the dramatic, atypical quality of these events that makes them especially revealing windows on lost social and mental landscapes. They become the occasion for reflection on and documentation of a society's (or a community's) rules, habits, and needs; they leave deep written traces that the routine of everyday life does not always provide.[9] In the case of the Great Stink of 1880, a new perspective on familiar histories can be found in a peculiar, unpleasant phenomenon that was, in the end, transient, but for a period of several weeks was all-important, preoccupying the inhabitants—both mighty and lowly—of a great metropolis.

COMPLAINTS

What exactly did it smell like in Paris during the Great Stink of 1880? Here the richness of the historical record and the representational power of language leave something to be desired. Rendering smells in words is nearly always an exercise in analogy—something smells "like roses," "like rotten eggs," "like burning rubber." Few adjectives exist to describe the precise component qualities of odors, beyond vague allusions such as "bitter" or "sweet."[10] In 1880, Parisians abstained even from this amount of description, instead evoking the odors' *effects* ("sickening," "nauseating," "suffocating") or qualifying them simply as "foul," "disgusting," and "horrible." "Putrid" and "fetid," two adjectives frequently used during the episode, begin to evoke at least a range of olfactory sensations, but the available evidence goes no further.

Nevertheless, one can infer a good deal from the *causes* identified by contemporary observers as generating the odors. In the case of the Great Stink of 1880, these included defective cesspits, the illegal dumping of cesspits' contents into the city's sewers, and the suburban solid waste treatment plants circling the capital. It is reasonable to conclude that the air of Paris in the late summer of 1880 somehow smelled intensely and unpleasantly like the one substance that these alleged causes had in common: human excrement.

The Great Stink of 1880 began not in Paris at all, but in the western suburb of Nanterre, where a waste treatment plant had become notorious for spreading unpleasant odors over the adjoining towns. Residents complained so insistently that on May 14, 1880, the prefect of police of the Seine department ordered the plant's operating permit temporarily suspended. However, this order seems to have been honored primarily in the breach, as local authorities continued to receive complaints of malodorous activity at the plant. Finally, nine neighboring towns—Nanterre, Rueil, Bezons, Saint-Germain-en-Laye, le Vésinet, Croissy, Montesson, Houilles, and Argenteuil—took the plant's operator, the Compagnie parisienne de vidanges et d'engrais, to court for violation of its original license and of the May 14 suspension. The judge found against the company, and ordered the plant shut down permanently; because the towns were unable to prove actual damages instead of merely hypothetical damages, they were denied the monetary awards they sought. Nevertheless, the ruling found convincing evidence not only that the waste treatment plant's odors caused "considerable depreciation" in local property values, but also that "illnesses and even deaths [had] increased rather notably" since the plant had begun operation in 1879.[11]

A small victory had been won for the olfactory sensibilities of the population, but it turned out to be short-lived. The suspension and subsequent shutdown of the Nanterre plant caused the Compagnie parisienne, which enjoyed a near monopoly in Parisian *vidange* (cesspit emptying) services, to transport the waste that would have been treated in Nanterre to other plants in the northern, eastern, and southern suburbs. It was also alleged that some of the resulting surplus waste was simply dumped into the Paris sewers.[12]

In the heat of July, during the suspension of the Nanterre plant's license, complaints about intolerable odors began to arise within Paris itself.[13] Shortly after the final shutdown of the plant in August, the complaints in Paris intensified, particularly in the north-central districts of the ninth, seventeenth, and eighteenth arrondissements. "Fetid emanations," residents claimed in the third week of August, were spreading through the city, particularly in the evening hours, and positively "stinking up" their neighborhoods.[14] By the end of the month, the odors had become an almost daily fixture in the Parisian press. Newspaper coverage of the increasingly unpleasant assault on the capital's nostrils typically appeared under one of two headlines: "The Odors of Paris" or "The Parisian Infection." (The French word *infection,* as will be discussed in chapter 6, has multiple meanings, including both "foul odor" and "disease transmission.") From late August through the month of September and into early October, these two labels came to designate a full-fledged public sensation, an object not just of private annoyance and complaint but of public policy, official debate, and rancorous accusations.

Here again, odorless words cannot possibly render accurately the full sensory experience of persistently revolting smells. However, a selection of testimony from Parisian daily newspapers[15] on the oppressive stench throughout the duration of the ordeal does convey a sense of the depth of popular feeling on the subject, and of the texture of the phenomenon that Parisians were forced to endure. Such evidence also provides insight into the underlying fears and expectations triggered by the experience.

The tone of outrage was fairly consistent from the earliest complaints through to the waning of the odors; such a smell was apparently not something to which one simply became accustomed. "Horrible miasmas," one newspaper reported on August 22, were "infecting certain districts" of the city; "never before has the infection of Paris been so great."[16] In early September, after two weeks of clamor, it was reported that "pestilential emanations . . . are turning Paris into a locus of infection" and that "the foul stench sweeping down on Paris has provoked a general outcry . . . [and] public lamentations."[17] By the end of the month, with the arrival of cooler weather, the odors had by all accounts lost none of their intensity, and some Parisians wondered if they would ever end: "All [last] night we fell prey to these fetid exhalations. In vain we hermetically sealed our windows; we couldn't sleep a wink all night. This morning, at seven o'clock, the remains of a pestilential mist still hung in the air. It was not until nine or ten o'clock that we had any relief. This torture is becoming unbearable. What, even in autumn, with a clear sky and a cool, dry breeze, which seems to herald winter? [Will it last] our entire lives then?! This can't go on!"[18] Finally, deliverance arrived in the early days of October, and although arguments continued into the following year over the assignment of blame for the odors, new complaints ceased.

Out of the wide array of allegations reported by the popular press over the course of two months, a set of central themes emerges. Furious and fearful, formulated in the heat of the moment, the various claims and reports seem outlandish at times, mutually contradictory at others. The smells, according to aggrieved residents, soured milk instantly, turned iron blue and red, and attracted (or even generated) swarms of large green flies. It is difficult to sort through and make sense of such claims, each of which seems to raise the stakes set by the previous ones, and all of which defy easy categorization. Nevertheless, it is possible to discern a core of common anxieties at the heart of the complaints, which together constitute a remarkable documentary record revealing not just beliefs about disease-causing odors, but also perceived relationships between body and environment in the late nineteenth-century city.[19]

The complaints point in three principal directions: the smells were intolerably disgusting; they represented a poison within the air of Paris; and they were capable of (or actually in the process of) causing widespread disease and death. The fact of profound disgust, to begin with, was contested by no one; it often manifested itself in feelings of nausea or suffocation. One reader complained in a letter to the editor of the newspaper *Le XIXe Siècle,* that "every evening around nine o'clock, for the last two months, the northeast wind brings us an asphyxiating stench."[20] Another resident was assaulted on the way to the Comédie-Française for an evening at the theater: "A horrible mist of nasty odors hung in the thick and heavy air. It was an infection to turn one's stomach."[21] In late September, after "a week of respite," one Parisian found to his disgust that the odors had "reappeared with a vengeance," as a "fetid mist" engulfed him while he rode in a horse-drawn carriage: "[The] coachman . . . slowed the carriage to a walk. He held the reins with one hand only, while the other held his nose."[22] Such seemingly banal (or even humorous) anecdotes suggest the extent to which disgust permeated everyday life in Paris during the Great Stink of 1880.

The stench was not only profoundly unpleasant; it was also poisonous—that is, it represented a dangerous chemical vitiation of that most essential and life-sustaining of elements: air. This vitiation took many forms, all of them potent and ominous. One family, "as a demonstration" of the noxious powers of the stinking air, placed a basin full of water on its balcony. "After a half an hour, the water was already fetid; and it's even worse for the milk."[23] Such acute contamination gave rise to other strange phenomena as well. The newspaper *Le Gaulois* reported on September 11 that "several neighborhoods of Paris were invaded by a considerable quantity of large green flies, which bothered both people and horses." The invasion was reported to be especially heavy in the Temple quarter, "where the odors are truly unbearable."[24] A reader wrote to the editor of *Le National* to complain about the powerful stench: "We were poisoned during the night, to the point that many people on our street fell sick with fevers, and got sores on their lips. I was working with some galvanized iron springs, and the poison was so violent that they turned blue, black, and red from the gases."[25] The multiplicity of effects—soured milk, green flies, mouth sores, colored metal—was proportional to the strength of the poison. One can sense in the complaints a feeling of helplessness and diffuse dread, as if the very ground was collapsing underneath the residents' feet; but instead of moments, this earthquake lasted for weeks on end. The possibility that the air itself—the most vital medium of life—was contaminated through and through undercut the prevailing nineteenth-century understanding of health as a delicate balance among elements in the body and in the surrounding environment.

The disgusting and poisonous odors of 1880 were also felt to be potentially or actually deadly. Illnesses and deaths were attributed to the Great Stink both by medical and scientific authorities and by lay observers, and predictions of imminent epidemics were made on a regular basis. The link between disease and what were commonly referred to as "pestilential" odors was direct and almost instinctive, as if something so unpleasant simply must have been a health hazard. Of course, the belief that foul-smelling emanations from decaying organic matter spread disease was central to the doctrine of miasmatism, which traced its lineage back to Hippocrates, and which served as a broad framework for understanding health and sanitation in France and elsewhere during most of the nineteenth century. The perceived connection between bad odors—or, more generally, "bad air"—and disease was both strong and durable.[26] In 1880, however, the conviction that the Great Stink would spread disease transcended miasmatism, and was shared even by those who explicitly rejected such vague, old-fashioned etiologies.

During August and September of 1880, Parisians occasionally reported specific illnesses (in themselves or in family members) that they blamed on the foul smells. In addition to the fevers and sores reported above in one neighborhood, the newspaper *Paris-Journal* printed this angry letter: "I have three children, who have had the fever for two months now—as have we parents too. If they die, it will be the fault of the city council and the engineers."[27]

Most often, however, the claims were more general, warning of an overall deterioration in the health of the population or pointing with alarm to purported recent increases in mortality caused by the odors. The press accused the local government, in its refusal to commit resources to remedial action, of "speculating on the health of the population . . . exploiting the mortality of poor little children," and "condemn[ing] to death several hundred Parisians, both young and old."[28] Commentators invoked expert opinion and especially the hard proof of statistics to bolster their warnings. "All doctors agree" and "the death statistics prove" that these odors cause disease, they argued.[29] Le Siècle editorialized: "Due to the poisoning of the air, an epidemic could break out any day now. One of my colleagues assures me that *child mortality has tripled*."[30] The Prefecture of the Seine department issued weekly reports on vital statistics, which served as the ostensible basis for many of the claims about the health effects of the Great Stink. According to *Paris-Journal*, "The salubrity of Paris is truly compromised, and for proof we need only look at the mortality tables compiled every week by the local prefecture."[31] Moreover, a direct connection was posited between localized odors and geographical differences in mortality within the city: "In the presence of this fearsome mortality, we must therefore look for [its] cause. . . . This cause is none other than the pernicious influence of the fetid emanations with which the atmosphere of certain quarters of Paris is saturated. The proof of this is the fact that it is precisely in those quarters where the disgusting exhalations are felt that infant mortality is highest."[32] Infantile diarrhea was singled out as the principal illness by which the mortal influence of the Great Stink expressed itself statistically, but some observers also argued that the odors spread typhoid fever and dysentery; even cholera and smallpox were mentioned.

It is difficult to find in the annual statistical compilations any clear echoes of the unequivocal assertions made at the time regarding the health effects of the Great Stink of 1880. More Parisians died in 1880 than in either 1879 or 1881, but the number of deaths increased in 1882 beyond the 1880 level. Deaths from typhoid fever were slightly higher in 1880 than in 1881, but far lower than in 1882; deaths attributed to infantile diarrhea were significantly higher in both 1881 and 1882 than in the year of the Great Stink. A month-by-month breakdown of deaths in the city for 1880 and 1881 shows no mortal upsurge during or immediately after the wave of foul odors. A possible correlation with the Great Stink seems to appear in the monthly

The Great Stink of Paris

deaths from infantile diarrhea, but the disease increased even more sharply in the summer of 1881, in the absence of remarkable odors.[33]

By all accounts, the various arrondissements, quarters, and even streets of Paris suffered unequally from the odors of 1880. The geography of the Great Stink casts some of the claims made at the time about its causes and consequences in a different light. Mapping each instance in which specific places were mentioned in complaints about the odors (Fig. 1) shows that few areas of the city were completely spared the ordeal. Nevertheless, complaints concentrated on the Right Bank, and the north-central districts (especially the ninth and eighteenth arrondissements) were hit particularly hard by the smells.[34]

The uneven geographic spread of the Great Stink provides another lens through which to evaluate the assertion that deadly diseases struck with particular intensity "precisely in those quarters where the disgusting exhalations [were] felt."[35] Here again, however, the available statistics fail to bear out the claims of the doomsayers at the time.[36] If anything, fewer residents of the ninth and eighteenth arrondissements died during and immediately after the Great Stink of 1880 than in prior or subsequent months, or in the corresponding months of 1881. Deaths from typhoid fever and infantile diarrhea in these two districts likewise showed no disproportion in the year of the Great Stink; for the most part, in fact, these figures were markedly lower in 1880 than in the following two years.

Obviously, commentators in the midst of the odors of 1880 could have had no inkling of what would happen to death rates from particular diseases in the future. Nevertheless, it is difficult to see any substantial quantitative corroboration—even based on what was apparent at the time—for the belief that deadly diseases were on the rise during the Great Stink of 1880. This makes the rock-solid conviction of many contemporary authorities all the more remarkable; in 1880, they positively knew, on a gut level, that disgusting smells were sickening and even deadly, and all available evidence would necessarily be interpreted in light of that certainty.

The turbulent social history of Paris in the nineteenth century might lead one to expect the Great Stink of 1880 to have a clear and sharp class dimension. The city's social geography preoccupied many observers at the time, and was felt to pose a potential danger at all times to the existing political order. The June Days of 1848 and the Paris Commune of 1871 had shown how class conflict could erupt into revolutionary violence, and had left deep traces in the national memory. The spatial segregation that divided Paris into bourgeois central and western districts and working-class

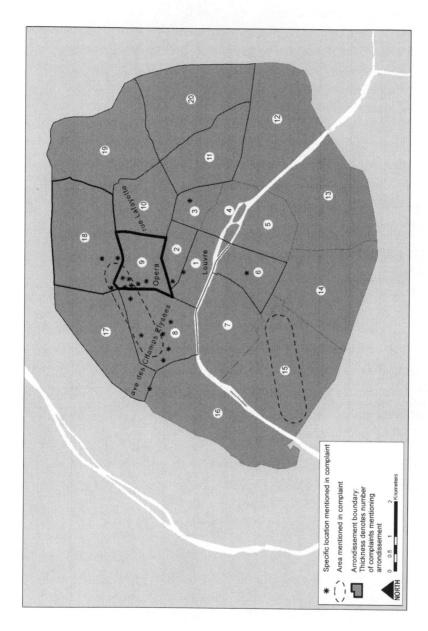

Fig. 1. Complaints about foul odors in 1880 covered most of Paris but were concentrated in the north-central districts of the city. Map courtesy of Cartographic Modeling Laboratory, University of Pennsylvania.

eastern districts and suburbs had been underway for decades; it was only accentuated by the massive public works programs undertaken during the Second Empire, which increased rents in the center of the city and accelerated the influx of working-class migrants from the provinces.[37] Moreover, a tradition of mutual fear and antagonism colored relations between worker and bourgeois. In particular, as Louis Chevalier has memorably shown, the respectable Parisian bourgeois in the nineteenth century felt besieged by a filthy, sickly, disgusting army of criminals and vagrants, who represented as much a threat of bodily as of political harm.[38] Might the odors of 1880 be a manifestation in the olfactory realm of the repulsion felt by the bourgeoisie toward the working class?

The evidence on this question is much more difficult to assess, but such a straightforward explanation seems inadequate. After all, most complaints involved odors perceived in the observer's own home, street, or neighborhood, and none specifically identified working-class residential districts as *sources* of the odors. Although the eighteenth arrondissement (where many complaints clustered) housed a predominantly working-class population, the same cannot be said of the ninth arrondissement, whose population was more socially mixed. Moreover, quite a few complaints came from areas with overwhelmingly bourgeois populations, including the eighth arrondissement and the avenue des Champs-Elysées.[39]

This latter fact raises an intriguing possibility: did bourgeois Parisians complain more often and more vociferously about the Great Stink of 1880, not because of the perceived social origins of the smells, but simply because of a special sensibility shared by the members of this particular class? Did other Parisians experience, but tolerate, phenomena that disgusted and outraged the bourgeoisie? The available evidence is either silent or equivocal on these points. It may be that complaints simply emerged wherever the odors were most intense, or that some combination of objectively strong smells and subjective sensitivity explains the distribution of the complaints. But examining the causes of the Great Stink of 1880, as identified by various observers at the time, can help shed light on the nature of the anxiety provoked by the experience.

CULPRITS

Nearly every aspect of the existing system of human waste disposal was a source of concern for Parisians in 1880. Cesspits under residential buildings, the drainage and transportation of their contents, the suburban treatment plants that turned waste into fertilizer and other chemical by-products, and the sewers of the city all operated defectively and hazardously, according to the complaints about the Great Stink. While few observers gave them all equal weight, these four aspects of waste disposal—cesspits, *vidange*, treatment plants, and sewers—were widely agreed by experts and laypeople alike to be the chief causes of the foul late-summer odors.

It was easy to find fault with the cesspit system, and many did. In theory, latrines emptied urine and feces directly into these impermeable containers, which stored them safely underground beneath each residential building, while ventilation pipes carried the malodorous fumes up above the rooftops, to be carried away inoffensively with the wind. In practice, the pits themselves often overflowed or leaked odors into the houses above; defective construction or installation also allowed their contents to leach into the surrounding soil or groundwater. The ventilation pipes, even when they were intact, too often merely carried their stench to adjoining houses or neighborhoods. When the ventilation pipes leaked, sickening gases could creep into the lodgings above and poison unsuspecting residents.[40]

Few Parisians were satisfied with the work of the cesspit cleaners, or *vidangeurs,* who were paid a fee by property owners to empty out each building's pit and cart its contents to suburban dumps or treatment plants. By law, the work had to be done at night in order to minimize inconvenience to residents and neighbors. Aside from the sheer smell produced by the entire operation and the annoyance of daytime *vidanges,* which evoked frequent complaints in some neighborhoods, it was alleged that the workers too often took advantage of the cover of darkness and the absence of police surveillance to illegally dump their cargo into gutters or into sewer outlets in the streets. This clandestine practice poisoned the entire network of sewers and, by extension (through manholes and ventilation outlets in the underground galleries) the very air of the city itself. Many Parisians long outraged by these abuses blamed them for the wave of offensive odors in 1880.[41]

Obstructions and inadequate water flow in the sewers was thought to compound the problem of illegal *vidanges,* as foul-smelling and hazardous material accumulated and stagnated in the sewers rather than being flushed out harmlessly and odorlessly through the system. In 1880, the sewers of Paris—one of the jewels in the crown of Baron Haussmann's massive rebuilding program in the 1850s and 1860s—were not the primary destination of human waste in the city. Rather, they acted in part as storm drains, collecting rainwater, institutional waste, nontoilet household wastewater, and miscellaneous refuse—in other words, that which would otherwise accumulate in the streets. The harsh winter of 1879–80 had piled unusually large amounts of snow in the streets of Paris. This caused a major snow removal problem as well as buildups of garbage and *vidanges* that could not be carted to their proper disposal sites. As a result, unprecedented quantities of snow, human waste, and miscellaneous refuse were dumped into the sewers, blocking normal flow and creating logjams whose scent could be smelled in the streets above.[42]

Finally, blame for the Great Stink of 1880 was laid at the doorsteps of the numerous suburban waste dumps and treatment plants that served as the final destination for the majority of Parisian excrement at the time. The plant operators' careless practices and disregard for neighbors' well-being was notorious in the suburban towns where they were located, but in 1880 the entire city joined in the chorus of denunciation. Under certain atmospheric conditions, the "exhalations" arising from the large stockpiles of human waste (despite the tall chimney stacks mandated by law for safe ventilation) could be smelled for miles around—not only in the adjacent suburban towns, but even as far as Paris itself. A petition to the Paris City Council from residents of the ninth and eighteenth arrondissements in September 1880 protested: "When the wind blows from the east, residents of [our] neighborhoods are extremely bothered by the bad odors that are given off by the waste dump in Bondy and which penetrate even into the most securely closed-off apartments. These intolerably fetid emanations could become, in the event of an epidemic, a real danger."[43] Especially after the final shutdown of the Nanterre plant in early August 1880 and the consequent overloading of the other facilities, this "belt" of waste dumps and treatment plants in the northern, eastern, and southern suburbs came to be seen as a noose encircling Paris, radiating "infection" inward to an aggrieved population.

Just as it is impossible more than a century later to know exactly what the odors smelled like or what the entire experience felt like, there is no way in retrospect to judge definitively the true role played by the various potential causes implicated in the Great Stink of 1880. All of the factors discussed above (and doubtless many others as well) were certainly capable of generating unpleasant odors in 1880. However, a fully convincing explanation would, in theory, need to identify a factor or factors that underwent significant change or increase between August and October of 1880. On the one hand, the harsh winter and heavy snowfalls might indeed have caused obstructions and buildups of *vidanges* and other refuse in the sewers; the

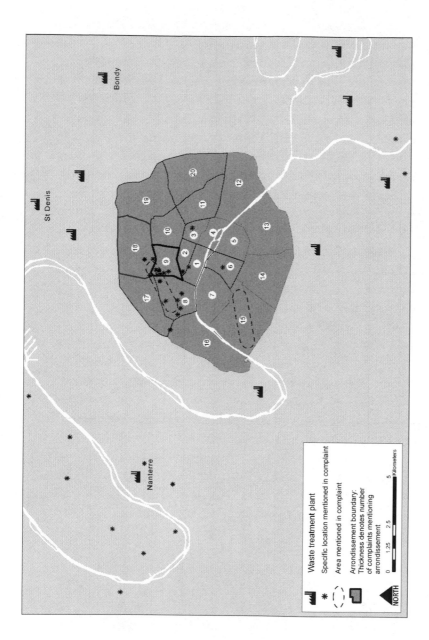

Fig. 2. Many observers blamed the Great Stink of 1880 on an unusual and persistent northeastern wind carrying odors from suburban waste treatment plants to the city. Map courtesy of Cartographic Modeling Laboratory, University of Pennsylvania.

heat of August might in turn have caused this ripe mass to exude its foul smell into the city above through the various sewer manholes and ventilating air shafts. On the other hand, the suspension in May and final closure in early August of the Nanterre waste treatment plant indisputably caused large amounts of human waste to be diverted to other plants or dumps in the suburbs. Numerous reports signaled an unusual prevalence of northerly and northeasterly winds in the Paris region during the late summer of 1880, and as some suggested, odors from dumps and plants in the northern and northeastern suburbs might have "come down rue Lafayette" or otherwise spread to the north-central districts of the city.[44]

Mapping the complaints of 1880, this time including suburban complaints and the locations of principal waste dumps and treatment plants, again tells a suggestive but far from definitive story.[45] (Fig. 2.) It is possible to interpret this map as supporting the treatment plant thesis, with complaints grouped near the end of the rue Lafayette thoroughfare that leads toward Bondy as well as in the eighteenth arrondissement near Saint-Denis and Aubervilliers. Likewise, there were numerous complaints from towns around Nanterre (complaints that led to that plant's closing), and in areas that were (at least on occasion) downwind from plants in Billancourt, Thiais, and Maisons-Alfort. But this map scarcely explains everything. Why so few complaints in the newspapers mentioning the tenth, nineteenth, and twentieth arrondissements, closer to Bondy than the ninth and eighteenth? One might expect zones of gradually decreasing intensity of odors radiating outward from the sources, but this does not seem to be the case here.

Even a much larger sample of complaints from newspapers would be an idiosyncratic and imperfect indicator of the actual severity and geographic distribution of the Great Stink. A published complaint, after all, reveals a combination of factors, brought together in a single place and time: the existence of odors, the perception of them as intolerable, an inclination to complain publicly, and access of some kind to the press. In 1880, the voices that arose from this combination told uniformly and angrily not just of discomfort, disgust, and illness, but also of demands for accountability.

DEMANDS

If the conviction that foul smells spread disease was time-honored "common knowledge," another recurring theme in the complaints about the Great Stink represents a response that was much newer in 1880. The aggressive insistence that the government, experts, local officials—anyone at all in a position of authority—*do* something about the disgusting odors was anything but familiar in the early years of the Third Republic. New expectations regarding the urban environment and new political realities combined to produce a climate in which certain complaints brought with them calls for remedial action.

The Great Stink of 1880 began with demands from residents of Nanterre and surrounding towns that a waste treatment plant be shut down because of the odors it gave off. They complained to their town councils, who in turn joined in legal proceedings against the plant's operator, claiming damages on three grounds: that the "nauseating emanations" from the plant rendered the air "unbreathable"; that residents had moved out, tax receipts had declined, and property values had depreciated because of the plant's presence in the vicinity; and that since the plant's opening, illnesses and deaths had increased markedly in the area.[46]

A month later, in mid-September, it was Parisians' turn to demand official intervention. Newspapers began referring to the odors as a "souvenir of the local administration." "When an entire population complains, quite justifiably," *Le Soleil* lamented, the government is "content merely to order an investigation." "What are our local officials waiting for before they act promptly and effectively?" asked *Le Gaulois*. The theme of government responsibility for prompt action runs throughout the press coverage of the Great Stink:

> Why no action?
>   It is incumbent upon our local officials, on the administration of the Seine department, [to recognize their] duty and responsibility to take charge of such a state of affairs.

Some accused the government of being more concerned with "moral disinfection"—that is, an anticlerical agenda of rooting out church influence in schools and other institutions—than with the actual physical well-being of the population. Others denounced secrecy and lack of communication in government circles.[47]

Especially galling was the fact that, as the odors had struck during the traditional period of summer vacations, prominent officials left the capital in the middle of the Great Stink for various (presumably pleasant-smelling) holiday destinations. While Parisians suffocated, "our local officials are in the countryside, inhaling to the point of intoxication the sweet scent of freshly cut hay," *La Lanterne* remarked acidly.[48] Prefect of Police Louis Andrieux,

The Great Stink of Paris

whose administration oversaw certain public health–related functions in Paris at the time, deserted the city for the fashionable Alpine resort of Aix-les-Bains, prompting more sarcastic jibes from the press:

> And what is M. Andrieux doing in the midst of this universal clamor on the part of Parisians?
>
> M. Andrieux has fled this vast center of pestilence, where he should have stayed to ward off the perils that threaten the public health!
>
> M. Andrieux is taking the waters at Aix-les-Bains, giving himself over to the exquisite joys and sensual pleasures of a summer vacation.
>
> M. Andrieux will return, no doubt, when Paris comes down with cholera![49]

Aside from casting personal discredit upon individual officials, the complaints reflected a seemingly widely shared outrage that such an intolerable sensory calamity would not just occur, but be allowed to continue for weeks on end, with no end in sight, no sign of remedial measures being undertaken, and nobody taking responsibility for the public welfare.

In an editorial in *Le Figaro* entitled "The Plague Victims of Paris," Georges Grison fulminated against governmental inaction, ridiculing the appointment of a high-level commission to study the odors. "We don't need commissioners, with their pens tucked behind their ears; we need workers armed with brooms and shovels." Administrators had fallen into the habit of considering themselves the masters of the citizenry, instead of its servants, Grison wrote. He targeted all levels of government for blame, from cabinet members to the city councilors who spent their time renaming streets while the city rotted: "Hah! messieurs, they all deserve the same name: *Plague street* [*la rue Pestiférée*]. What, when you come back from your meetings . . . to the neighborhoods that elected you to represent their interests, don't you even smell the infection that prevails there?"[50] Diatribes such as Grison's hint at a new perception of the proper relationship between the government and the governed in a democratic republic. The people's representatives owed their electors not just a general duty to defend the public interest, but an immediate, everyday obligation to secure their well-being and respond to their needs. This ethos of responsibility and responsiveness to constituents underlay the outcry over the odors of 1880.

It was not only the press that demanded action and accountability from the government. Residents of Paris on at least three occasions circulated petitions that called for local authorities to protect the public from the noxious stench afflicting the city. The petitioners beseeched the city council and the Prefecture of the Seine department to clean out the sewers and to transport the capital's bodily waste far away into the countryside, where it would no longer be "a scourge for the Parisian population."[51] Although it is unclear how many people signed these petitions or whether their demands played an important role in shaping the official response to the odors, the mere fact of the petitions is significant. It suggests a certain degree of citizen initiative aimed at enforcing the new imperatives of democratic government: accountability to constituents and responsibility for cleansing the urban environment of disgusting influences and everyday health hazards.

It is not hard to detect political grudges in some of the more virulent critiques of official inaction in the Great Stink of 1880. Indeed, in an atmosphere of continual accusations and recriminations, and in a political culture that cultivated heated factional animosity (which occasionally turned violent, either spontaneously or in the ritual context of dueling),[52] it might be reasonable to interpret as run-of-the-mill partisanship the drumbeat of vituperation directed at the government over the lingering stench in Paris. Le Figaro, for example, which printed Grison's biting editorial, was traditionally hostile to the opportunist republicans who dominated the government in 1880.

Several commentators, however, remarked that concern about the odors and anger at governmental inertia transcended the usual political cleavages and rivalries. Indeed, newspapers representing widely divergent political camps joined in a unison of criticism, as even "republican nostrils" were "painfully afflicted" by the odors.[53] The staunchly prorepublican Le Soir called the situation "grave" and the "infection of the sewers ... undeniable," and urged the departmental authorities to assume their responsibilities.[54] In fact, one wag referred to the Great Stink as the only matter "that currently has the privilege of provoking complete harmony among newspapers that are utterly divided on all other points."[55] This is not to say that the criticism was not political, however—far from it. What all the critics shared was the conviction that elected officials bore a special responsibility to their constituents to get rid of the dangerous smells. This consensus across the political spectrum signals the most enduring political development of this era in France: the fragile but definitive victory of the republic.

Faced with such loud and sustained demands, the authorities had no choice but to respond in some fashion. However, amid confusion and uncertainty over the nature of the problem, the various governmental bodies and agencies concerned could neither speak with a single voice nor formulate a clear plan for intervention. The result was a combination of dismissiveness, defensiveness, and blame shifting; even the scientific and medical experts who were consulted gave conflicting opinions. Nevertheless, a majority of these experts—including the most prominent among them—agreed on one conclusion that stood at the time as the government's final statement on the matter: the foul odors of Paris were indeed a threat to public health.

Official bodies at various levels, from neighborhood board to cabinet ministry, weighed in on the question of the odors during the Great Stink and in the ensuing months. At the level of the administrative districts or arrondissements of Paris, public health committees were charged with investigating complaints regarding possible health hazards within their districts. Unpleasant odors always figured prominently among the subjects of investigation, but only on the scale of individual lodgings or buildings. Tenants typically complained about inadequate sanitary facilities or building maintenance, and the health committees decided on a case-by-case basis whether a particular problem was severe enough to warrant officially enjoining the landlord to make improvements. In 1880, some of the district health committees never even discussed the odors of Paris, focusing instead (as they did every year) on individual reports of odors and other problems resulting from poorly installed or maintained toilets, inadequately ventilated apartments, and accumulated garbage.[56]

The health committee of the sixth arrondissement, however, did address the Great Stink directly. It found that the odors came from multiple sources: from the soil, from the sewers, from cesspit ventilation pipes, and from the suburban waste dumps and treatment plants. The committee's discussion called attention to the exceptional frequency of northerly winds in the late summer of 1880, and of their tendency to transport the "gases" from the plants of the northern suburbs "through the rue Lafayette to the ninth and tenth arrondissements." There was some debate in scientific circles, the report acknowledged, over whether such gases provided a hospitable environment for "those lesser organisms that have been blamed for the spread of epidemic diseases." However, the committee concluded that under any circumstances, the gases were dispersed in the air in quantities too small to pose any real danger; moreover, the city's weekly mortality statistics showed a general tendency toward *improvement* during the period between July and October 1880, the report said. As a result, the committee concluded, the health effects of the bad smells had been "exaggerated."[57]

The conviction that the odors of Paris were dangerous and even deadly was stronger among the members of the city council. On July 27, 1880, even before the press had seized upon the public complaints, council member Jules Roche demanded to know what the Prefecture of Police was doing to alleviate the odors, which he called "a perpetual danger to health."[58] The council debated the matter at length in early October (after its summer recess), interrogating officials from various departmental offices in order to determine the causes of the odors and find out who was responsible for remedying them. Coming under particularly critical scrutiny from the council members were Prefect of Police Andrieux and the director of public works, Adolphe Alphand. Roche and his colleagues challenged the administrators to defend their record of inaction and resolve the problem once and for all.

Andrieux replied that the press and the public had "singularly exaggerated" the seriousness of the odors, which he blamed on "a special atmospheric state" caused by the succession of a harsh winter and a hot, stormy summer: "I acknowledge that disagreeable odors have appeared. . . . The persistent inconvenience that has been remarked on is undeniable, but . . . there is a big difference between the true situation and certain assessments which would actually lead one to believe that the plague was about to break out in Paris." Andrieux hastened to "reassure the population" that such claims were unfounded. Furthermore, he insisted he had acted as vigorously as his position allowed in enforcing existing ordinances. Every time that a violation of the regulations governing waste treatment plants had been brought to his administration's attention, he claimed, an official report was filed and the operator brought before the courts. He could scarcely be blamed for the fact that the existing law provided for only nominal fines and penalties, Andrieux added. Moreover, he had sent an official circular to all suburban mayors urging them to file their own reports of violations and to call in police inspectors when needed.[59]

As far as the state of the sewers and the system of cesspit emptying were concerned, Andrieux disclaimed all responsibility. He deflected all questions on such matters to Alphand, whom he called "the great sweeper and cleaner of Paris" and whose duties included the surveillance of waste disposal inside the city limits. (Under the elaborate administrative system that deprived Paris of a mayor and divided the capital's government between the Prefecture of the Seine department and the Prefecture of Police, the departmental public health council was appointed by and reported to the prefect of police, who was also responsible for the regulation of potentially hazardous industries such as waste treatment plants; meanwhile, the prefect of the Seine department and his director of municipal public works were in charge of garbage disposal, sewers, water supply, and regulation of cesspit-emptying crews.) "Everything that was in my power to do, I have done," Andrieux concluded: "In this entire affair, the responsibility of the Prefecture of Police is as negligible as are its powers under the law. I repeat, we are powerless, and we could not have done any better than we have done."[60]

For his part, Alphand presented a more aggressive defense, claiming not only that the odors were harmless to human health, but also that the campaign of outrage and criticism in the press was politically motivated and orchestrated. The director of public works compared the city's official mortality figures for the second half of September—"that is, after the appearance of these emanations which they would have us believe are pestilential"—with the figures for early August, which were notably higher. Alphand also blamed unusual meteorological conditions for having brought about the odors, as weak northeasterly winds transported the fumes from the waste treatment plants of Saint-Denis and Aubervilliers "between the hills of Montmartre and Belleville" and "down the great corridor formed by the rue Lafayette into the ninth and tenth arrondissements." Furthermore, Alphand argued, it was entirely unreasonable to expect a metropolis such as Paris to be sweet smelling: "One cannot prevent odors from being generated in an agglomeration of two million residents, sweating, eating, etc., not to mention animals of all kinds. I must add that Paris is not only a city of wealth and fashion, but also an industrial city; and factories always give off more or less disgusting odors. But between that and a great poisoning, there is a big difference." Making no apologies and no concessions, Alphand finished with a dramatic flourish, saying that if the present allegations resulted in his firing, he would leave "head held high, with a clear conscience, and, I hope, with everyone's esteem."[61]

Several council members rose, if not actually to defend Andrieux and Alphand, at least to distance themselves from some of the claims of the extreme alarmists. Nevertheless, a consensus prevailed on the council that the administration needed to do much more to enforce existing regulations and protect Parisians from foul smells. A resolution was passed demanding that the prefects of police and of the Seine department "apply rigorously" the rules governing the cleaning of sewers, the clandestine dumping of cesspit contents into the sewers, the regular disinfection of all cesspits, and the operation of all waste treatment plants—with any plant found in violation to be closed.[62]

The Conseil général de la Seine, the equivalent of the city council for the Seine department as a whole (including suburban towns), also rehearsed in turn the allegations and recriminations surrounding the Great Stink of 1880. For the suburban representatives, the problem was nothing new, even if their neighbors inside the city limits of Paris noticed it for the first time only that summer. Waste treatment plants, they argued bitterly, continued to befoul the air of surrounding towns with impunity despite years of persistent complaints and open violations of their operating licenses. Council member Benjamin Raspail attacked Prefect of Police Andrieux for failing to crack down on the facilities and the "permanent poisoning" they caused, despite his repeated promises to do so and despite the continual complaints of residents. Raspail accused Andrieux of being either a hypocrite or a "bad administrator" by failing to use the powers of his office while claiming to pursue a rigorous surveillance of all treatment plants.[63]

The worst offender, in Raspail's view, was the Hautes-Bornes waste treatment plant in Arcueil, south of Paris, which for years had been spreading typhoid fever and other diseases as well as the "dreadful odor" of its "horrible emanations" to surrounding towns, and even as far as the Luxembourg Gardens in Paris. Agricultural workers begged their employers not to send them to work near the Hautes-Bornes plant, where the "suffocating" summertime stench made them vomit, and the local school medical inspector reported that the plant's operations seriously compromised the health of children at a nearby nursery school. According to Raspail and other critics, the Nanterre plant had been closed because of the complaints of certain wealthy and influential individuals who lived nearby, whereas the Hautes-Bornes plant was protected from the same fate because its owner and its directors (including Andrieux's former deputy) were politically well connected themselves.[64]

Andrieux defended himself before the Conseil général in much the same way as he had before the city council. He insisted that he had done, was doing, and would continue to do everything in his limited powers as prefect of police to enforce all regulations governing waste treatment plants.[65] Andrieux could also point reassuringly, as he had before the city council, to a report he had commissioned from the departmental public health council on the health effects of the pervasive odors in the Paris region.

On September 2, 1880, in the middle of the Great Stink, Andrieux asked the health council to study the question of the odors and report back to him. The council named a subcommittee to examine the problem in detail and prepare a report. Among the six members of the subcommittee—and its chief expert witness—was the engineer and public works director Alphand. Perhaps unsurprisingly, the report fully vindicated both Andrieux and

Alphand, and absolved the departmental administration of any responsibility for the unpleasant odors. According to the health council, there were "various" causes to which the unpleasant odors could be attributed, chief among them being "the abnormal atmospheric situation" that had prevailed in the Paris basin during the late summer. The weather conditions both increased the intensity of and facilitated the spread of odors from cesspits, sewers, and waste treatment plants. The health council hastened to add that the odors were (though bothersome) largely harmless. "We must begin," the report read, "by reassuring public opinion regarding the effect of sewer emanations on mortality and on the spread of epidemic or contagious diseases."[66]

Attributions such as "M. Alphand informed us that . . . ," "The Director of Public Works assured us that . . . ," and "As M. Alphand observed to us . . ." are scattered throughout the council's report. Moreover, the principal testimony on which the subcommittee based its report was Alphand's, which the council voted to have reprinted in its entirety alongside the report in the government's official daily publication, the *Journal officiel*. The report's three final recommendations urged the prefect of police (1) to ask the prefect of the Seine department to energetically pursue and prosecute those who clandestinely dumped cesspit contents into the sewers, (2) to pass on to the appropriate body the council's proposal to tighten the legislation controlling waste treatment plants, and (3) to ask the inspectors of those plants and other dangerous industries to bring to his attention any potential health hazards observed in their regular visits. These recommendations were accompanied by several reassuring pronouncements both in the report and in Alphand's appended testimony:

> Let us hasten to repeat . . . that the emanations coming from . . . these plants, disagreeable and uncomfortable though they may be, do not transport miasmas far and wide, as some people have claimed. . . .
>
> There is no parallelism between the extent of the foul stench and the extent of mortality. . . .
>
> An eminent scientist informed us that . . . the odors of Paris . . . can offend our sense of smell, [but] do not ever give rise to miasmas that could harm the public health.[67]

The report even cited the work of France's most prominent scientist, Louis Pasteur, to prove that disease-causing germs could not stay alive in the gases emitted from the chimneys of the waste treatment plants. Pasteur himself, however, had yet to be heard from directly.

In the press and in the deliberations of these official bodies, then, both expert scientific opinion and everyday empirical observation were invoked to bolster opposite assertions: foul-smelling excremental emanations did, or did not, spread disease. Whom to believe? Amid the lively debate on whether the Great Stink of 1880 was merely unpleasant or truly dangerous to public health—following the seemingly definitive but conflicting conclusions of the arrondissement health councils, the city council, the Conseil général, and the departmental health council—one prestigious body would end up having the last word.

The Science of Emanations

On September 28, 1880—toward the end of the Great Stink, as it turned out—the central government entered the fray. The minister of agriculture and commerce named an eleven-member commission to study the causes of the "infection" of Paris and to recommend remedial measures. Among the commission's members were two leading authorities who had yet to weigh in on the Great Stink: Louis Pasteur and Paul Brouardel. Pasteur was already an internationally renowned figure in 1880, though his fame would certainly increase considerably in the ensuing years, and Brouardel was one of his staunchest allies in the medical community, professor of public health and forensic medicine at the Paris medical faculty and preeminent authority in late nineteenth-century French public health.[68]

The commission held twenty-one plenary meetings between September 30, 1880, and June 20, 1881, in addition to numerous subcommittee meetings, and issued a lengthy final report in 1881. Its strategy was three-pronged: subcommittees were named to investigate in detail all potential causes of the Great Stink inside the city itself—including the cesspit system and the sewers; all suburban industrial establishments that might have spread odors to the city, including the waste dumps and treatment plants; and the advisability of continuing to allow the Paris sewers to empty into the Seine downstream from the city. The final report detailed an exhaustive array of sites and practices that were potential or actual causes of odors, ranging from tanneries and slaughterhouses to tar distilleries and, of course, cesspits. It concluded, cautiously, that all of these factors, and many more, were jointly responsible for the odors of 1880, and that it was impossible to discern the exact proportions in which each cause contributed to the total effect.[69]

The commission went to great lengths to emphasize one vital point, in the ambiguity of which can be found one of the essential meanings of the Great Stink of 1880: *some—but not all—odors are hazardous to human health*. In the commission's view, both elements of this assertion deserved equal weight: not all odors are harmful, but (equally importantly), some odors are in fact harmful. The tone of the report suggests that the commission knew some might find it difficult to accept that intensely foul smells were innocuous: "Very unpleasant odors, extremely offensive to one's sense of smell, can be harmless to the body, and odorless emanations can, on the contrary, be very dangerous."[70] The commission's phrase evoked a witty maxim (attributed to the eminent veterinary scientist and Pasteur ally Henri Bouley) frequently used to spread the message of germ theory: "tout ce qui pue ne tue pas, et tout ce qui tue ne pue pas"—Not everything that stinks kills, and not everything that kills stinks. This motto of the new public health was easily comprehensible to a lay audience, emphasized the novelty of the bacteriological approach to health and illness, and clearly distinguished its scientific character from the old inferences of miasmatism. From now on, only experts trained in the new medical sciences and backed by laboratory methods were in a position to arbitrate what was safe and unsafe, harmless and hazardous.

Given this new orthodoxy, and in light of the commission's caution and equivocation over identifying the specific causes of the Great Stink of 1880, the report's unambiguous assertion that "these odors . . . can pose a threat to public health" is especially remarkable.[71] For some reason, the commission felt it important to emphasize the danger of some foul smells while simultaneously insisting, in effect, that "not everything that stinks kills." Because the association of odors with disease laid the foundation for the uproar over the Great Stink of 1880, the scientific elaboration of this link deserves detailed exposition. The process by which the odors of Paris were implicated in the spread of disease reveals unexpected layers of meaning in ostensibly straightforward scientific texts, casting new light on a period of decisive change in French medicine and society.

The development of the germ theory of disease dramatically altered the scientific environment within which the Great Stink of 1880 unfolded. Around this time emerged the first suggestions that the salvation of mankind from the scourge of illness lay in the new science of bacteriology. Between the mid-1870s and the mid-1880s, among other advances, the first microorganisms responsible for specific diseases were isolated and identified (including those of anthrax and typhoid fever, which were to figure centrally in the discussion of the odors of Paris), and new kinds of vaccines were first developed from attenuated strains of pathogenic microbes. The most famous actor in these dramas was Louis Pasteur, the chemist turned microbiologist, whose research promised to reveal the hidden truths of disease and held out the hope of previously undreamed of preventive and therapeutic breakthroughs.[72] To say that Pasteur's opinions on the Great Stink of 1880 carried considerable scientific authority is an understatement; when he spoke, it was not only fellow scientists who listened. If there was something like an oracular source at which scientific truth could be sought at that time, particularly where microbes were concerned, it was Pasteur's laboratory on the rue d'Ulm.

While others speaking out on the odors worried about cholera, typhoid fever, infantile diarrhea, or other diseases associated with possible fecal transmission, Pasteur's primary contribution to the work of the ministerial commission was to discuss some of the implications of his recent work on anthrax. Among the most breathtaking advances in bacteriology during those formative years was Pasteur's famous anthrax vaccine demonstration at Pouilly-le-Fort in the spring of 1881. The dramatic experimental performance stands out as a landmark in the development of modern medical science, and its success paved the way for the wider acceptance of the germ theory of disease, and of the attenuation of pathogens as a practical strategy of vaccine development.[73]

Beginning on May 5, 1881, a group of animals consisting of twenty-four sheep, one goat, and six cows were vaccinated twice, two weeks apart. Two weeks after the second vaccination, these and an identically comprised group of unvaccinated animals were inoculated with a virulent strain of anthrax. On June 2, a crowd of journalists, scientists, dignitaries, and curious observers gathered for the great event, the theatrical demonstration of bacteriology's boundless promise. The onlookers were astonished and awestruck at the spectacle that greeted them: twenty-one unvaccinated sheep and one goat dead, three other sheep mortally ill, the six unvaccinated cows showing noticeable symptoms, and all vaccinated animals apparently in perfect health. (In fact, one vaccinated goat died the next day, but it was found that she was pregnant, and her death was attributed to the prior death of the fetus inside her.)[74] These results certainly changed the course of science, and the mute testimony of the dead animals spoke volumes about the promise of attenuated vaccines. (Fig. 3.)

Far less well known than the Pouilly-le-Fort trial is Pasteur's anthrax ex-

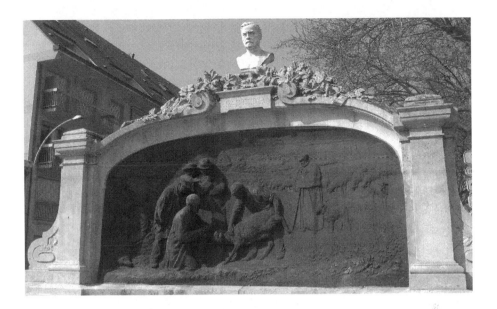

Fig. 3. This monument in Chartres commemorates the research undertaken on nearby farms that led to Pasteur's successful demonstration of an anthrax vaccine on sheep at Pouilly-le-Fort in 1881. Photo by author.

periment at Rosières the previous autumn, which he cited in the final report of the ministerial commission on the odors of 1880. (The experiment began on October 8, 1880, just after the end of the Great Stink in Paris; its results were published in January 1881, shortly before the commission issued its report.) A farm in that village, near the city of Senlis north of Paris, had been suffering severe livestock losses to anthrax over the years. There seemed to be particular "deadly zones" on the farm, which, it was thought, corresponded to areas where dead animals had been buried. Along with his collaborators Charles Chamberland and Emile Roux, Pasteur devised an experiment to test a theory about the duration of anthrax virulence. The results were reported both in the proceedings of the Academy of Sciences and in the commission's report as evidence for the possible spread of disease-causing germs in fecal emanations.[75]

Pasteur, Chamberland, and Roux began by having seven healthy sheep led from the farmer's flock to one of the so-called deadly zones, where the cadavers of sheep killed by anthrax had been buried a full twelve years earlier. No grass grew on the surface of the site, and the animals ate nothing while they stayed there. The healthy sheep were left at the site for a period of several hours, then led back to the sheepfold with the rest of the flock.

This procedure was repeated with the same sheep every day for nearly seven weeks. Two of the seven experimental subjects died of anthrax in late October and early November, while the control sheep remained healthy. The two animals' deaths, Pasteur concluded, could not be explained by the usual mode of transmission of anthrax—the ingestion during feeding of virulent spores: "We are dealing here with a momentary stay on the surface of a site where for twelve years no animals who had died of anthrax had been buried, and the sheep who were the subjects of the experiment did not graze on the site; *the germ of the disease therefore can only have penetrated their bodies through the well-known habit that sheep have of continually sniffing the ground.*"[76] The startling but inescapable conclusions were that the spores of anthrax bacilli could conserve their virulence for as long as twelve years, and that these virulent spores could somehow migrate not just to the surface of the ground above the old cadavers, but even into the air above that ground, where they could be inhaled by new victims.

Yet Pasteur did not stop there. The immediate relevance of his experiment, he insisted, reached far beyond a previously unknown danger to livestock. The farmer's family, as it happened, kept a kitchen garden near the deadly zones of the farm, and regularly consumed its produce. Pasteur, Chamberland, and Roux asked the farmer whether there had been any cases of anthrax in his family: "The farmer answered: " 'Not to my knowledge. Only I myself have had a malignant pustule, which healed, as you can see from the scar,' " he told us, pointing to his face. *It may be presumed that, if the vegetables consumed at the farm had not been cooked, things would have happened differently, and we would perhaps have found victims of the terrible disease there.*"[77] The danger, it turned out, was more insidious and far-reaching than it first appeared. If one combined the ostensibly proven danger of emanations with the potential danger of other imaginable means of transmission, the chain of death might quickly extend beyond sheep, and even beyond the boundaries of the farm itself. Not only farmers, but potentially all human beings, were at risk from the unseen and long-lived creatures Pasteur had found. "Change the living conditions of the farm's animals even slightly, as we have just done," he argued, and you will kill some number of them. Their bodies will in turn pose a threat—"by whatever mode of transport, direct transmission or indirect by flies"—to other animals and even human beings: "witness the example of the farmer himself."[78]

The report of the Rosières experiment, obscure and historically unremarkable when compared with the dramatic import of Pouilly-le-Fort the following spring, nevertheless raises several puzzling questions. The most obvious one is that of Pasteur's basic conclusion itself: that is, his contention that he had scientifically proven the transmissibility of anthrax to living animals by means of *emanations* from the ground where cadavers had been buried long before. The two sheep in question, it is important to remember, became sick not by grazing on the deadly ground, but merely by sniffing the air above it.[79]

It is possible to imagine other scenarios by which Pasteur and his colleagues could have explained the two sheep's demise; more to the point, one could imagine contemporaries not finding the circumstances at Rosières to be directly relevant to the Great Stink of 1880 in Paris. Pasteur's conclusion—that germ-filled emanations, whether malodorous or not, threatened to sow pestilence within their deadly zones of influence—may seem somewhat far-fetched in light of the subsequent development of germ theory, which highlighted airborne droplets, fecal-oral transmission, and waterborne infection as the principal routes by which most infectious diseases are spread. Yet for some reason, the idea of contagion through emanations carried compelling explanatory appeal at the time. Why would Pasteur and others go to such great lengths to prove the danger of germs in emanations? One clue may lie in another of Pasteur's breakthroughs, this one from two decades earlier, which in some respects represents the very birth of germ theory.

In a legendary confrontation with naturalist Félix-Archimède Pouchet between 1860 and 1864, Pasteur definitively laid to rest the scientific doctrine of "heterogenesis," or spontaneous generation.[80] Pouchet and others claimed that microscopic life could arise either from inorganic substances or from nonliving organic debris under certain conditions. Pasteur, on the other hand, was convinced that life could originate only from life, that tiny germs were present on dust particles in the air, and that media rendered sterile would forever remain so (no matter what their chemical composition) absent contact with existing microorganisms. Pasteur devised an elaborate series of demonstrations to prove these contentions and effectively refute spontaneous generation.

Liquid media in flasks of various configurations were boiled and then briefly exposed to the ambient air in various locations: Pasteur's laboratory at the Ecole normale supérieure, the basement of the Paris observatory, and at altitudes of 850 meters in the Jura plateau and 2,000 meters on an Alpine glacier. In related experiments, flask necks were shaped to prevent contact between the liquid and atmospheric dust, even when the neck was unsealed. Microbes grew on the media exposed to airborne dust, in varying quantities depending on location and altitude, and failed to grow where contact with dust was prevented. In 1864, an Academy of Sciences commission pronounced in favor of Pasteur in his dispute with Pouchet; spontaneous generation was discredited, and the groundwork was laid for the pioneering work on germ theory that would follow in the ensuing decades.

Two of the important lessons learned from Pasteur's work on spontaneous generation were that germs were always present, invisibly, in the air, and that they were present in varying concentrations in different kinds of air. There were more germs in the air of Pasteur's laboratory than in the observatory, for example, and more at an altitude of 850 meters than at 2,000 meters. Whereas miasmatic thinking drew upon a certain kind of common sense in linking emanations from foul-smelling substances with the spread of disease, proponents of germ theory could now invoke scientific proof as well as that same common sense to show that microbes were in the air, and in some airs more than in others. In the late 1870s and early 1880s, researchers at the Montsouris Observatory in Paris conducted a series of extensive and well-publicized studies measuring the concentration of microbes in air taken from various locations around the city.[81] The powerful and durable impact of the spontaneous generation debates could explain at least in part the insistence with which Pasteur and others sought to find deadly germs in the air of Rosières—and Paris—in 1880.

In both of those instances, the leap from observed phenomena to potential threat was large and instantaneous. How and why did Pasteur, for example, move from the death of two sheep to the scenario of an epidemic barely avoided? The Rosières narrative adopts what would ultimately become the central stylistic device of contagionist rhetoric. Scientific demonstration of transmission, and even of resultant illness, was not enough. The contagionist agenda demanded that the stakes be raised, that the specter of mass calamity and vaguely ominous plagues be projected to the population at risk—that is, to everyone. The fact that anthrax was extremely rare among humans did not prevent Pasteur from scaring his readers with the prospect of disaster narrowly averted by sheer luck. In the future, one might reasonably infer, luck would not be enough, and only the expertise of scientists would be capable of preventing a catastrophe. The analogy to the danger of fecal emanations in the sewers—explicit in the governmental commission's report on the Paris odors, which quoted extensively from the Rosières study—intensified the ominous tone of Pasteur's warning.

The chemist-turned-microbiologist Pasteur, of course, was no physician, and anthrax was not a serious human health threat. (Neither was rabies, which accounted for Pasteur's greatest medical achievement, a vaccine effective on human beings, in 1885. Because of its lengthy incubation period, dramatic symptoms, and nearly 100% case-fatality rate, however, rabies enjoyed more cultural visibility than did anthrax.) In part, this focus on animal diseases was due to the extraordinary difficulty of experimentation on human subjects at the time, although questions have recently been raised over whether Pasteur did in fact experiment on human beings in his work on the rabies vaccine.[82] His ally Paul Brouardel, however, was a leader among French physicians and an expert on human diseases. The one that preoccupied Brouardel during the Great Stink of 1880 was a disease that was widely believed to be spread by fecal matter: typhoid fever.

As chairman of one of the ministerial commission's three subcommittees, Brouardel took the opportunity offered by his section of the report to warn of the transmissibility of this scourge by fecal emanations. The Germans Karl Eberth and Edwin Klebs succeeded in isolating the bacillus responsible for typhoid fever in 1880, but even before that it was widely believed that feces played the crucial role in the transmission of the disease. The precise nature of that role, however, was unclear. In Brouardel's mind, it was no longer a matter of doubt that typhoid could be spread by airborne means, through emanations from human excrement. He cited many cases proving such transmission as part of the commission report, including one from his own personal experience: his friend Isidore Geoffroy Saint-Hilaire, director of the Paris zoological garden, was away from home when the ventilation pipe of his cesspit broke, and leaked emanations into one of the rooms of his house. Two ladies and three children were staying in rooms adjoining the one where the leak occurred. "Around midnight, the two ladies and two of the children were awakened by stomach pains; they began vomiting, and a window had to be opened because of the infection of the air."[83]

The four afflicted residents recovered. Once again, however, the threat of emanations proved to be more severe than initially suspected. "None of those who were ill that night experienced any further effects," Brouardel continued. "Only an eight-year-old child had slept through the night without incident; a week later he had a serious case of typhoid fever." Direct contagion, he contended, could be ruled out in this case: Geoffroy Saint-Hilaire had lived in the house since its construction, no other cases of typhoid fever had been discovered in the area, and none of the children in question had had any contact with other children. "It would be difficult to argue that the broken ventilation pipe was not the cause of this young child's typhoid fever."[84] Only the foul gases escaping from the cesspit could account for the transmission of typhoid fever to the young boy.

This anecdote was accompanied in the commission's report by an exhaustive list of further examples, drawn both from the medical literature and from word of mouth. Brouardel invoked William Budd of Bristol, Charles Murchison of Edinburgh, Franz von Gietl of Munich, and other authorities to show that "for doctors of all countries, *the propagation of typhoid fever through the air is now uncontested.*"[85] Henceforth, particularly in large cities, all feces, toilets, cesspits, and sewers were to be considered potential sources of infectious emanations.

The alarm sounded by Pasteur and Brouardel found echoes among other scientists and physicians in Paris during the Great Stink of 1880. Prominent chemist Henri Sainte-Claire Deville granted that the "nauseating" quality of the odors did "not necessarily make them harmful"; he warned, however, that they could "borrow from their sources the germs to which typhoidic and choleriform diseases are attributed these days." Adrien Proust, professor at the Paris medical faculty and member of the Academy of Medicine, agreed that diarrheal diseases, dysentery, "and perhaps typhoid fever" were spreading "under the influence of these emanations." Notwithstanding the position of the departmental public health council (which considered the odors unpleasant but relatively harmless), some local physicians in Paris and surrounding towns felt certain that just as a swamp could engender certain deadly fevers, the "concentrated miasmas of decomposing animal and excremental matter" were responsible for "the extension, if not the production, of certain epidemics."[86]

A peculiar hybrid of miasmatism and germ theory, this science of emanations was uniquely situated to make sense of the odors of 1880. Microbiology (led by Pasteur) and the new microbe-oriented public health (with Brouardel among its most prominent spokesmen) were being built in part on their novelty, and on their difference from what had come before. The claim that foul-smelling emanations spread disease is quintessential miasmatism. The old sanitary science equated unpleasant smells with pathogenic influences, especially in the urban environment. As English health reformer Edwin Chadwick famously remarked in 1846, "All smell is disease."[87] This was the old theory of disease that Pasteur and his followers were in the process of overthrowing in 1880. One would hardly expect to find outspoken advocates of germ theory going out of their way to call attention to the public health danger of unpleasant odors. And yet that is precisely what happened in the commission's report.

A potentially confusing web of historical trajectories must be disentangled in order to properly understand the distinction between miasmatism and germ theory in 1880. In the long run, it is clear that a predominance of miasmatic perspectives on common diseases in the mid-nineteenth century was eventually displaced by a consensus in favor of bacteriological explanations in the early twentieth century. By 1900 to a considerable extent, and even more thoroughly two decades later, microscopic organisms had become the presumed causal agents of most human disease. Although the microbes associated with many diseases had yet to be found in those early decades—and the discoveries that had been made had provided extremely limited therapeutic and prophylactic benefits—it was commonly expected that microbiology would eventually find both causes and cures for a wide variety of illnesses. The long-term view of the triumph of germ theory has prompted some observers to read into late nineteenth-century public health discourse an inherent and inevitable battle between conservatism and progress, miasmas and germs.[88]

However, this dichotomy distorts the situation as it must have looked to participants and observers in the debates of 1880. In the midst of the initial flurry of bacteriological discoveries—the "golden years," one historian has called them, in which the microbial causes of major diseases were being identified "at the phenomenal rate of one a year"[89]—advances in germ theory certainly attracted attention, and some scientists and physicians (including Pasteur and Brouardel) had already cast their lot definitively with the new approach to disease. Nevertheless, for most observers, there was no clear and practical distinction between miasmas and microbes as causes of disease; the difference was for the most part semantic, intellectual, or speculative, and made no apparent difference in the everyday effort to prevent or cure human disease. Miasmatism, with its focus on malign emanations from marshes and putrefying organic matter, denotes less a specific medical doctrine than a language in which observed disease phenomena could be discussed and addressed, as well as a tendency to look for health threats in particular places.[90] In the lingua franca of the late 1870s and early 1880s—both inside and outside the medical world—the word "miasma" could denote any disease-causing influence, and the less commonly used "germ" (germe in French), while associated by some with recent scientific discoveries of pathogenic microorganisms, could be used generally to indicate the "seeds" or origins of disease. Although one can identify distinctive styles associated with miasmatism and germ theory, they were not mutually exclusive schools of thought, and their terminology often overlapped in discussions of specific diseases or public health policies.

When the Great Stink struck, then, the advocates of germ theory seized on the problem as evidence of the hidden danger of pathogenic microbes, while others perceived the problem through the lens of an amalgam of expectations and predispositions. Neither committed to nor opposed to germ theory per se, they were influenced by the long-held conviction that foul odors were dangerous and somehow spread disease, but demanded convincing evidence before determining that any particular substance or practice was conclusively harmful or safe. It was against this backdrop that doctors, hygienists, government officials, journalists, and ordinary citizens understood and debated the Great Stink of 1880. Whenever new circumstances arose, the cognitive default option was to fit them into preexisting templates. The use of certain terms such as "miasmas" and "germs" should not necessarily be taken as evidence of a skirmish in a greater etiological conflict.

Nevertheless, determined advocates of germ theory such as Pasteur and Brouardel did enter the debate over the odors of Paris, and the question remains: why would the leaders of the new scientific public health insist on the danger of certain odors, and seize on the Great Stink of 1880 to promote their cause? Given the aims of the bacteriologists, it might seem more reasonable either to downplay the danger of foul odors in the city or ignore the problem entirely, focusing instead on hidden health threats that had hitherto escaped public notice. Indeed, some experts did claim that the odors of 1880 were harmless. These voices of moderation agreed that the odors were unpleasant, even intolerable at times, but they refused to grant them the power to spread disease. The public health council of the Seine department and Adolphe Alphand, the director of public works, argued that there was no real increase in mortality during the Great Stink in Paris, and that in any case such odors could not cause serious illness. The council's report, as was common among observers on both sides of the issue, spoke simultaneously of "miasmas" and "germs" of disease when it claimed that the odors were attributable to the suburban waste treatment plants, which were incapable of projecting miasmatic influences over a great distance; moreover, the report concluded that the plants' practice of heating waste products during treatment killed disease-causing microbes.[91] Nevertheless, the predominant view at the highest levels of French science and medicine held that—regardless of whether one identified miasmas or germs, or both, as the cause of disease—the disgusting smells of 1880 were potentially lethal. Dr. Hippolyte Marié-Davy, responding to the public health council's report exonerating the odors, put it this way: "I persist in thinking that these emanations are prejudicial to public health; I persist in considering these foul gases to be the most active propagating agents of contagious diseases."[92]

Pasteur, Brouardel, and their colleagues lent their prestige to the alarmists rather than to the voices of reassurance. They used the distress over the Great Stink of 1880 as a platform from which to pursue their project of reshaping the nation's health policy and educating the population regarding the true causes of disease. But this begs another question: why, in the course of demonstrating that the odors of Paris could indeed spread disease, insist on the fact that "not everything that stinks kills, and not everything that kills stinks"? Paradoxically, the miasmatic belief that foul-smelling emanations cause illness, modified by this clever slogan, actually demonstrated the urgent need for a new science of public health built upon the foundation of germs. Germs, it now seemed, were everywhere; they proliferated even underground, in the vast network of the sewers, and in the air above, transported miles from their original source on the wind and in sinister vapors. Though they could not be seen, they could be smelled—but not always. To get the better of them, or even to understand the first thing about where they were and how they behaved, one needed a cadre of scientifically trained experts who could identify and ultimately neutralize them.

The puzzle of the Rosières study and its relation to the Great Stink only deepens when one consults Pasteur's original laboratory notebooks. The notes for the "deadly zones" experiment correspond to the published study in every respect but one. The sentence concluding that because the sheep in question did not graze on the site, "the germ of the disease therefore can only have penetrated their bodies through the well-known habit that sheep have of continually sniffing the ground" (le germe de la maladie n'a pu pénétrer dans leur corps que par suite de l'habitude bien connue qu'ont les moutons de flairer sans cesse la terre) appears in the lab notebooks as follows: "therefore, the sheep can only have placed their noses in the ground on the surface of pit no. 1" (les moutons n'ont donc fait que pouvoir placer leurs nez dans la terre a la surface de la fosse n° 1).[93] In the original French as well as in the English translation, "sniff the ground" is not synonymous with "place their noses in the ground." The latter involves physical contact, while the former does not.

Why the change from "place their noses in" to "sniff"? There are several plausible explanations. It may have been an empirical revision: Pasteur and his collaborators may have decided upon reflection or discussion that the animals did not in fact touch the ground with their noses. It may also have been a simple stylistic revision: where "place their noses in the earth" is awkward, "sniff the earth" is smooth and concise. It is also possible, however, that Pasteur edited the phrase in order to amplify the experiment's resonance beyond the question of sheep and anthrax. In 1880 and 1881, neither the medical profession nor the general public were paying much attention to bacteria and their dangers. Pasteur and his allies found themselves compelled to sound the alarm about germs in the most dramatic manner possible in order to convince policymakers and the general public of the urgency of bacteriological research. In the Great Stink commission's deliberations and in other discussions of public health dangers around this time, a diffuse and generalized threat—one that could attack a victim who merely sniffed the air, for example—might have been seen as more alarming than one that required direct physical contact. This reading is consonant with the tone of the Rosières study's closing paragraphs, in which Pasteur energetically, almost lyrically, conjures the fearsome specter of an epidemic averted by sheer luck.

For advocates of germ theory, both the anthrax outbreak in Rosières and the Great Stink of 1880, rather than representing the miasmatic prejudices that science could prove groundless, embodied the ever-present danger of unseen pathogens. The odors of Paris appeared first in one place, then another, then disappeared only to make themselves felt even more intensely some time later in yet another part of the city. The acuteness of the sensation, when combined with the elusiveness and invisibility of the phenomenon, only served as a reminder of the fact that the threat of germs was ubiquitous; the danger was compounded by the fact that the presence of germs did not always signal itself to the senses. Moreover, the fact that not all odors were dangerous established the necessity of scientific expertise to distinguish the harmless nuisances from the true hazards.

More was at stake, however, in the Great Stink of 1880 than professional imperatives and scientific prestige. The conviction that the putrid stench was an imminent danger owed its prevalence to many factors outside of science itself. Beyond the question of whether odors truly contained germs or could spread disease, Parisians confronted grave anxieties about the growth of their city, the disposal of their waste, and the challenge of integrating millions of consuming and excreting bodies into a republican polity and a civilized culture.

In [the first half of the nineteenth century] Paris looked around and was
unable to recognize itself. Another, larger city had overflowed into the
unaltered framework of streets, mansions, houses and passageways, piling
man on man and trade on trade, filling every nook and corner, . . . packing
the suddenly shrunken streets and the now overpopulated gothic graveyards,
resurrecting and overloading the forgotten sewers, spreading litter and
stench into the adjacent countryside.

—LOUIS CHEVALIER, *Laboring Classes and Dangerous Classes*
in Paris During the First Half of the Nineteenth Century (1973, 45)

On a fundamental level, one must look for the causes of the Great Stink of 1880 in the brutal fact of the physical growth of Paris during the mid-nineteenth century. During the half century preceding the Great Stink, the city had grown in population from less than 800,000 to more than 2.2 million.[94] It was the second most populous city in Europe, behind London (which was much larger in area). In 1860, seemingly on the verge of implosion, the city of Paris annexed several suburban towns, thereby adding a sizable poor and working-class population to the city and expanding its spatial reach outward. The largest population growth over any single census period in the century took place during the time of the Great Stink, between 1876 and 1881. For olfactory purposes, what this explosive growth meant was both a vastly greater total output of human waste and a geographic expansion of the population outward, ever closer to the dumps and treatment plants whose vicinity had previously been semirural and sparsely inhabited.

The city's growth also provoked crises in housing, in water supply, and in sewage disposal. During the Second Empire, Napoleon III and his prefect of the Seine department, Georges Eugène, Baron Haussmann, attempted to remake the very physical fabric of the capital in an ambitious campaign of demolitions and slum clearance accompanied by the construction of wide new boulevards, spacious parks, aqueducts, and sewers. In one of the most wide-ranging urban public works programs of all time, what has become known as "Haussmannization" seemingly turned Paris into an immense construction site, displacing tenants from the crowded central districts and causing rents in the city to rise dramatically. Critics at the time and since have exposed financial irregularities in Haussmann's rebuilding program, ridiculed the drab architectural monotony of the new streets, lamented the expulsion of the working class from central Paris, and protested against the strategic aims that called for wider streets to prevent barricades and facilitate troop movements in the event of political unrest.[95]

Alongside the corruption and the cynical political calculus, however, a particular vision of the modern city animated the work of Haussmann and his engineers. Public health figured centrally in this vision. Metaphorically, the sick city beset by revolution and epidemics needed to be healed, and mild treatments would not do. As one architectural historian has pointed out, surgical metaphors became "firmly embedded in the unconscious analogies of urban planning": "After the prolonged pathology, the drawn-out agony of the patient, the body of Paris, was to be delivered of its illnesses, its cancers, and epidemics once and for all by the total act of surgery. 'Cutting' and 'piercing' were the adjectives used to describe the operation."[96] Health concerns inspired the metaphorical surgeons Napoleon III and Haussmann on a more literal and immediate level as well. Both the emperor and the prefect were (or claimed to have been) directly motivated by "hygienic science" in the formulation of their plans.[97] The four major arenas of the Paris public works programs in the Second Empire—street building, parks, sewers, and water supply—were all explicitly touted as public health measures. The wide new streets and spacious squares brought air and sunlight into the overcrowded quarters where disease had flourished. The Bois de Boulogne, the Bois de Vincennes, the Buttes-Chaumont, and other parks were intended as the "lungs of the city," purifying the Parisian air. New aqueducts, reservoirs, and water mains greatly expanded the supply of fresh water into the city, and more than 600 kilometers of new sewer lines drained the streets of impurities.[98] From the realm of metaphor to the everyday world of practical details, the transformation of Paris was fundamentally conceived as a work of *assainissement*—"sanitation" or "cleansing."

Urban hygiene and sanitation reforms were certainly an important aspect of the Haussmannization that gave birth to the modern sewers of Paris. But there was more to it than that. Haussmann and his patron, Napoleon III, aimed above all to remake the topography of the city, to refashion its image by substituting order for disorder, uniformity for haphazard accretion, and a classical ideal of beauty for the Gothic mix of filth and splendor that marked the Old Paris.[99] And the beautification was not meant to be simply visual.

Chadwick, the great British sanitary reformer, was reported to have said to Emperor Napoleon III on the subject of the massive public works program he had entrusted to Haussmann, "Sir, it was said of Augustus that he

The Great Stink of Paris

found Rome brick and left it marble. May it be said of you that you found Paris stinking and left it sweet."[100] Freedom from offensive odors was now not just an ideal of civilized individuals, but a more or less officially recognized goal of the modern state, and a demand that citizens were in turn beginning to make of the state.[101]

Haussmann's Paris represented a radically new ideal of the modern city, entirely apart from the actual physical changes wrought in the city's physiognomy during the Second Empire. Although the famously autocratic prefect's rebuilding program encountered fierce political resistance and the greater part of the city maintained its previous appearance, Haussmannization succeeded in projecting new norms of spatial order onto the urban environment—in "giv[ing] modernity a shape."[102] What emerged from the Second Empire was not so much a capital city physically transformed as an ideology of transformation that held out the prospect of a chaotic, filthy environment ordered and cleansed.

The scale of Haussmann's intervention set an important precedent, and helped usher in a new conception of public space and of state responsibility for controlling the urban environment. From the monotonously uniform façades of the new buildings and the broad perspectives offered by the wide new boulevards to the grand new public parks and the vast sewer network, Napoleon III and Haussmann laid the groundwork for a new modern metropolis, a place in which no aspect of political, social, or even sensory life lay beyond the reach of state power and state responsibility. The control of urban space, street by street, in this volatile city had proved critical to the survival and fall of political regimes for nearly a century. But after the mid-nineteenth century, more was at stake in this effort than avoiding or quashing popular uprisings. Geographer David Harvey has highlighted the "dramatic shift from the introverted, private, and personalized urbanism of the July Monarchy to an extroverted, public, and collectivized style of urbanism under the Second Empire," which brought with it a "sense of proprietorship over public space" that forever altered the relationship between citizen and city.[103] Henceforth, the physical environment of Paris was everyone's affair. In 1880, in the aftermath of Haussmann's autocratic precedent, and with a newly democratic, reform-minded republican regime in power, Parisians in the early Third Republic did not hesitate to express their anxiety and anger when they saw (or smelled) danger in the streets.

The empire's legacy, etched in the very stone of the city, was never far from the surface in debates over the Great Stink of 1880. To progressive, positivist republicans, it was unthinkable that a corrupt, authoritarian regime could have done more to improve the city's health than a modern, democratic one. "The odious, execrable previous government cleaned Paris up, [while] . . . the current, admirable government is stinking it up," complained the newspaper *Paris-Journal*.[104] In addition to spending "enormous" amounts of money to complete the "hygienic" work of Haussmann's street-building program, a petition to the city council asked in late September, couldn't local authorities "sacrifice some money, if necessary, to prevent half the city from breathing poisoned air?"[105] One newspaper went so far as to bring Baron Haussmann himself out of retirement as an expert commentator on the Great Stink. Haussmann blamed the odors on the dumping of unauthorized waste into the sewers, and on an insufficient water flow within the sewers. Perhaps predictably, he proposed an audacious solution on a grand scale: the construction of an entirely new canal system that would bring water from the Loire River near Nevers in central France north to the capital, vastly increasing the water supply available for the city's sanitation.[106] Haussmann's presence lingered on in Paris—not only in the new boulevards and parks, but even in the mental associations that seemed to link his name automatically with any phenomenon relating to the physical appearance (and even smell) of the city. If Paris fell victim to a pervasive stench, one immediately thought of Haussmann, and asked his opinion. And if there was a single area in which Haussmann's legacy catalyzed dispute and controversy during the Great Stink of 1880, it was underneath Paris, in the sewers.

The Underworld

Simultaneously a triumph of sanitary engineering and "the direct continuation of the sick person's intestines," the Paris sewers provoked equal measures of admiration and loathing in the late nineteenth century.[107] Although the city's first covered sewer dated from the fourteenth century, and by 1850 there were 143 kilometers of sewer lines underneath the capital's streets, the Second Empire marked the golden age of sewer construction. Under Haussmann's administration, existing sewers were rebuilt and 630 kilometers of new lines added, multiplying the extent of the sewer network more than fivefold.[108] Only rainwater, street debris, and miscellaneous refuse were welcome in the sewers, however; human excretions continued to follow the itinerary that led to the cesspit, the *vidange* cart, and finally the waste treatment plant. It was not until the mid-1870s that city officials proposed to evacuate all human waste through the sewers, which would empty out either into the Seine downstream from Paris or on the fields of sewage farms in the Saint-Germain forest west of the city.[109]

The battle that resulted was fierce, and raged until the eve of World War I. City engineers, convinced that the cesspit system was antiquated and unsanitary, and faced with the intractable problem of waste disposal for the ever-growing numbers of Parisians, determined that the safest thing to do with the city's urine and feces was to evacuate it through the sewers. This proposal became known as the *tout-à-l'égout* system: "everything into the sewers." The system would require every building in the city to add pipes connecting each toilet to the sewer line under the street. It would also require a huge increase in the amount of water supplied by the city to each building in order to ensure that all solid wastes were carried through to the sewer network, as well as a greater volume of water in the sewers themselves to ensure a constant flow.

Among the very few defenders of the ungainly cesspit system were Parisian landlords. Doggedly resisting any kind of change, they feared the major expenses that the retrofitting of their buildings and the increased water supply would bring. Moreover, proposed ancillary municipal ordinances that would require a minimum ratio of toilets to inhabitants in each residential building did nothing to endear landlords to the *tout-à-l'égout* plan. The cartel of cesspit-emptying companies, who faced the total loss of their livelihood, also fought the project tooth and nail.[110]

The reasons for the opposition of leading scientists and hygienists, however, are less immediately obvious. Certainly, these men felt no fondness for the existing cesspit system. Yet they insisted that to allow human excrement to circulate freely underneath the city, exposed in many places to the very air breathed by Parisians, would be to court disaster and invite epidemics. The likelihood that microbes responsible for contagious diseases were present in the city's solid waste, combined with the fact that sewers were underfoot everywhere and connected in countless places with the world above, horrified many authorities. Even *tout-à-l'égout* proponents spoke of "creating a dark city [*une cité ténébreuse*] underneath the living Paris into which would flow the wastewater and excretions of its 70,000 houses, 2,000 factories, and streets." How could responsible men of science, one physician opposed to the plan asked, consider innocuous "the slow and permanent circulation of fecal matter in the sewers—that is, under our feet, under our streets, in the middle of Paris, between each row of houses"?[111]

During the Great Stink of 1880, even without the *tout-à-l'égout* system in place, many Parisians insisted that the foul odors enveloping the city were coming from the sewers, and for proof they pointed with disgust at sewer vents and manholes:

> Horrible emanations are coming from every sewer opening. . . . Pass by place Saint-Sulpice, or rue du Cirque, or rue La Boétie, or rue Saint-Arnaud, and you will be struck by the sickening scents coming out of the . . . sewers.[112]

> Out of this mass of horrible muck [that the circulating current in the sewers leaves behind as residue] comes . . . asphyxiating emanations. You need only pass next to a sewer manhole to be convinced of this fact, which is *as plain as the nose on your face.*[113]

The ministerial commission on the odors of Paris, though it acknowledged sundry possible causes for the stench, also focused considerable attention on the sewers and on the dangers of the *tout-à-l'égout* system, which it unequivocally denounced. "It would be imprudent at the very least, in the current state of science, to accumulate in the sewers . . . matter that contains the germs of various contagious diseases," the commission concluded.[114]

For its opponents, the plan to bring together the totality of the city's human waste in the sewers, then dump it on suburban sewage farms or "filtering fields" (*champs d'épuration*), was foolhardy and potentially disastrous. In effect, it would turn all of Paris into the apartment of Brouardel's friend Geoffroy Saint-Hilaire at the Jardin des Plantes: through the openings in toilets and sewer vents and manholes, each dwelling and each street would be on the receiving end of emanations from the excrement of all Parisians—thousands of whom were at any given time suffering from diseases known to be spread fecally. Perhaps nobody expressed the anxiety caused by such a possibility as evocatively as did Brouardel himself, in his contribution to the ministerial commission's final report: "When the sewers receive fecal matter, they can become the vehicle that transports and propagates the poison [of typhoid fever] and they may be considered . . . as 'the direct continuation of the sick person's intestine.' "[115] The entire city would be turned into a vast circulatory network for poisonous, contagious excrement—both above and below ground, thanks to the role of emanations. One need hardly be a professor at the Paris medical school to contemplate such a prospect with abject horror.

Perhaps most revealing of all is the alternative system touted by Pasteur, Brouardel, and others fearful of sewer emanations. Instead of the *tout-à-l'égout,* they proposed a separate, self-contained, airtight disposal network leading from each toilet (with a secure, airtight hinged opening) to ultimate deposit far from civilization, where waste could be harmlessly released. Pasteur called the tout-à-l'égout plan "not in accordance with the findings of modern science" and warned that an accumulation of the "germs contained in sewage" could invite epidemics. He himself favored the separate closed circuit, leading from Paris to the sea, "where [these germs] could no longer cause harm." Both the indoor and outdoor air of the city would be protected from contamination, and the English Channel would serve as the final resting place for the bodily waste of Paris.[116] Safety and progress lay in transport and disposal without reaching any of the human senses.

In the end, the strenuous objections of Pasteur, Brouardel, and other opponents were not enough to kill the tout-à-l'égout plan, though its final victory was a long time coming. After having been initially approved by the Paris City Council in 1876, the new system received a legislative go-ahead from the parliament only in 1894. The number of houses in Paris connected directly to the sewer exceeded the number of houses with cesspits only in 1903, and on the eve of World War I nearly 26,000 cesspits remained in use in the City of Light.[117]

Warnings of the danger posed by sewer emanations were usually hypothetical, based on what could happen or what might happen if germ-filled excretions were evacuated into the sewers or if the tout-à-l'égout plan became a reality. But suddenly, in the waning days of the Great Stink of 1880, the death of four sewermen transformed overnight what had been a vague and generalized fear into a terror of deadly immediacy. In the early morning hours of September 26, 1880, a crew of ten employees was cleaning a section of sewer line under the boulevard Rochechouart near the rue de Clignancourt, in the eighteenth arrondissement, when five of their number failed to answer a call to join their co-workers above ground for a rest break. The neighborhood firemen who rushed to the rescue dragged to the surface four dead bodies and one sewerman near death. Seventeen-year-old Louis Prot survived, but the odors of Paris now had their first martyrs: Bertrand Bourillon, 50, the crew chief; Joseph Para, 42; Constant Garnerat, 32; and Camille Richard, 22. Bourillon was married, with six children; Para was a widower, with two children; Garnerat and Richard were unmarried.[118]

The tragedy began around ten o'clock Saturday evening, September 25, with a routine sewer cleaning operation under the boulevard Rochechouart. One team of five workers shoveled accumulated sand and other debris from the sewer into buckets, which their co-workers carried up to the surface for removal. The night's work proceeded without incident until 4:30 Sunday morning, when the crew chief banged three times on a manhole cover, the customary signal for the workers underground to come out for a rest break. This time, there was no response. When the crew chief went down to investigate, he was forced to turn back by an intense odor in the sewer, and ran to the local fire station for help. Although one of the rescuers himself nearly passed out from the odors, his helmet and the buttons of his jacket turned red and black by the fumes, all five bodies (including that of Louis Prot, who was barely breathing) were eventually recovered and brought to the surface. One of the victims was found lying face down in a pool of sewage.[119]

A crowd quickly gathered in the street above to see what the commotion was about. When they heard the news, they had no doubt at all what had caused the catastrophe. They immediately accused the *vidangeurs* who at the time of the deaths had been emptying the cesspit at number 17 rue de Clignancourt, just off the boulevard Rochechouart. The *vidangeurs* fled the scene as soon as they learned of the tragedy, doing nothing to allay the neighbors' suspicion that they had illegally dumped the cesspit's contents into the sewer. The workers were arrested the next day, and chemical analysis found clear traces of fecal matter both in the sewer line adjacent to the house and in the pipe that evacuated the building's household wastewater into the sewer. This latter finding suggested that the cesspit cleaners had established an illegal connection for their pump in the wastewater pipe. Prot, the accident's only survivor, remembered only that he smelled a "strong odor of *vidange*" before losing consciousness. Most experts agreed that the waste from the cesspit entered the sewer either shortly before or at the same time that the sewermen collapsed; the fumes then overcame the unfortunate workers, either because they found themselves between the waste deposits in front of them and a sewer vent behind them or because a temporary dam set up to retain water flow within the sewer during cleaning had just been removed. Whatever the case, the sewermen were suddenly asphyxiated by a strong concentration of gases, and Prot's four co-workers were killed instantly.[120]

The deaths in the boulevard Rochechouart sewer occurred on September 26, 1880, when the Great Stink was still very much on the minds and in the nostrils of many Parisians. Few hesitated to draw a direct link between the calamity underground and the olfactory ordeal above. How could there be any more dramatic proof that the odors afflicting the city were not only unpleasant but also deadly? The same newspapers that had attacked Alphand and the local administration almost daily throughout the Great Stink seized

The Great Stink of Paris

on the disaster to press their case that the disgusting odors were coming from the sewers; the odors were not in fact harmless, as Alphand and others had claimed; and the *tout-à-l'égout* proposal was the height of folly, posing a very real threat to the health and safety of anyone subjected to the foul fecal emanations that would be spread throughout Paris. *L'Illustration* called the dead sewermen "martyrs for no good reason." The *Gazette des tribunaux* was full of righteous indignation, mocking Alphand's declaration that the odors of Paris were not coming from the sewers: "Yesterday's accident on the boulevard Rochechouart proves [him] wrong. . . . Sewage emanations are, thus, not inoffensive, as partisans of waste disposal through the sewers claim. . . . These emanations contain gases that are very dangerous for those who breathe them. What will they be like when all the cesspits of Paris empty directly into the sewers? . . . Yesterday's accident contains a lesson, which the administration ignores at its own peril."[121] The deaths of the four sewermen only reinforced the perception that the mysterious subterranean world of the sewers was threatening and dangerous. The prospect of the constant circulation of human waste underfoot, under every house and street—with its disgusting and deadly emanations—was especially frightening to many Parisians.

It is a stranage paradox that the sewers of Paris could inspire such acute dread and still be a popular tourist attraction. Beginning with the international exposition of 1867, guided tours through the new sewers of Haussmann's Paris became an all-but-mandatory stop on the itineraries of visitors to the capital city. As the Larousse encyclopedia observed proudly in 1870, "Everyone knows that no foreigner of distinction wants to leave the city without making this singular trip." Visitors marveled not only at the impressive engineering achievement the sewers represented, but also at their "enchanting, otherworldly aspect" and even their remarkable odorlessness. Historian Donald Reid has called attention to the curious and lasting ambivalence that characterized Parisians' attitudes toward the sewers. On the one hand, they feared the dark subterranean world and associated it with crime, prostitution, and subversion as well as with stench and disease; on the other hand, they mastered their fears (or at least held them in abeyance) by visiting the sewer galleries and marveling at the civilization and cleanliness they symbolized. If the old sewers of the July Monarchy immortalized in Victor Hugo's *Les Misérables* represented the city's underbelly of transgression and disorder, Reid notes, the new sewers of the Second Empire reassured the bourgeoisie that "their order reigned below" as well as above ground, in the rectilinear and controlled urban environment of Haussmann's administration.[122] While visits to the sewers may indeed have helped Parisians as well as tourists confront their fears of the underworld and its foul, disturbing emanations, those fears did not disappear entirely; they merely sank beneath the surface, only to reemerge with fierce intensity when the air above became tainted or when the air below turned deadly.

THE POSITIVIST REPUBLIC

The French state too was undergoing fundamental transformations when the Great Stink struck. Although the Third Republic had been in existence for a decade in name and in form, a truly republican government was actually in its infancy in 1880. A fractious group of monarchists joined occasionally by Bonapartists had dominated the regime since it was founded on the ruins of the defeated Second Empire during the Franco-Prussian War in 1870. But after a constitutional crisis in 1877 paralyzed the government, and after the cryptomonarchist General Patrice MacMahon finally resigned as president in 1879, a coalition of moderates durably committed to the republic came to power. Perhaps understandably (given the nine decades of political ferment, upheaval, and revolution that the nation had endured), their fear of disorder and instability was as deep-seated as their distrust of the clergy and their positivist faith in scientific progress.[123] Moreover, epidemics and revolution had been closely linked in the political mythology of Paris at least since the cholera epidemics of 1832 and 1849.[124] The prospect of an impending epidemic in 1880, as heralded or even spread by noxious odors, was clearly unsettling, and the preservation of order along with (or by means of) an enhancement of democracy was a paramount concern for the republicans newly arrived in power.

Just how critical a turning point the Third Republic had reached when the foul odors invaded Paris in 1880 is suggested by several key events that took place that very summer. On July 13, the National Assembly finally voted a full amnesty for those who had been arrested and deported for taking part in the Paris Commune of 1871. Although nothing could erase the bitter memories on both sides of the popular uprising and its bloody suppression, the amnesty announced an official reconciliation that was designed to "cauterize" the still-unhealed wounds of the era. The republican regime now felt itself strong enough and confident enough to reintegrate the rebels of 1871, just as it had survived the machinations of monarchists and Bonapartists for a decade. Simultaneously, after much hesitation and sharp debate, parliament proclaimed July 14 the official national holiday. The anniversary of the taking of the Bastille in 1789 not only linked the regime historically with the revolutionary tradition, but it also provided the occasion for popular celebrations of the republic in every city, village, and hamlet in France. From its very first staging on the day after the amnesty of the Communards, the *quatorze juillet* proved to be tremendously successful both as joyous popular celebration and as enactment of republican legitimacy.[125]

Meanwhile, one more event marks that political season in France as especially noteworthy. Two months after the amnesty and the first Bastille Day, on September 23, 1880—in the midst of the Great Stink in Paris—Minister of Education Jules Ferry replaced the more moderate Charles de Freycinet as prime minister, ushering in an unprecedented period of imperial expansion overseas and of aggressive secularization at home. In fact, the immediate cause of Freycinet's replacement by Ferry was an anticlerical policy measure: Freycinet had hesitated to authorize a set of governmental decrees prohibiting unauthorized religious groups—including the Jesuits—from being involved in education in any way whatsoever. The plan had begun as a law that narrowly failed to pass both houses of Parliament, and Ferry (unlike Freycinet) was willing to brave the vigorous conservative and Catholic opposition by implementing the plan through official decree, in order to pursue the secular republican agenda.[126]

The new government did not pursue any radical new measures to combat the stench in Paris. In fact, beyond the commission reports and the continuing battle over the *tout-à-l'égout,* state intervention and specific policy initiatives relating to the Great Stink of 1880 were remarkably less vigorous than the public outcry and demands for action might lead one to expect. Neither did the popular response to the odors change noticeably after the new government took office. In short, there was no direct causal link between the stench and political change. What does appear to be the case is that both changes in the political landscape and reactions to foul odors in Paris testify to ongoing, deeper, less immediately visible changes in French culture and society.

That Ferry—the father of free, mandatory, secular education in France—first came to power in September 1880 points to the emerging predominance of a certain set of issues within the political class in France rather than a direct connection with the Great Stink in Paris. These issues included not only secularization and colonialism, but also a lasting commitment to the republican form of government, responsiveness to the concerns of the electorate, and a thoroughgoing positivism that instilled in an entire generation of social reformers a profound faith in progress through science and education.[127]

Meanwhile, a parallel shift in attitudes and expectations had reshaped the French electorate itself. Although it is easy to exaggerate changes in public opinion based on relatively meager evidence, reports of the popular response to the Great Stink of 1880 are ample and consistent enough to demonstrate that, at least in Paris, citizens had come to expect a new responsiveness and accountability from their government under the republican regime. Henceforth, not even the air was exempt from constituents' demands and potential recriminations. Not only did Parisians complain about the sickening odors and demand some kind of action from their elected officials, but they also linked their demands explicitly to the democratic self-image of the republican government.

On September 4, 1880, the Parisian daily *Le Siècle* (generally sympathetic to the republican cause) vented its anger at official inaction, claiming that infant mortality had tripled in Paris since the odors had begun. Meanwhile, the newspaper observed indignantly that Prefect of Police Andrieux had recently left Paris for his vacation in Aix-les-Bains, "where the air is more pure," leaving behind the millions who could not afford such holiday travel, and whose health was at grave risk:

> How can this be? Now that we are in a republic, now that all civil servants are answerable to public opinion, now that Paris has an elected city council, will such urgent complaints—when the health of two million people is at stake—not be heard?
>
> We can't believe it. If the prefect of police, if the prefect of the Seine department and the public health council continue to do nothing, we will insist that the Paris city council convene a special session. Not to act is to condemn to death hundreds of Parisians, young and old alike.[128]

Here, it is the existence of an accountable, democratic regime—and not simply the presence of the intolerable odors—that makes the authorities' failure to act so galling and unacceptable.

A week later, *Le Siècle* continued its campaign to goad the government into action. The newspaper bemoaned the "monarchical" habits of public silence and dissimulation that continued to plague the French administration: "The first obligation of a republican government is . . . to maintain constant communication with the public, which is the only real sovereign power." The editorial went on to urge readers "in the infected areas" to contact their city councilors and to demand a special council session to deal with the deadly odors.[129]

Even those Parisians whom one might expect to have been impervious to the republican agenda of accountability joined in the chorus. A noble-woman whose name was withheld but whose title was given as "Duchess" wrote an angry letter to the editor of Le XIXe Siècle about the foul smells. In 1880, the French nobility—whether wholeheartedly monarchist or not—was still largely hostile to republicanism. But instead of invoking the Great Stink as proof of the inability of a republican regime to properly govern France, the disgusted duchess demanded the responsiveness that elected officials implicitly promised their constituents. "What is our *elected* city council thinking of?" she asked. "Has there ever been a more municipal matter than this one?" If public money was needed to clean the city up, so be it; she was willing to pay her share. "Bleed us," she wrote (in a pun equating excessive taxation with bloodletting as medical treatment), "but asphyxiate us no more."

> If Paris had stunk this badly under the empire, what rage would have been un-leashed against M. Haussmann and against the city council that was appointed by the government!
>
> At least we have a free press. . . . Let your complaints pierce the fetid air that is enveloping us. And if our administrators, engineers, [and] public works directors have no noses, let them realize—at their own expense—that they do have ears.[130]

Even the nobility looked to elected officials and government experts, via the pressure of public opinion, for solutions to the sensory ordeal plaguing Paris. (Fig. 4.)

Having matured politically under the Bonapartist regime of the Second Empire, the republican generation led by Ferry and by Léon Gambetta stood for a combination of democratization and secularization that both evoked the republican tradition and held out the promise of what Philip Nord has called "a new relationship between constituent and representative." When Gambetta called in 1869 for "a government of public opinion," he signaled that responsiveness to popular concerns had assumed as central a place in the republican program as had secularism, freedom of the press, freedom of association, and universal public education. Wedded to positivism and its promise of limitless progress through rationalism and scientific expertise,

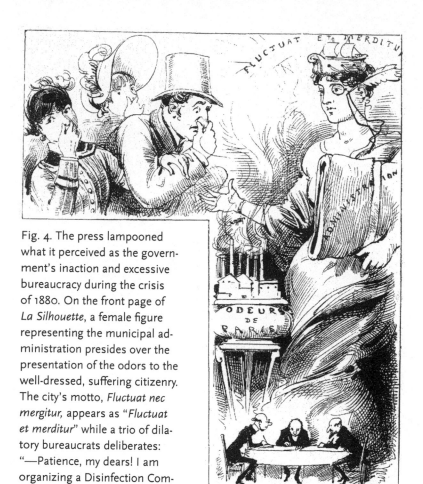

Fig. 4. The press lampooned what it perceived as the government's inaction and excessive bureaucracy during the crisis of 1880. On the front page of *La Silhouette*, a female figure representing the municipal administration presides over the presentation of the odors to the well-dressed, suffering citizenry. The city's motto, *Fluctuat nec mergitur*, appears as "*Fluctuat et merditur*" while a trio of dilatory bureaucrats deliberates: "—Patience, my dears! I am organizing a Disinfection Committee charged with forming a commission which will name a subcommittee which will elect a Council which will organize a bureau which will choose a delegation which will designate a reporter. . . . And when all of this is in place . . . /—We will all be dead! /—Indeed; but you will no longer be uncomfortable."

Ferry's generation intended simultaneously to serve and to shape the will of the people. The new republican representative was to be both accountable to his electors and "master of the situation, the people's pedagogue no less than its spokesman."[131]

THE THIRD REPUBLIC STANDS AS AN ENDURING PARADOX in French political history. Perpetually unstable, continually under attack, it remains the most long-lived of all regimes since 1789. The government of the early Third Republic was certainly not perfectly responsive to citizen concerns—far from it. However, what the confluence of events and opinions surrounding the Great Stink of 1880 suggests is that the French state was significantly and newly attuned to public awareness of problems concerning the physical infrastructure of everyday life, and determined to bring the secular, specialized expertise of scientific knowledge to bear on remedying those problems. For the positivist republicans of France, however, large-scale state intervention in any area of civilian life (with the notable exception of education) was anathema. Remedies for social problems lay in the self-made revitalization of the individual citizen, encouraged and perhaps initiated by the state, and made possible through an amelioration of the milieu in which that citizen lived and worked, and in which children were raised and educated. The state's role would remain limited to providing schooling, mobilizing scientific expertise and advice, and moral uplift, while any financial involvement in aid for the poor and needy would have to come from private charities.

This vision of improvement through philanthropy with government encouragement can perhaps be seen most clearly in the quintessential social reformer of the early Third Republic, Jules Siegfried. Siegfried, whom one historian has called a "professional paternalist," came from a Protestant family prominent in the Mulhouse textile industry, but made his name in the commercial and shipping center of Le Havre. As member of the chamber of commerce, then city councilman, mayor, member of parliament, and several times cabinet minister, Siegfried played a founding role in many reform organizations in Le Havre and nationwide. With missionary zeal, he agitated for the moral and physical uplift of the working class through hard work, sobriety, education, and improved housing. In Le Havre, he led a group of businessmen who built *cités ouvrières* (on the model of earlier experiments in Mulhouse) in which poor families paid low rents (credited toward eventual ownership) for clean, sanitary housing units, with even private courtyards and gardens in some cases. Siegfried also founded a workingmen's social club to provide education for adults and an alternative to the sociability of the cabaret. As mayor, in 1879, he also created the first municipal board of health in France; in Siegfried's view, the deplorable morbidity and mortality of Le Havre's working class was inseparable from the environment of ignorance, immorality, and unsanitary housing out of which it arose. Removed from their accustomed milieu of filth and depravity, cultivated, educated, and surrounded by fresh air and cleanliness, the hard-working poor would surely rise above the poverty, disease, and despair into which they had been born.[132]

The legacy of Haussmann's audacious administrative reach joined with Ferry's positivist republican ideology to produce a new relationship between the state and the physical fabric of Paris. What emerged was a political landscape in which the integrity of the urban environment was a paramount concern and popular demands for action could not be ignored. The fearful clamor over the Great Stink of 1880, however, was about more than just politicians' responsiveness to the everyday concerns of constituents. The thoroughly contaminated, unbreathable air of Paris threatened the biological future of the local population and, by extension, of the nation itself. Cleansing the tainted environment was less a plank in a political platform than a matter of dire necessity, even of survival.

2

The Sanitarians' Legacy,

or How Health Became Public

When Napoleon I went into his final exile in 1815, the science of health in France—"hygiene"—was an abstraction, an ideal, a set of recipes for healthy bourgeois living. By the time his nephew took power in 1848, "hygiene" had gone "public," and had grown into a quantitative, empirical domain of rigorous local investigation—the gritty science of filth, slums, and deviance. This new science could lay claim at midcentury to its own institutions, its own professional journal, and its own recognizable set of characteristic problems and methods.

Paris in the early nineteenth century has long been known as the birthplace of modern clinical medicine,[1] but it can also legitimately lay claim to the same title for the science of public health. What are often considered the early classics of public health literature—Johann Peter Frank's *A Complete System of Medical Police* and Edwin Chadwick's *Report on the Sanitary Condition of the Labouring Population of Great Britain*—emerged from Vienna between 1779 and 1819 and from London in 1842, respectively. Both of these influential texts survive today as landmarks in the early attempts to establish a scientific—and political—field of inquiry concerning the health of populations. Frank laid the theoretical groundwork for an enlightened and totalizing system of governmental monitoring of and intervention in the health of the citizenry. Chadwick shone the harsh light of exhaustive quantitative and qualitative investigation on the wretched slums of Britain and their inhabitants. But in between those two cities and those two dates, a dedicated group of French physicians and reformers managed to build a fundamentally new structure for the study and improvement of "public hygiene" that transcended the impact of a single publication. Frank's compendious treatise survived primarily as a dead letter, often invoked but never translated into policy on a sustained basis in any country. Chadwick's report, in contrast—the first such empirical inquiry in Britain—durably influenced debate and policy on health and "the social question," but as even its author acknowledged, it was not entirely original in its inspiration or in its method; its roots lay in Paris.[2] A more plausible birthdate for "public health" might be 1829, when a group of prominent physicians in Paris founded the first professional journal devoted exclusively to "public hygiene and forensic medicine," the *Annales d'hygiène publique et de médecine légale.*

Regardless of which country claims paternity over the modern science of public health, it has long been acknowledged that the French hygienists of the early nineteenth century constituted a uniquely energetic, pioneering, and prolific group of (self-proclaimed) experts, who certainly believed they were forging a new body of scientific and medical knowledge. And even though the history of public health has not enjoyed as much prestige nor attracted as much sustained attention as has the history of medicine, scholars since Erwin Ackerknecht in 1948 have found themselves repeatedly drawn to the pathbreaking labors of the early nineteenth-century Paris hygienists.[3] The systematic empirical and quantitative study of public health and the establishment of the intellectual groundwork for the assumption by local and national governments of responsibility for health-related public works (among other advances) have been credited to these pioneers.[4] That which endures as the legacy of this "school" nearly two centuries later must be carefully distinguished, however, from its significant medium-term impact on public health science and policy just half a century later, in the full flower of the Bacteriological Revolution.

Ann La Berge's definitive study of the Paris hygienists has shown their "mission" to be fundamentally about their "method."[5] Through their cultivated skepticism of received wisdom, their rigorous empiricism, and their aggressive (for the time) pursuit of quantification, they sought not just incremental advances in sanitary policy, but also an entirely new foundation for public health knowledge. The precise form of that knowledge ultimately mattered less than the fact that it would be scientific—rooted in empirical observation, methodically gathered, quantitatively analyzed, and systematically integrated into policy deliberations. Other scholars have generally concurred in identifying the same methodological innovations as the key contribution of the early Paris hygienists to the development of public health. Some have emphasized the pioneering role of Alexandre-

Jean-Baptiste Parent-Duchâtelet, the diligent firsthand observer of sewers and prostitution;[6] others, like William Coleman, have preferred to call attention to the work of Louis-René Villermé, the first social scientist to document in a rigorously quantitative fashion the direct correlation between poverty and disease.[7] Nearly all historians have agreed, however, that the early nineteenth-century French public health movement transformed primarily the method of public health investigation rather than the content of health-related knowledge.

From a twentieth- or twenty-first-century perspective, this conclusion is quite sensible. After all, the most significant breakthroughs in disease prevention—from the identification of insect vectors and healthy carriers to the connection between cigarette smoking and lung cancer—came in the first half of the twentieth century, as did much early research based on knowledge of specific microbial pathogens responsible for specific diseases. However, the legacy of the early sanitarians looks quite different when viewed from the perspective of 1880 or 1900. To the disease detectives and policymakers of the early bacteriological age, the most significant contributions of Villermé, Parent-Duchâtelet, and their colleagues were *both* methodological and substantive. Late-century medical authorities marked their distance from their predecessors in some respects, but they clung to a vocabulary and a focus on certain danger zones derived in large part from those same forefathers. Seen in the hindsight of a half century rather than nearly two centuries, the legacy of the *Annales d'hygiène publique* and the movement it represented consisted of a set of durably established styles, habits, and recipes for reform. They include most notably:

- a methodological commitment to firsthand empirical investigation and, where possible, quantitative analysis of data;
- a tradition of affiliation with and investigation through institutions such as local health councils and journals such as the *Annales;*
- a nearly obsessive focus on human waste and its disposal (or, more generally, on the threat of contamination in the urban environment);
- elaboration and promotion of a collective hygiene based on bodily separation and aeration;
- a tone marked by acute disgust and pervasive moralism;
- faith in technocratic regulation rather than prohibition of putative health hazards;
- the conviction that the improvement of health conditions depends on the civilization of certain subpopulations.

The conventional view of the early French sanitarians, then, continues to be valid, but it must be supplemented along these lines in order to recapture their legacy as it appeared to their successors in the last quarter of the nineteenth century. This chapter surveys in their broad outlines these central elements of the prevailing disease prevention strategy in the era of the July Monarchy (1830–1848). What emerged during this period was an increasingly widely recognized sanitary imperative, which regarded the reordering of both the physical (especially urban) environment and the moral underpinnings of French society as equally and simultaneously urgent—even inseparable from each other. Two elements that have been mostly neglected so far are emphasized here: first, the extent to which the indictment of disgusting substances and behaviors as health hazards was part and parcel of the moralization strategy (rather than, say, the result of simple empirical discoveries); and second, the vital importance of an ideology of civilization—as an inevitable historical process and as an immediate reform project—underlying all hopes for sanitary improvement.

SKEPTICAL EMPIRICISM AND THE INVESTIGATIVE IDEAL

As La Berge and others have abundantly demonstrated, the early Paris hygienists and their *Annales* secured a place in history primarily through their "application of scientific or empirical method to the study of public health problems."[8] One might agree or disagree that, for example, emanations from sewers caused disease, but henceforth it was impossible to maintain that reliable knowledge on such questions could be ascertained without some combination of skeptical testing of existing theories; direct observation; investigation in situ, in person; and quantitative analysis of relevant data.

A carefully cultivated mistrust of conventional wisdom served as a cornerstone of the emerging hygienic knowledge. No orthodoxy was too sacred to be tested, no truth too self-evident to question. The iconoclastic Parent-Duchâtelet led the way in this regard, seeming to take an almost malicious pleasure in dismantling received knowledge. The horse-rendering plant and waste dump at Montfaucon in northeastern Paris had spread many deadly diseases through its foul emanations for years—according to neighbors, physicians, and other concerned Parisians—when the contrarian hygienist entered the fray in 1835. Protests had reached such a fever pitch that the government had agreed in principle to relocate the plant, but each proposed location generated new concerns and new complaints. An untenable, universally denounced situation seemed fated to endure indefinitely, as long as every alternative generated more alarm than the inertia-fueled status quo. (Montfaucon was finally closed in 1849.)[9]

Parent-Duchâtelet, ostensibly the protector of the public health, took up a quixotic crusade not to forbid but to allow the proposed relocation of the plant from Montfaucon to a property on the banks of the Seine between Paris and the north-central suburb of Clichy. Furthermore, in case there was any confusion regarding his underlying agenda, Parent-Duchâtelet left out of the title of his report any reference at all to Montfaucon or the safety of such plants, calling it instead "On the Obstacles Which Medical Prejudice Presents, in Some Circumstances, to the Sanitation of Cities and to the Establishment of Certain Industries." More than the particulars of the case at hand, it was the battle against groundless "prejudice" in medical thinking that preoccupied him. Only careful investigation could reveal, he thought, which environmental influences were harmful to human health and which were harmless (even if unpleasant).

Parent-Duchâtelet saw prejudice—that is, the reflexive denunciation of occupations, practices, locations, or substances as pathogenic in the absence of any systematic investigation of their actual health effects—as a serious obstacle to progress in public health. Even the most eminent medical authorities in France fell prey to this tendency, in his view. Among those opposing the relocation of the Montfaucon plant to Clichy, for example, was at least one professor from the Paris medical faculty who had been a mentor to Parent-Duchâtelet during his student days. Even personal loyalty had to be set aside, however, as duty bound the hygienist to maintain his scientific skepticism: "Here we are judges," he wrote, "and before such an obligation, all friendship must be silent, all consideration must give way." He hastened to add that he had been motivated only by the search for truth "and never by the desire to give offense."[10]

As specialization had begun to restructure medical practice, Parent-Duchâtelet insisted that the emerging discipline of public health be accorded as much respect as any other branch of medicine. Recognized experts ought not question one another's expertise across the boundaries of specialties. And yet, Parent-Duchâtelet complained, too many physicians considered any public health question to be fair game for uninformed opinion and speculation. Opponents of the new horse-rendering plant raised the prospect of various calamities—neighbors suffocating in unbreathable air, rats overrunning nearby farms, local water supplies irreparably contaminated—but the core of their objections involved the spread of disease from the accumulation of putrid matter in the large new plant. After patiently and painstakingly rebutting each of the allegations made against the proposed plant, Parent-Duchâtelet reserved his harshest criticism—and an uncharacteristic vehemence—for those who claimed the plant would surely generate contagious diseases or "putrid and malignant fevers" in its vicinity. Addressing himself rhetorically to his former mentor, a surgeon, the hygienist conceded that the passage of time and lack of practical experience had eroded whatever surgical expertise he had gained as a medical student: "If today, then, I were to give my opinion on . . . which cases require immediate amputation, [or] on the advantages and disadvantages of circular amputation . . . ; if I were to meddle in a discussion of the state of the hernial sac in recent versus old hernias; on the position of the epigastric artery in the former and in the latter, what would our colleagues say? You can guess their response: Stick to your own affairs, they would tell me, and *do not put so many lives in jeopardy with your half-knowledge.*"[11]

Could one not legitimately say, asked Parent-Duchâtelet, that in the present case, the roles were reversed? Did his own years of study, research, and (above all) observation on precisely these specialized questions not entitle him to address the same reproach to his former teacher? Here the hygienist's careful, scientifically dispassionate tone slipped momentarily. In response to the assertion that the proposed plant would generate "intolerably foul odors" and "harmful miasmas," Parent-Duchâtelet snorted, "What? You have resorted to ignoring everything that can be accomplished by forced ventilation?" He ridiculed the would-be experts' failure even to visit a single existing horse-rendering plant. "Do you know what is happening in some of [these] manufactories?" he asked. "And if you don't know, why do you allow yourself to make contrary assertions?"[12]

Parent-Duchâtelet's reproachful anger continued to rise as the second person he rhetorically addressed seemed to refer less and less to the project's opponents in general, and more and more to his former professor in particular:

You say that the proposed establishment will become . . . a veritable hotbed of infection. . . .

Alongside your frightening words . . . you have only forgotten one thing: that is, to give the proof of everything that you are asserting, *not based on what the ancient authors say . . . but based on your own observation.*

As for me . . . I remember you promoting the virtues of direct observation of diseases and of [all] natural phenomena; I have not forgotten that you always recommended this observation as the source of all true science, and as the only means for gaining positive knowledge about the causes and the nature of diseases[;] I have followed your precepts in the study of public health.[13]

The hygienist's creed did not bar dissent and debate, but it did emphatically reject speculative or theoretical reasoning in the absence of empirical observation. In the short term—and even in the long term, as this book shows—Parent-Duchâtelet's attempt to sever the link between putridity and disease was doomed to fail. More important in this context, however, is his confidence in promoting a new empiricist epistemology in the would-be science of public health. Evoking the direct observation that lay at the core of pathological anatomy—which he studied at the foot of this unnamed mentor, after all, in the heyday of the "Paris clinical school"[14]—reinforced his claim to scientific legitimacy and linked public health to the innovations that made the city the world's medical mecca in the first three-quarters of the nineteenth century.

Empirical skepticism alone was not enough, however. Just as central in the formation of a disciplinary identity for public health was the promotion of energetic, sustained, firsthand local investigation—no matter the personal sacrifices entailed. Reliable knowledge could be generated, many hygienists firmly believed, only by experiencing putatively pathogenic influences personally, with one's own senses and one's own body. The scientist himself could in effect become experimental subject. Here too Parent-Duchâtelet led the way. Long before Haussmann's prodigious public works and long before *tout-à-l'égout,* the hygienist viewed the sewers of Paris as marvelously "useful monuments" and at the same time as a potentially grave health hazard. Only careful firsthand investigation could reliably guide public policy on such an important question: "I have not been content merely to read what has been written on this matter, and to question workers and employees superficially[.] *I wanted to see everything for myself* at different times and under different circumstances; *I have spent time in all of the places I describe* [here;] I have had frequent conversations with all of those who are . . . responsible for our sewers, from the most distinguished academician to the lowliest of the workers; I have been present more than once during their labors; I have asked them for information both in the sewers and in their homes."[15]

In the end, Parent-Duchâtelet concluded that most sewer workers enjoyed good health, but that they and the sewers themselves nevertheless required constant surveillance and oversight in order to guard against the very real danger of noxious emanations. Perhaps more important than these findings, however, was the means by which they were arrived at: "I have surmounted without hesitation the repugnance and the dangers [that are] inseparable from such research; I have sacrificed my time, and my money, and my comfort; I can scarcely recount the procedures I have had to go through, the fatigues I have experienced, and the setbacks I have had to endure."[16] Professional self-promotion was clearly at work here; the wretched pathos of this passage certainly aimed to enhance Parent-Duchâtelet's status as a man of science and as a public servant. One can also sense in the hygienist's voice a strong resentment toward the prevailing complacency and passivity of his colleagues, who were of course all too willing to offer confident opinions.

Even more important than these personal agendas, however, was the recognition of a new standard by which to judge public health knowledge: the more involved and painstaking the research, the more valuable the findings. When Parent-Duchâtelet upbraided his opponents for their "medical prejudice" in opposing the proposed new facility in Clichy, he faulted them above all for not bothering to "go see what was happening"—that is, to examine the health and mortality situation in detail in the neighborhoods near Montfaucon and near the proposed new location. Had they taken the trouble to do this research, which was "more unpleasant and less profitable than visiting patients, and which require[d] real courage," they would have seen clearly how superior the Clichy proposal was to the status quo at Montfaucon.[17]

Parent-Duchâtelet was not the only hygienist touting suffering as the necessary pathway to useful knowledge—far from it. The same cultivation of personal sacrifice infused the single most influential text to emerge from the early nineteenth-century public health movement in France: Villermé's *Tableau de l'état physique et moral des ouvriers employés dans les manufactures de coton, de laine et de soie.* The Academy of Moral and Political Sciences asked Villermé and fellow hygienist Louis-François Benoiston de Châteauneuf to assess the "moral and physical status" of the French working class. While Benoiston de Châteauneuf focused on central France and the Atlantic coast, Villermé visited the textile-industry centers in the north and east of the country. What distinguished his inquiry above all was its investigative method. Not content to survey, to ask questions, to read documents, or to consult with experts, Villermé insisted on living his research: "Such was the care I desired to put into my investigation, that I followed the worker from his workshop to his home. I went inside with him, I studied him among his family; I sat with him at his meals. And I did more: I saw

The Great Stink of Paris

him both at work and at home, I saw him at play and observed him at his meeting-places." The resulting two-volume, 900-page treatise stands not only as a pioneering public health document, but also as a monument of nineteenth-century social investigation. By inserting himself into the textile workers' milieu, "interrogating poverty without humiliating it, [and] observing bad behavior without irritating it," Villermé aimed to produce an unflinching portrait of a social group regarded by many of his peers as threatening and mysterious.[18]

Villermé's dedication to his work was legendary. "Standing the night watch, enduring fatigue—no price was too high for him to pay in order to discover the truth," one colleague avowed in frank admiration. Another reached back to an incident early in Villermé's career in order to capture the hygienist's single-minded tenacity. During his tenure as a military surgeon during the Napoleonic era, he found himself in charge of a hospital in which "fevers of bad character reigned." Villermé insisted on keeping the hospital's windows open to maintain ventilation, but prejudice and folk wisdom proved difficult to overcome; each time he entered the hospital, he found the windows closed again. Finally, in the face of the patients' "clamor and threats," Villermé had the window panes broken once and for all.[19] The committed hygienist would let nothing stand in the way of progress.

The ideal championed by the likes of Parent-Duchâtelet and Villermé of personal involvement and sacrifice in the service of public health eventually became enshrined in the lore of the discipline. By 1877, a leading hygienist looking back over the past half century could only marvel at the transformation of the discipline; what had long been "the art of pompously dispensing banalities" had made itself into "an applied science"—"practical, one could even say utilitarian" in nature. Its success was due above all to the rise of this investigative ethos in the nineteenth century: "Today . . . it is in the workshop, [it is] in the middle of the factory, it is by living with the workers that the physician gathers the raw material of public health; the latter being the art of applying the . . . other sciences, we must familiarize ourselves in the most minute detail with everyday life in all classes of society, in order to be able to combat the many anti-hygienic conditions with the resources of chemistry, physics, and . . . biological knowledge."[20] Long gone were the days when useful knowledge in public health flowed from systems and theories; henceforth, the hygienist was expected to get up from his desk and find knowledge in the field, surrounded by the very health hazards and sick people who were the objects of his investigation. It was, literally, a dirty job.

Just as central to the development of "hygienism" as this investigative ideal was the tendency to see all health problems in spatial terms. In the hygienists' worldview, disease simply inhered in the arrangement of bodies in space, from the geographic macrolevel of the planet or continent to the moral microlevel of domestic sleeping configurations. No danger seemed more pressing in Paris throughout the first half of the nineteenth century than that posed by the city's rapid population growth. A flood of rural migrants to the capital strained its limited sanitary infrastructure to a frightening degree, and the city's housing supply could not keep up with the influx of newcomers. As a result, hygienists and other bourgeois observers worried, there were too many Parisians crowded into each residential building, too many in each apartment, too many in each room. Healthy, civilized living seemed incompatible with such overcrowding. It was even suggested by as authoritative an observer as Villermé that the agglomeration of people in large industrial communities in and of itself caused immorality and a host of attendant ills.[21]

Crowding could cause a multitude of evils. As early as 1822, hygienist Claude Lachaise decried the lack of sunlight in congested dwellings on narrow streets, calling its effect on workers' health "similar to the wilting of plants"; he specifically cited "intermittent fevers, scrofula, scurvy, dropsies, arthritis and rheumatism" among "a multitude of other illnesses" as effects of living in such close, dark quarters.[22] In 1828, a mysterious epidemic of swollen feet broke out in Paris. The illness seemed to afflict primarily the working class and soldiers garrisoned in the city, and triggered "a more or less intense irritation of the digestive passages" along with a severe inflammation of the soles of the feet. The Paris health council (an advisory board comprised largely of physicians, charged with investigating local causes of and remedies for disease in the capital)[23] sought out the roots of the outbreak, and came across something in its research that, if not a smoking gun, was at least a highly suggestive correlation. The council had "reason to believe that low-ceilinged . . . dormitories where air . . . cannot renew itself, must have contributed greatly to the development of the disease in the barracks." Moreover, the same cause came under suspicion in the civilian component of the epidemic, as it was "among people living in small apartments with low ceilings, situated in narrow streets, that it has been most frequently observed."[24] A more precise explanation of the strange syndrome's causal mechanism was superfluous in the presence of an apparent correlation with a universally recognized health threat—that is, living in extremely close quarters.

Villermé's 1840 *Tableau* found cause alternately for great optimism and deep pessimism in the arrangement of working-class bodies within French cities. While remarkable progress had been made in the quality of housing available in many neighborhoods, too many one-room lodgings "crowded with beds, trunks, chairs, looms, tools, in which [families] sleep, work, cook, and take their meals" continued to fester in "narrow, dark, dirty streets." Even more ominously, a moral/sanitary segregation had divided up many cities. While "honest workers" chose to live in newer houses located in less crowded neighborhoods (even if they had to pay more for the privilege), "those of blameworthy conduct and morals withdraw into the same streets [and] the same houses, almost always the dirtiest [and] the most unhealthy."[25] Faced with such conditions, a hygienist might view the glass as half-empty or half-full, but none could miss the clear correlation between ample bodily space and health on the one hand, and between crowded quarters and disease on the other.

When he revisited the question ten years later, improvements in working-class housing loomed less large in Villermé's mind. In a study of the benefits and drawbacks of *cités ouvrières* (workers' housing projects designed by social reformers) published in the *Annales d'hygiène publique,* he focused less on the advantages of recently undertaken projects than on their defects—and on those of the existing housing stock. His description of the prevailing conditions in many urban neighborhoods hints at the environmental determinism that colored hygienists' perceptions of the relationships among residential configurations, moral well-being, and physical health: "Each household disposes of only a single room, small, low-lying, dark, humid . . . often below street level or in attic space, glacial in winter, oppressive in summer, and with no horizon other than a dismal wall a few feet away; on muddy, narrow, unhealthy streets, in houses falling into ruins, with dilapidated floors and stairways covered with a slippery layer of filth! Fortunate are those who do not also . . . have to confront the encumbrance [of] work-related equipment, dirty pallets with just a straw mattress and tattered blankets, and the promiscuous pell-mell of ages and sexes piling up and pressing upon one another."[26] Seen from the perspective of Villermé and his fellow hygienists, the pressing of buildings together on a narrow street, the pressing of apartments together within dilapidated buildings, and the indiscriminate pressing of bodies together in a bedroom were all of a piece. Excessive crowding simply denied human bodies the minimal requirements for physical and moral survival.

Physicians and health reformers were not the only bourgeois Parisians concerned about overcrowding in early nineteenth-century Paris. One can see this same growing horror at human-spatial disproportion in the fiction and political literature of the period. Pamphleteers, novelists, political agitators—all feared (in an increasingly physical and immediate way) the sickly and criminal "dangerous classes" that such an environment fostered.[27] Balzac pointed out that the inability of the sunlight to penetrate the capital's narrow streets not only made "any daring pedestrian who ventures to walk from the Marais to the quais . . . have the feeling that he has been groping through cellars all the way," but also preserved the perennially damp and stagnant street muck. Garbage carts could not even gain access to streets some of which were only five feet wide, like the rue du Tourniquet: "So in rainy weather the blackish waters promptly washed against the base of the old houses on this street, carrying down the garbage deposited by each household beside the corner posts." Balzac called another nearby neighborhood an "unhealthy pile hemmed in on all sides by tall houses," and described the adjoining narrow streets as "damp thoroughfares where the thronging people are stricken with rheumatism."[28]

"How ugly Paris seems after one has been away for a year! . . . How one stifles in these dark, damp, narrow corridors!" exclaimed the "Vicomte de Launay," pen name of Delphine de Girardin (poet, playwright, novelist, and journalist of modest renown). "And thousands of people live, bustle, throng in the liquid darkness, like reptiles in a marsh."[29] The image of barely human creatures piled one upon the other, wallowing in filth pervades much of the literature of the period. Utopian socialist Henri Lecouturier contemplated the view of Paris from the heights of Montmartre, "the congestion of houses piled up at every point of a vast horizon," and saw little reason for optimism: "Seized with sudden fear, one is reluctant to venture into this vast maze, in which a million beings jostle each other, where the air, vitiated by unhealthy effluvia, rising in a poisonous cloud, almost obscures the sun. . . . A haggard and sickly crowd perpetually throngs these streets, their feet in the gutter, their noses in infection, their eyes outraged by the most repulsive garbage at every street corner. . . . There are alleys, too, in which two cannot walk abreast, sewers of ordure and mud, in which the stunted and withered dwellers daily inhale death."[30] In a finite space, multiplied beyond an acceptable population density, humankind effectively descended beneath a minimal standard of humanity, and became like doomed animals, an appalling affront to a society that considered itself at the historic apogee of civilization.

The Great Stink of Paris

The scientific literature on public health rarely examined exactly how overcrowding caused disease, since the emerging hygienic method often lent itself better to establishing the correlation itself than to speculating on its causal mechanism. The question was raised periodically, however, and eventually hygienists ambivalently pointed toward an environmental etiology that in many ways resembled contagionism but could never be reduced to such a vulgar doctrine.[31] By 1876, on the eve of the great bacteriological breakthroughs in etiology, Léon Colin was able to explain "the pathogenic influence of human agglomerations" to readers of the *Annales* by referring to "the miasmas of overcrowding." For too long, complained Colin, hygienists had denounced overcrowding almost out of habit, without bothering to investigate its empirical particulars: which diseases were actually caused by crowding, and how?[32]

Colin's lengthy study aims to find a middle ground between common-sense miasmatism and a contagionism dressed up in respectable clothing. For example, nobody could deny in 1876 (or 1776 or 1676, for that matter) that smallpox was contagious. Overcrowding, therefore, certainly exposed more people to the contagiousness of smallpox, but Colin's review of the evidence showed that crowded conditions per se did not seem to intensify or aggravate smallpox epidemics. On the other hand, diseases such as typhus, typhoid fever, dysentery, puerperal fever, and "hospitalism" (*la pourriture de l'hôpital,* or septic fever) seemed to not only correlate with but positively to depend on severely crowded conditions in order to thrive and spread: "Whereas the morbid germs [*germes morbides*] emitted by a single smallpox patient or convalescent will be sufficient to result in contagion around him, normally a certain number of typhus patients are needed in order to propagate their affliction; and isolated cases of typhus remain, in general, sterile." The same was true, Colin argued, for typhoid fever, and "one of the most absolute rules of hospital hygiene" was the "dissemination" of typhoid patients throughout the wards. Similarly, the crowding together of too many injured people or birthing women in a hospital ran the risk of producing a "surgical or puerperal miasma" capable of spreading uncontrollably.[33]

Most curiously of all, overcrowding was even capable of conferring the property of contagion on banal, noncontagious diseases. For example, Colin suggested, dysentery—even the variety that resulted "from a simple drop in temperature"—could become contagious if enough of its victims were gathered together at the same time, as was the case with soldiers' "camp dysentery." The sheer quantity of "pathological secretions" and the difficulty of burying or otherwise disposing of them safely intensified the disease's "malignity" and endowed it with an unusual "contagiousness" (*contagiosité*).[34] In effect, this classic prebacteriological culprit, overcrowding, allowed the hygienist to negotiate (hesitantly) a new potential version of miasmatism, one that emphasized the existence of a seemingly specific principle or "germ" capable of spreading contagion under certain unhygienic circumstances. Already in 1876, as the emerging science of microbes was just beginning its conquering assault on the realm of etiology, key elements of the Old Regime were being retooled, and showed signs of being flexible enough to survive the revolution.

CLEANSING PUBLIC SPACE

Overcrowding produced other effects too, of course. The most visible—and tangible, and "smellable"—were the various kinds of filth generated by an increasingly densely packed urban population. Beset by the problem of refuse and its disposal for centuries, Paris nonetheless confronted a new kind of crisis in the early nineteenth century, when the offal of everyday life accumulated to an unprecedented degree. Certain substances threatened health especially acutely, in the emerging hygienic view: human excrement, for example, remained utterly nonpareil as a contaminating danger in the city. But hygienic alarm was not limited to the specific properties of individual substances; it was the daunting volume of all organic matter produced, consumed, and excreted by nearly a million Parisians—uneaten foodstuffs, animal hides, carcasses, dung, all human bodily fluids and solids—that worried contemporaries.

As usual, Parent-Duchâtelet was in the forefront of the hygienic campaign for improved waste disposal in Paris. One of the first to sound the alarm about the dangerous "infection" of the city's (pre-Haussmann) sewers, he campaigned to have them dredged completely, and observed the operation firsthand when it was finally undertaken. The system's small pipes and insufficient slope had allowed residues of waste matter to accumulate, and the city's explosive growth exacerbated the problem to an alarming extent, as Parent-Duchâtelet pointed out in an investigation of a section underneath rue Amelot near the Bastille: "In a short time, [the sewers] contracted such a degree of infection that it bothered the neighborhood's residents, who complained to the [municipal] administration. . . . None of the attempts [to alleviate the blockages] was successful; most of the workers involved in these projects were asphyxiated, [and] some of them lost their lives." Here it is noteworthy that the neighbors' complaints are linked seamlessly to a real, verifiable danger to health. This infection (that is, stench) truly killed. Parent-Duchâtelet, never one to sound the public health alarm lightly, warned that the sewers represented an "imminent peril" to the population before they were dredged. Remedying this emergency clearly amounted in his eyes to one of the first major victories of the newly self-conscious discipline of public health—or at least of his own personal activism.[35]

The menace of filth could not be contained only by better sewers, however. The population implosion in Paris triggered increased demand for certain potentially noxious trades, even as it drastically reduced the amount of space available for those trades. Parent-Duchâtelet saw this problem coming as early as 1822, when he proposed concentrating "all of the dirty and disgusting professions exercised in Paris" along the banks of the Bièvre River, which at the time (it has since been covered) wound its way languidly toward the Seine past the Gobelins and the Jardin des Plantes in southeastern Paris. Tanners and hide-dressers had long before been forced by royal ordinance to relocate from the Seine to the Bièvre, and Parent-Duchâtelet argued that other offensive occupations (dyers and hatters, among others) ought to join them there. Counterintuitive as it might seem to concentrate many dangerous trades in one small area of the city, the hygienist claimed that it would end up working in the interests of all parties concerned. The manufacturers would be able to cooperate with one another to ensure that their water supply and other needs were being adequately met, while the quarters they left behind would find themselves considerably improved by the departure of the offensive neighbors. Because the Bièvre had long been a refuge for such unpleasant industries, its immediate vicinity was already undesirable, and would remain so whether these other trades relocated or not. Recent efforts to divert water from the Ourcq basin to the capital could benefit all parties; the potential health catastrophes promised by rapid urbanization could actually be transformed into progress, Parent-Duchâtelet hinted, if only authorities with the appropriate expertise were involved in public decision-making.[36]

Even public urination swelled the puddles and streams of dangerous filth that seemed ubiquitous in Paris. Both the practice and complaints about it were so common that in 1850, a police ordinance forbade this "bad habit" on all streets with public urinals—and on other streets, prohibited urinating on public monuments, on sidewalks, and against storefronts. The *Annales d'hygiène publique* applauded this overdue measure, which "public salubrity and morality" "fervently demanded."[37] Filth in public space was inevitably and inseparably both a moral and a sanitary problem. Of course there was nothing dangerous about urination per se—as long as it was done in the proper places and circumstances. Exposed and uncontained, it contaminated both minds and bodies.

While the accumulation of miscellaneous refuse in the sewers and the proliferation of objectionable occupations certainly worried hygienists in the early nineteenth century, there was one sanitary problem that transcended all others in their eyes: excrement. The handling and disposal of human waste preoccupied scientists, administrators, and residents alike, and concern only intensified as urban population density grew. Parisians simply could not tolerate the accumulation of excrement underneath every apartment building and its transport in carts through the city's streets—but in the absence of any widely accepted alternative, they were stuck with their cesspits and *vidange*. "The maintenance and emptying of cesspits has forever been a considerable burden and a source of discomfort for the inhabitants of Paris," Parent-Duchâtelet observed with a mix of understatement and exasperation.[38]

Some hygienists dissented from the prevailing view by claiming that the dangers of cesspits and their emptying had been overstated, and could be readily managed with new techniques and equipment. However, even these reassuring voices sounded a note of great caution when discussing what could happen when *vidange* was undertaken without proper precautions. "The stinking emanations" liberated during the operation, one doctor warned in 1844, "are not only . . . disagreeable . . . ; they sometimes precipitate the gravest accidents, and can even cause death": "I saw a small child succumb in this manner; born the previous day, he had a vigorous constitution; I left him in perfect health, and the next day I found him lifeless: a cesspit had been emptied during the night; those who were in the same room as the child suffered greatly from the bad odor; [the baby] did not stop crying all night; nothing could comfort him; as morning neared, his voice became weaker and weaker, and he expired shortly after dawn." The body showed a generalized purple tint, especially remarkable in the face. Examined on autopsy, the baby's brain, lungs, heart, and liver were "engorged with black blood."[39]

"Not only disagreeable"—the refrain resonates throughout the sanitary literature. The denunciation of a very real health hazard was central to the campaign for a more civilized treatment of human waste. In fact, so closely were sensory taints identified with pathogenic contaminants that it is

The Great Stink of Paris

almost impossible to imagine a prohibition against disgusting substances based solely on politeness or sensibility. "If the sense of smell alone was disagreeably affected by the disgusting procedure of a *vidange,* then there would doubtless be a matter worthy of our attention; it would be, however, only an inconvenience; but the emanations act upon the health of the workers, [and] even result in grave dangers for them." This hygienist, writing in 1848, reprised Parent-Duchâtelet and others in calling for the closure of the waste treatment plant at Montfaucon on the grounds that new treatment methods would allow more material to be handled more safely at other locations.[40]

Although most early nineteenth-century hygienists were based in Paris, and the capital seemed to distill all sanitary dangers into their most concentrated form, French public health reformers did not entirely neglect the provinces. What they found there was no more encouraging than was the situation in Paris. Adolphe Chevallier reported in 1832 on a tour through a handful of towns in southern France, and lamented (of all things) the *lack* of cesspits. Excrement was disposed of in the streets, and street cleaners could not keep up with its collection. Whether or not the resulting emanations by themselves *caused* epidemics, Chevallier had no doubt that under certain circumstances, they "served as vehicles for the propagation of diseases."[41] Other reports from provincial towns in the 1830s and 1840s traced local epidemics to all-too-common rural manifestations of filth and contamination, including the careless accumulation of animal waste and the washing of clothes and consumption of water from streams and ponds contaminated by human waste and animal cadavers. The investigating doctors often noted that informed intervention—whether to refute popular beliefs in contagion or to remove the sources of contamination—proved quite effective.[42]

The sanitary obsession with filth—that is, uncontained human and animal waste and corpses in public space—persisted beyond the initial heyday of the movement in the 1830s and 1840s. Debates flared and new discoveries were proclaimed around the edges of the problem; for example, the "putrid exhalations" from a depository of baskets used by fishmongers were reported to have contributed to the deaths of eighteen young children from "chronic enteritis" in a single building in 1850.[43] Doubts were expressed periodically (and more frequently beginning in the 1860s) regarding the pathogenic properties of miasmas and putrid emanations.[44] Nevertheless, the prevailing consensus among hygienists was captured by Ambroise Tardieu (pioneer of forensic medicine in France) in his 1862 *Dictionary of Public Hygiene and Salubrity* under the entry "putrid emanations": regardless of whether their noxious effects came from mineral-like products, from slow combustion, from miasmas resulting either from fermentation or putrefaction, or even from the same mechanism as that of any other strong odor, "it is nonetheless obvious that we must seek to mask, to cut short, to modify, or finally to eliminate phenomena of putrefaction in the vicinity of inhabited areas."[45] This imperative remained "obvious" when microbes arrived on the scene and began to transform the landscape of medicine and public health in the 1870s and 1880s. Its very obviousness would prove to be something the bacteriologists could not ignore.

OPTIMISM AND TECHNOCRATIC REGULATION

The unrelenting, decades-long litany of sanitarian fire and brimstone directed at filth can obscure at least in part one very important corollary ideology very dear to the hygienists: a sincerely optimistic faith that enlightened technocratic regulation could and would protect the public's health from the many morbific influences threatening it. It is this bedrock belief, as much as any specific breakthroughs in disease prevention or public works projects, that has undergirded the ambition of public health professionals (and the confidence placed in them by governments and the general public) ever since. While modern sewer systems, water supplies, and "magic bullets" such as diphtheria antitoxin and vaccines certainly bolstered the reputation of public health as a science and as an arena of government activity, the discipline's claim to authority largely predated those advances (with the exception of the original vaccine against smallpox).

Parent-Duchâtelet envisioned a leading advisory role for hygienists in local government, as with his 1822 proposal to concentrate all offensive industries along the banks of the Bièvre River: "At a time when the population of Paris is growing at an incredible rate, and when manufactures are multiplying every day, it is the duty of enlightened magistrates to prevent the overcrowding of residents in a single location, and especially the accumulation of manufactures, as it has been observed that through such accumulation alone, otherwise harmless establishments can become extremely dangerous."[46] His conviction had only deepened when he argued for the relocation of the Montfaucon waste dump and horse-rendering plant in 1835. When it came to the unpleasant but absolutely necessary functions of city life, the prevailing knee-jerk prohibitionism ended up perpetuating the unacceptable status quo—of which Montfaucon was Exhibit A. Meanwhile, private industry was busy devising new ways of treating various kinds of waste, which could benefit the public if only the authorities would allow them to implement their discoveries.

The hygienist's role was not to discover new sanitary techniques, but rather to evaluate and report on them, and to advise government bodies accordingly. More often than not, Parent-Duchâtelet reported promising results: "The fruitless attempts made for such a long time to remove from Paris the hideous and repulsive spectacle with which Montfaucon confronts us have convinced most of the commissions [which have considered the matter] that we needed to consult the arts and industries in order to achieve a real change. . . . The docile arts did not take long to show what they are capable of when skilled hands know how to apply them for the benefit of society."[47] "Already the problem of instantaneous and complete sanitation of fecal matter has been resolved," Parent-Duchâtelet continued, his reforming zeal perhaps pushing him toward hyperbole. Furthermore, he reported, recent demonstrations of new techniques for the disinfection and disposal of horse carcasses had shown promise in addressing the other component of Montfaucon's notoriously contaminating stench. "Parisians can see before them," he concluded, "a time when the greatest source of infection that may have ever existed, which had been on their doorstep for two centuries, will disappear."[48]

Montfaucon festered for another fourteen years after those words were written, and the events of 1880 would ultimately remind all Parisians that the problem of waste disposal had not been resolved with the closure of that fell holdover from the ancien régime. However, neither the longevity of Montfaucon nor the Great Stink of 1880 shook the faith of hygienists and others in sanitary progress. If anything, such affronts only added further fuel to the determination to remain vigilant; optimism never justified letting down one's guard.

Periodic investigations in the *Annales d'hygiène publique* of the safety of cesspits and *vidange* struck a similar note of optimism amid warnings about potential hazards. A survey of *vidangeurs* (conducted through their employers) found them not to be significantly unhealthier than other workers. Another review of new technologies in the field—improved disinfectants, a so-called odorless *vidange*, plumbing that divided liquid from solid wastes—predicted significant safety improvements in the future. Nevertheless, both warned that careful professional attention to the industry was imperative because of its inherent dangers.[49]

In light of all the anguished Parisian hand-wringing regarding the deleterious effects of urbanization and overcrowding, it is perhaps surprising to find that global proclamations concerning the health of the French population were remarkably sanguine during this period. Villermé himself seemed to recognize the irony: "Although in the cities there are still too many narrow, dirty, and dark streets, where a large number of families live . . . in a single room crowded with beds, trunks, chairs, looms, [and] tools, in which they sleep, work, prepare their food, and take their meals; it is nonetheless true to say that in general workers' lodgings are no longer those kinds of windowless, unfurnished huts, receiving daylight only from the doorway. You even see many built in a sanitary manner, comfortable, and situated on wide and clean streets." Ask any elderly worker, Villermé continued, and he will tell you that he is better housed (and his lodgings much better furnished) than he was thirty years ago. The problem was that the exceptions to this general trend were highly localized, concentrated, and glaring. Workers of questionable moral character invariably gravitated toward and clustered in the most unsanitary neighborhoods, where they reinforced the worst traits in one another; "honest workers," on the other hand, fled these filthy slums as fast as they could.[50] If progress was global, pathology was quite local—and hard to ignore.

An 1840 Academy of Medicine report on epidemics in France concurred that the big picture looked bright indeed. Long gone were the days of overcrowded cemeteries spreading their foul stench in the middle of large cities; gone too the murderous, long-lasting epidemics of the Middle Ages and the ancien régime that decimated the populations of entire regions. Next to them, even the horrible "cholera-morbus" (Asiatic cholera) paled into near insignificance. "What is more," the academy's report added, "we neutralize with disinfectant agents the miasmas that still threaten us"; new scientific discoveries in this field promised further advances. The report credited the improved health of the population to "the combination of civilization and the progress of the [natural] sciences," which together gave birth to the science of "public hygiene": "As we advance, the gravity of epidemics diminishes in proportion to improvements in public hygiene. The widening of streets, the cleaning and maintenance of public spaces, the isolation of graves, the draining of swamps, etc., have destroyed—or at least rendered much less murderous—the epidemic disasters that terrified our ancestors." There remained much still to be done, of course, as the academy's report acknowledged. Most of the sanitary improvements had been undertaken in cities, by urban interests, under the advisory guidance of urban scientific experts. "As a result, epidemics now come to us most often from the countryside." Like Villermé, the academy found localized pathology amid generalized progress, but saw the danger zones in the nation's vast rural landscape rather than in particular urban neighborhoods. "It is thus a duty for us to unite our efforts with those of our predecessors in order to improve the sanitary status of our compatriots, and to make the enlightenment of hygiene penetrate into our least enlightened regions."[51] The confident meliorism of the middle third of the nineteenth century called upon hygienists to pursue the forward march of civilization into hitherto unconquered territory. The battle for health would henceforth be fought, it seemed, in the dim refuges of the dissolute stratum of the urban working class and in the "least enlightened" pockets of deepest, darkest France—la France profonde.

"CIVILIZATION"

What exactly was this civilization to which hygienists attributed impressive long-term improvements in health? Did it mean a superficial refinement in manners, as opposed to a set of fundamental shared values, as has been suggested by the (frankly Francophobic) German opposition between civilisation and Kultur?[52] The word is as versatile as it is imprecise, but it is possible to gain insights into its particular, grounded meanings in the mid-nineteenth century by taking a closer look at its invocation in the context of public health. What emerges from such an examination is the outline of civilization as a historical phenomenon comprising a combination of economic and cultural development. The touchstone of a teleological view of human progress, civilization was seen as both an all but inevitable historical process and an imperative responsibility to be actively pursued by enlightened servants of the public interest.

Villermé in particular believed in civilization as an explanatory variable in the study of public health. The concept fulfilled a useful role in his work: for one thing, it allowed him simultaneously to sustain two seemingly contradictory arguments, that the health of the French population had improved markedly with urbanization (along with its attendant economic and social changes) and that sanitary conditions were abominable in many French cities. More broadly, the abstraction "civilization" supplied a crucial connection between the economic and moral domains; in effect, Villermé contended, economic progress could not bring about improved health unless it was accompanied (as it ought normally to be, in the telos of civilization) by moral progress.[53]

Villermé's first approach to the question, in 1833, posited the declining severity of deadly epidemics as proof of civilization's beneficial effect on health: "Everywhere we see epidemics diminishing in frequency and intensity, as barbarism fades away, [and] as arts and institutions develop . . . and serve more people." (Anticipating the objection that the previous year's devastating visitation of cholera weakened his thesis, he argued that the disease attacked the indigent above all—"that is, those who participate the least in the advantages procured by the various industries.") More varied agriculture (including the planting of potatoes, "not subject to scarcity"), better communications between distant lands, improved housing and clothing, new industries, and better government all contributed to this remarkable sanitary progress, as Villermé saw it. Another disclaimer provides further clues as to the specific constituent elements of civilization: "Finally, I do not confuse in my assertion ordinary epidemics, which [vary] depending on sudden variations in temperature or other sensible qualities of the air, on diet, on housing, on certain mores, or on any other known circumstance, with altogether exotic epidemics, which appear only at long intervals, and which nothing seems to be able to facilitate or . . . eliminate." If the argument was to hold water, then (and assuming that human agency could not influence temperature variations), the ingredients of civilization most relevant to the prevention of epidemics included diet, housing, and "certain mores." The validity of his thesis, Villermé maintained, could best be gauged by tracing the history of outbreaks of a single disease—smallpox, for instance, which he claimed was more deadly among the native populations of the Americas and of the Russian Far East than among what he called "policed peoples" (les peuples policés).[54]

In the same article, Villermé offered some specific historical examples of civilization's salubrious effects. Viareggio on the Tuscan coast had languished "in a deplorable state of poverty and barbarism" and suffered "since time immemorial" from periodic attacks of epidemic fevers. After the drainage of the local swamps in 1741 through a system of locks with mobile gates, the fevers disappeared, and the town became "one of the most healthy, most industrious, and richest" in the region, while the inhabitants enjoyed unprecedented "health, vigor, longevity, and moral character." The same phenomenon could be observed in Zeeland in the Netherlands, and in many other places where the intensity of periodic fevers had progressively diminished; more generally, it accounted for the greater prevalence of epidemic disease in the countryside than in cities. "This miracle, I repeat, is that of civilization," Villermé commented.[55] The juxtaposition of long-term economic changes and specifically identifiable public policies in Villermé's analysis leaves some lingering doubt about the extent to which civilization could be actively sought or encouraged by health-minded reformers among his readers in 1833. However, the article's conclusion makes it clear that he expected decision-makers to heed his findings directly, not simply to pursue laissez-faire policies and wait for economic development:[56] "One directly useful finding, one lesson whose application is easy, is the diminution of the frequency and intensity of epidemics by the progress of civilization. . . . Let us vow that this lesson will be put to use . . . by governments, by public administrators, and by all those whose duty or position calls them to work toward the happiness of mankind."[57] Villermé refrained from providing specific policy recommendations, perhaps feeling that to do so would unnecessarily bog his overall project down in partisan political battles. However, he left no doubt that the road to health was one that needed to be paved by enlightened administrators, elected officials, and scientific experts.

Seven years later, after the publication of his monumental *Tableau*, Villermé was summoned by the Academy of Moral and Political Sciences along with his colleague Benoiston de Châteauneuf to visit Brittany and investigate in detail the living conditions of the population. The resulting portrait mingled the ethnographer's sincere respect with the despair and disdain of the modern man of science. Timeless, tradition-bound, stubbornly resistant to change, Bretons stood as a race apart within France, "holding on with a religious respect to their institutions, their mores, their dress, and their language, as they maintain in their [physical] traits the still recognizable characteristics of the race to which their ancestors belonged." On the one hand, their attachment to an unchanging way of life preserved the Breton traditions, institutions, and love of the land; on the other hand, it also made "the bad eternal and the better impossible."[58]

Villermé and Benoiston's lengthy investigation of the state of Breton civilization deserves careful attention for two reasons. First, it is the relatively neglected stepsibling of Villermé's 1840 *Tableau*, as the two partners followed up on their initial mandate from the academy and carried it into previously uncharted territory. Second, in the aftermath of the revolutions of 1789 and 1830, Brittany represented the absolute self-defining Other for secular, urbane, and scientific-minded Frenchmen. The prevailing way of life there became, in essence, the very antithesis of Frenchness. As much as urban health hazards preoccupied reformers like Villermé and Benoiston, the fact that there existed on home soil a population even more atavistic and resistant to progress than the urban working class was both reassuring and alarming; their remoteness diminished the intensity of their danger, while duty called for the light of public hygiene to be spread throughout the nation. A romantic respect for authenticity and tradition collided with a nascent civilizing imperative.

Housing conditions in rural Brittany simply appalled Villermé and Benoiston: "In order to get an idea of their destitution, you have to have entered into the home of a poor Breton peasant, into his dilapidated cottage whose roof slopes all the way down to the ground, whose interior is blackened by the continual smoke from the burning undergrowth which is the only fuel for his hearth." Life in such places was barely human. Furnishings were crude and sparse, and it could be difficult to tell the human beings and the animals apart: "It is in this miserable hut, where daylight enters only through the door and is snuffed out as soon as it shuts, that he lives with his family, half-naked, using for furniture only a poor table, a bench, a cauldron and a few wooden or clay utensils; for a bed, a kind of box with a bale of oats as a mattress and no sheets, while in the opposite corner of this dreary closet of a house, chewing its cud on a small pile of manure is the thin and scrawny cow which feeds the family with its milk."[59] The simplest distinguishing marks of humanity—clothing, beds, living apart from animals—were absent. How could one even begin to preach hygienic reform in such an environment? Here as elsewhere throughout the report, one senses Villermé and Benoiston torn among competing impulses: the urge to denounce such offensive subhuman habits, the need to preserve the scrupulous distance of faithful scientific observation, and a genuine compassion for the plight of the poor peasants.

Conspiring to perpetuate these abominable material conditions were the fatalism, ignorance, and powerful Catholic faith of those who endured them. Resignation to this lot in life was so deeply ingrained in the Breton people that it caused the hygienists to wonder whether these peasants would even consent to trade their diet or belongings for better ones if given the choice. The Breton accepts his fate as final and absolute, observed Villermé and Benoiston, quoting another contemporary observer to the effect that "he treats his poverty like a hereditary and incurable disease."[60] Isolation and lack of education led to a lamentable ignorance, which in turn gave free rein to all manner of superstitions. Many Bretons, the investigators reported, believed in ghosts, in the devil, in fairies, in sorcerers, and in a race of hairy black dwarves who took delight in doing evil. Local legends about various portents of doom or blessing abounded, and the water of certain springs and fountains was believed to heal previously incurable ills, including obsession with the devil. The other side of this coin was the sincere and abiding faith that gave Bretons an admirable strength of character. The intensity of religious observance might seem in the eyes of outsiders to border on the fanatical; when a son became a priest, for example, and visited his parents, he ate meals alone at table, served by his parents who bowed before him and addressed him henceforth with the formal pronoun *vous*. Ritual processions and sacraments served as a central organizing principle of daily life in Brittany. Yet behind the external observances burned what Villermé and Benoiston called "a true piety, a sincere faith," which allowed the afflicted to bear their burdens with courage and patience.[61]

There was one other thing that helped Bretons to endure so much suffering: alcohol. Women as well as men fell prey to "this degrading vice," and the endlessly repeated exhortations of teachers and employers had proven powerless to vanquish it. The two hygienists found the causes of this unfortunate habit not in an inherent character flaw, but in the Breton's "thick senses" (*des sens grossiers*), which responded only to strong stimulants, and in the need to forget momentarily the pains and privations of this earth. The problem was that "in Brittany, there is little civilization and much poverty"; with more of one and less of the other, drinking was bound to decrease: "More education and more wealth would without doubt introduce more propriety in the mores and more sobriety in the appetites. Furthermore, these shameful penchants . . . which the Breton owes more to his position than to his character, are counterbalanced by his admirable qualities, the virtues which do him credit."[62] In the end, then, the fundamental virtues of the Breton character redeemed a multitude of vices. However, Villermé's and Benoiston's gracious benediction did not solve the problem of hygienic reform in Brittany.

The hygienists' struggle with that problem triggered an ethical dilemma uncharacteristic of nineteenth-century reformers. What if civilization took more away from Breton society than it added? they wondered. Might the noble project of increased communication, education, and general integration of Brittany into the cultural life of the nation end up subverting all that was valuable in Breton culture to begin with? Concerned local observers asked Villermé and Benoiston whether their enterprise signaled the beginning of the end of Breton distinctiveness. Perhaps the local way of life was somewhat crude, they argued, and some age-old customs might appear strange, but they neither harmed nor threatened anybody. Their culture had been distinguished by "a great ignorance, which cannot be defended, but which has at least left sleeping in their hearts the ferment of passion and the fever of desire." They loved their country (that is, Brittany) and their language. If this culture disappeared, they asked the investigators, "what will replace it?": "Polite manners which will hide a lack of honesty beneath an excess of urbanity; more education, which will multiply the needs of a simple people previously content with very little, will cause [them] to trade the true wealth they possess for false [hopes] . . . and may even weaken that sincere faith which gives the poor enough resignation to tolerate their sort, and the rich enough charity to alleviate it." For all of the benefit in material comfort, the hygienists asked themselves, when bodies were better fed and better rested, would souls be better off too? Might the cultural loss outweigh the economic gain?[63]

The prospect of sowing avidity, ambition, and selfishness where contentment had previously reigned disturbed Villermé and Benoiston, but in the end, they could not bring themselves to believe that "to stay an honest man, one must always live in ignorance": "We hold civilization in high enough regard to believe that it can enlighten minds without corrupting them, procure well-being without sparking a thirst for gold, cleanse beliefs without weakening faith; finally, we have told ourselves that if there are evils that must be accepted, there are also good things that must not be resisted." Ultimately, the hygienists' faith in science and progress won out over their other competing impulses. The forward march of civilization, far from being halted, ought to be hastened: "We have [therefore] expressed our hope that civilization, which has already advanced along the coasts of Brittany, will soon extend its progress into the interior, in order to introduce among the populations living there the germs of the prosperity they lack, and to add to the pleasant qualities they already have . . . more employment, more widespread education, more active and intelligent industry, [and] greater affluence."[64]

Although few examined it at such length and with such eloquence, most French hygienists in the nineteenth century shared Villermé's and Benoiston's vision of a beneficent civilization lifting filthy peasants and urban workers up from squalor. (This vision's remarkable staying power is illustrated in detail in chapters 4 and 5.) Many of them emphasized the physician's key role as activist and educator, as in the report of a devastating typhoid fever epidemic in the tiny town of Prades in Ariège in 1838 (310 cases and 95 deaths out of a population of 750). Terrified residents blamed the influence of the moon and feared contagion, but the enlightened physicians sent to investigate reassured them by swallowing blood taken from patients' excretions and by sleeping in beds recently vacated by deceased victims of the disease. They also took pains to explain to the benighted peasants that the epidemic resulted not from lunar influence but rather from the prevailing wind direction bringing miasmas into the village. In many instances like this one, the reporter made clear, the physician's didactic role was as important as his therapeutic expertise.[65]

As early as the 1820s, prominent physicians François-Joseph Double and François Mêlier claimed to have proven statistically that education improved health. In 1827, Double compared annual mortality in two neighboring districts of the Loire department in south-central France. The death rate in the Forez plain was nearly twice as high as that of the mountainous district nearby, and there were more than three times as many septuagenarians in the mountains than on the plain. Double painted a bleak picture of life on the Forez plain: "The squashed, one-story adobe houses are poorly ventilated, and the constant dampness of the soil penetrates throughout them; the nonchalant, apathetic inhabitants push their lack of concern in matters of health to the highest degree; almost always sickly, they are always extremely susceptible to the intermittent fevers by which they allow themselves to be consumed." In contrast, their neighbors in the mountains were "more enlightened, more hard-working, and more dedicated to commerce," and they enjoyed better housing, better clothing, and a better diet. Physically, they were more "robust"; morally, more "pure." Although this stark contrast could not be attributed to a single factor, Double considered the lack of education in Forez—and the attendant "noncivilization" of its residents—to be a principal cause of the area's poor health. All of the department's other districts were better served by schools than was the Forez plain, and all were healthier too. Moreover, Double argued, other health-promoting influences such as economic expansion and the lifestyle it brought with it most often went hand in hand with improved education.[66]

A year later, in 1828, Mêlier was inspired by a map of France showing the differential prevalence of elementary education by department to draw up a similar map for mortality. The dark tints on Mêlier's map indicated departments with high annual mortality, while the lighter ones represented low mortality. The correspondence of the two maps was striking; in general, northern departments enjoyed better education and lower mortality, while southern departments ranked poorly in both respects; the Breton departments, however, were solid black on both maps, with the lowest educational levels and the highest mortality.[67]

More than forty years later, in the infancy of the Third Republic, as parliament prepared to consider a bill providing for mandatory public education, another hygienist evoked Mêlier's and Double's studies in order to demonstrate the sanitary—and political—advantages to be gained from the diffusion of education. Octave du Mesnil conceded that many factors other than education—including agricultural improvements, industrial advances, economic growth, and wider distribution of wealth—clearly affected overall population, mortality, and life expectancy in France: "To this I answer that it is impossible to separate these three terms: ignorance, poverty, and mortality; that the same population the teacher finds indifferent to the benefits of education, ignorance [makes them] resistant to the application of new methods, . . . to the use of improved machines in industry, [and] . . . to the observation of the rules of hygiene." Lest his readers in 1872 (the traumatic memory of the Paris Commune fresh in their minds) miss the implied political dimension of his argument, du Mesnil made it explicit: "To answer those who . . . object that education gives rise to envy, which becomes a danger to public order," he argued "that while education is the most active instrument of progress . . . it is at the same time the surest guardian of order, because it teaches [people] not to trust those absolute and radical doctrines which make violence a right and impatience a virtue."[68] Several historians have pointed out that in the French "cholera years" of the July Monarchy and Second Republic, disease and revolution fused in a two-headed threat to bourgeois order and political stability.[69] According to the party of hygiene, education (and civilization more broadly) was the weapon of choice to cut off both of these heads.

MORALIZATION AND DISGUST

In the hideous lairs which Paris hides away behind its palaces and museums . . . there lurks a swarming and oozing population that beggars comparison. There are crusts and wretched remnants all around. . . . [It is] a vile bohemian world, a frightful world, a purulent wart on the face of this great city.
—JULES JANIN, *Un hiver à Paris (1845)*

Other scholars have abundantly documented the central tendency of early nineteenth-century "hygienism" toward moralization;[70] further demonstration of this feature of the movement would be superfluous (though perhaps picturesque). However, it is worth insisting on the importance of the elaboration, through the hygienic literature, of a vocabulary and a grammar of disgust, which helped convey this moralizing agenda and which continued to shape the discourse of public health long into the bacteriological era. The "foul effluvia and pestilential vapors" of Paris,[71] Lille's filthy slums, workers who live in unspeakable "promiscuity," peasants who live surrounded by animal feces—all served as foils for hygienists and other medical observers (speaking on behalf of the respectable classes in France) to articulate by opposition the central tenets of modern, civilized bourgeois identity:

- cleanliness and order in public and domestic spaces;
- moderation and self-control;
- containment and disposal of bodily substances; and
- a progressive distancing of individual human bodies from natural functions, from animals, and from one another.

An 1840 report explaining the frequent dysentery epidemics near the town of Josselin in southern Brittany illustrates the seamless way in which material and moral causes combined to cause disease in the mid-nineteenth century. The investigating physician blamed primarily "bad fruit" and "variations of temperature" for the attacks of dysentery but felt compelled to point to accessory causes as well: "I must add that the country is wooded [and] humid, [and] that the inhabitants are smokers, drunkards, [and] unclean."[72] Under the flexible etiologies of midcentury, it was both self-evident and empirically proven that bad habits and hygienic neglect (as well as geology and a range of other possible contributing factors) could together create a susceptibility to various diseases, and that even seemingly minor precipitants (unusual weather, bad fruit) could cause the disease most appropriate to those conditions to burst forth onto the scene.

Beyond specific local etiologies, moralization also helped bourgeois observers rationalize the calamities that seemed to result from the poverty, inequality, and squalor to which industrialization and urbanization had given birth. Here is Villermé, for example, on the dangers of bringing together large numbers of workers in industrial centers:

Everywhere [you go] . . . the man condemned to labor earns his bread by the sweat of his brow; but also everywhere [you go], laziness, lack of economy, debauchery, [and] corruption inevitably produce poverty. . . .

Very commonly . . . manufacturing workers lack sobriety, economy . . . and morals, and quite often they are poor by their own fault alone.

This evil is not new, but it is [worse] than ever; it results principally from the typical gathering of workers together in large workshops . . . where the sexes and ages are mixed together, and from spending time . . . in large cities.[73]

This is the same Villermé who elsewhere linked civilization (that is, in large part, industrialization) with improved health, and along with Benoiston absolved dirt-poor Breton peasants of blame for their own destitution. In this formulation, agglomerations of population cause immorality, which in turn causes poverty. One recognizes here the deep ambivalence of the reformer whose science led him to indict poverty and inequality, but whose abiding commitment to liberal political economy prevented him from drawing the conclusions others might have drawn from the same evidence.[74] Again, material and moral causes of suffering are inseparably interdependent.

The preceding pages are replete with thoroughly disgusted descriptions of one health hazard or another. Disgust not only tended to assign blame for unacceptable and dangerous living conditions to those most endangered by them, but it also performed the critical function of conferring a moral valence on ostensibly neutral or value-free variables that might be linked to disease. What lessons could be learned, for example, or what practical conclusions drawn from an etiology attributing an epidemic to weather conditions? In and of themselves, excrement and goats are as value-neutral as the weather; but in practice, of course, they become disgusting—and anathema—when they are "out of place."[75]

Filth has perhaps always been pathogenic in this basic cultural sense, to the extent that members of a given community agree on its nature and its dangers. In nineteenth-century France, urbanization and other fundamental changes in the material conditions of life, the continually declining tolerability of certain bodily substances and sensory experiences, and the establishment of public health as a domain of expert knowledge made it necessary to define (or at least allude to) the means by which disgusting things caused disease. Some were content to infer a causal relationship from a proximal association, for example, between foul air and elevated infant mortality: "Paris is a great manufactory of putrefaction, in which poverty, plague and disease labor in concert, and air and sunlight barely enter. Paris is a foul hole where plants wilt and perish and four out of seven children die within the year."[76] Others struggled to capture the effect of filth in more precise scientific terms. In his 1835 study of Montfaucon, Parent-Duchâtelet compared the fecal odors of the waste dump with the animal odors of the horse-rendering plant. Both were horribly disgusting, but the scientifically minded hygienist could not leave it at that: "Even though the . . . putrefying animal matter spreads around the place itself a much more repulsive odor than does the fecal matter, its putrid odor disseminates and blends, so to speak, more easily in the air than that which comes from fe-

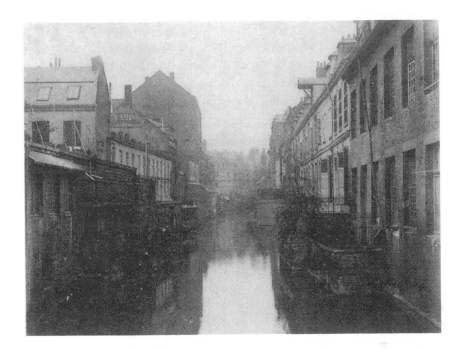

Fig. 5. The St.-Pierre Canal in Lille (Nord), early twentieth century. Photo courtesy of Bibliothèque municipale de Lille.

cal matter gathered together in great quantities. Thus, the odor particular to these latter materials will still be recognizable at several kilometers distance, whereas the odor of the former will cease to be noticeable at a few hundred paces."[77] He attributed this fact to the higher ammonia concentrations in feces.

The need to classify and detail potentially pathogenic odors intensified after etiological discussions began to shift during the 1870s in the direction of putative microbiological causes of specific diseases. In 1879, hygienist Jules Arnould tried to capture the danger in the canals of Lille (Fig. 5) by arguing that the question of disease specificity and the possible existence of "the germs of various diseases" in "these putrid waters" were beside the point: "*It is not good to breathe an air impregnated with putrid and malodorous emanations;* the lungs do not accept air such as this any better than the stomach accepts contaminated food." Even if a specific illness did not directly result, Arnould added, "other predispositions toward illness, which are simply gradually acquired deviations from normal nutritive processes," were likely.[78] In retrospect, Arnould's may seem a strained attempt to reconcile old-fashioned miasmatism with new discoveries in bacteriology.

However, even years later, after the definitive triumph of germ theory, the integration of the old sanitarian dangers (filth, odors, indirect contamination) into the new etiological framework remained an important item on the hygienic agenda. When Pasteur and Brouardel insisted in early 1881 that foul-smelling emanations could indeed transmit disease-causing microbes, their stand was not out of step with the mainstream of scientific thought, though in retrospect it seems to clash with the principal thrust of Pasteur's life work.

The same moral register of disgust was also brought to bear on a class of transgressions less immediately physical in nature. Apart from venereal diseases, alcoholic or sexual excesses and violations against modesty or propriety were linked to illness more indirectly than were odors or other physical threats. However, the fundamental problem of the concentration of large numbers of human bodies in a limited space invariably led commentators to suggest dark moral scenarios that had arisen or might arise in crowded, undisciplined conditions. Villermé warned of "orgies" if single male workers were housed in separate dormitories or apartment blocks under new workers' housing programs under consideration in 1850: "These men . . . are the workers who earn the best wages, have the least expenses, are the most lacking in economy, in sobriety, in morals, and ordinarily spend everything as they receive it, from day to day, in excesses, in debauchery, without any savings for tomorrow. Without a family to support . . . they have less to fear from abandoning themselves to intemperance."[79] With similar concerns uppermost in his mind, Villermé recommended that the new workers' housing projects, or *cités ouvrières,* be designed to give families "all of the conditions of air, sunlight, space, comfort, salubrity, and isolation that are compatible with their positions as workers and honest, hard-working married persons, who raise their children in the principles of religion and morality, and especially their daughters in modesty and self-restraint."[80] Although the sermonizing tone dominates passages such as this one, it is important to note that Villermé is not only preaching moderation and modesty to working-class families; he is also, with equal force, calling for local officials and philanthropists to create the conditions that will allow morality to flourish.

Hygienists' moralizing disgust reached a crescendo in descriptions of the working-class quarters of Lille gathered for Villermé's great *Tableau.* Even more than a century removed, one can glimpse in these passages the motive power of this kind of vividly disgusted expository style. There is a synesthesia of foulness that, set forth gradually, bit by bit, becomes physically overwhelming. In one description, quoted at length by Villermé, the departmental health council expressed its shock at the conditions it found in the lodgings of Lille's working classes: "It is impossible to conceive of the appearance of the homes of our poor if one has not visited them [in person]. The heedlessness in which they live brings upon them evils that make their poverty horrible, intolerable, murderous. Their poverty becomes their fate through the state of abandon and demoralization that it produces."[81] Again, the poor have themselves to blame for their poverty, which becomes self-perpetuating as it deepens the moral failings that were present to begin with.

Yet it was not enough to pronounce moral judgment, in the health council's view. It was understood that the moral and the physical were indivisible, and one had to experience (even if only vicariously) the very physical texture of this "demoralization" in order to fully grasp the enormity of the sanitary crisis facing cities such as Lille: "In their dark cellars—[rather,] in their rooms which one could mistake for cellars—the air never circulates, it stinks; the walls are plastered with a thousand kinds of garbage. . . . If there is a bed, it is only a few dirty, greasy boards; it is damp, putrescent straw; it is a rudimentary sheet whose fabric and color are hidden beneath a layer of grime; it is a blanket resembling a sieve. . . . The furniture is broken, worm-eaten, covered with bits of foulness." A Breton peasant might have felt at home in such a hovel. Light and air were seemingly barred entry: "The windows, always closed, have . . . panes but [they are] so black, so covered with smoke, that daylight could never penetrate them. . . . The floor of the dwelling is even dirtier than the rest; everywhere are piles of garbage, of ashes, of bits of vegetables gathered in the streets, of rotting straw; nests for all kinds of animals; the air is no longer breathable." The most lasting impression of the scene was olfactory: "One finds oneself fatigued, in these holes, by a stale, nauseating odor, [the] slightly acrid odor of filth, odor of garbage, odor of bodies, etc., etc."[82] The reporter's fatigue is apparent in the "etc., etc." with which this passage closes, as if he is gasping for breath and cannot muster up the strength to continue the description.

Not surprisingly, the residents of these dwellings were far from the picture of cleanliness and health. Their clothing was ragged, their hair unkempt; both were covered with the residue of the workshop. Their skin, though dirty, was recognizable as such on their faces, but on their bodies it was "painted—hidden, if you will—by the gradual deposits of miscellaneous exudations." The children were "discolored, thin, sickly, old—yes, old and wrinkled." "Their bellies were fat and their limbs emaciated; their spines were curved . . . their necks are . . . covered with [swollen] glands; their fingers are ulcerated and their bones swollen and softened; finally, these little unfortunates are tormented [and] devoured by insects."[83] The council's report summed up the situation thus: "Nothing is more horribly dirty than these poor demoralized [people]" (Rien n'est plus horriblement sale que ces pauvres démoralisés). The cumulative effect of such descriptions was, among other things, to reinforce the link between moral and physical health. Sanitary improvement was unimaginable without moral improvement.

If it was possible to match this latter description in detail and disgust, Villermé did it in his own exposé of conditions in the Lille neighborhood of rue des Etaques. Once again, the text deserves fairly extensive quotation simply because its power lies in its vividness, its specificity, and the unpleasant sensations produced by its cumulative effect. This working-class quarter somehow shoehorned 3,000 people into 24,000 square meters of three- and four-story apartment buildings. The poorest of the poor lived in the cellars and attics; the cellar lodgings could be reached only from the interior courtyard by a stairway, which usually substituted for a door and windows. Their vaulted stone or brick ceilings measured six to six-and-one-half feet tall at the peak of the vault:

> It is in these dark and dismal dwellings that a large number of workers eat, sleep, and even work. Daylight arrives for them an hour later than for others, dusk an hour earlier.
>
> Their typical furniture comprises, in addition to the tools of their occupation, a kind of cupboard or a board on which to place food, a stove, an earthenware chafing dish . . . a small table, two or three poor chairs, and a dirty pallet with a straw mattress and a tattered blanket.

Here Villermé feigns reluctance to continue, but duty compels him to shrink at nothing in his portrayal of this horrible underworld:

> I would prefer to add nothing to this detailed depiction of hideous things which, at first glance, reveal the profound misery of the unfortunate inhabitants; but I must say that, in several of the beds that I just mentioned, I have seen lying together individuals of both sexes and of very different ages, most of them without nightshirts and repulsively dirty.

A footnote here explains, "There are even spinning-mills where the color of the workers' bare feet could cause one to mistake them for negroes, so blackened are these feet by grime." The lurid exposé continues:

[In these beds] father, mother, old people, children, adults press together [and] pile up together. I will stop here . . . [ellipsis in original] The reader will finish the portrait, but I warn him that if he wants to make it accurate, he must not allow his imagination to recoil before any of the disgusting mysteries that are enacted on these impure beds, amid darkness and drunkenness.

To this slyly salacious hint, Villermé adds in a sober footnote: "Two physicians and a police sergeant told me they knew with certainty that incest is sometimes committed, and others informed me that they have heard workers accuse each other of this in their arguments." To add a final indignity to the description of housing conditions in rue des Etaques (and to emphasize the complete lack of modesty and self-control of the population), Villermé notes that there are sometimes only one or two toilets in a building housing hundreds of people, and "in the evenings, when the workers have just returned home, one commonly sees women coming out of the alleys, stopping over the gutter in the street, and there, in front of passersby and even jostled by them, do without shame that which they would never [otherwise] do in public."[84]

It is difficult to know which would be more offensive to mid-nineteenth-century bourgeois sensibilities: the idea of grimy, smelly incest in a pile of bodies or the sight of an adult woman urinating in public in plain view of (even while touching) passing pedestrians. This genre of social investigation is meant to disgust and to outrage, and examples such as this one are certainly vivid enough to succeed in this aim. Is it possible that bourgeois commentators such as Villermé (and their intended audiences) experienced, alongside their obvious sensory discomfort and nausea, a perverse kind of pleasure in such lurid—even pornographic—descriptions? Could wallowing in the minute details of such totalizing squalor simultaneously titillate, terrify, and reassure?[85] The depths to which this subhuman Other had sunk, after all, reaffirmed the elevated status (and moral worth) of the observer, even as it threatened the continued viability of the society that made possible both extremes.

The reader might think (or hope) that the dismal housing conditions represented the worst that neighborhoods such as those of rue des Etaques had to offer; but this was not the case. Determined to observe the working classes in the totality of their misery, Villermé followed them to their equally dreary, even more overcrowded bars and drinking establishments: "I wanted to penetrate into these places, where I saw, through the doors and windows, through a cloud of tobacco smoke, the inhabitants of this hideous quarter swarming together like ants in an anthill; but it was obvious that, despite the precautions I had taken to dress so as to make them less suspicious of me, my appearance in their midst would have aroused their surprise, [and] especially their distrust." He was forced to observe from the window, where he saw men and women crowded together, without enough places to sit down, all drinking beer or "the detestable distilled grain alcohol." In the streets, he saw many passersby stop at the grocer's shop for a drink on their way to the bar, and he overheard "even children saying the most obscene things." At this point, the accumulation of horror and outrage and disgust in rue des Etaques seems to have reached a point of excess even for Villermé, who abruptly added, "I can state clearly: *I have never seen at the same time so much filth, misery, and vice in a more hideous, more revolting setting.*"[86]

There are many obvious conclusions to be drawn from the hygienists' moralizing investigations, including the very simple one that bourgeois observers were struggling to confront for the first time the realities of poverty in an industrializing world of great wealth and equally great deprivation. However, it would be a mistake to conclude that these disgusted reactions and moral judgments are straightforward or merely natural, even if we twenty-first-century readers find ourselves un-self-consciously sharing in them. It is important to point out that certain elements of working-class and peasant lifestyles tended to arouse bourgeois emotions more readily than others. Close quarters, darkness, dampness, the "promiscuous" intermingling of bodies, foul odors, bodily excretions, and human proximity to animals or animal products—these were the most common triggers of bourgeois shock, rejection, and revulsion.

A HYGIENE OF BODILY SEPARATION AND AERATION

One can read backward from these bourgeois reactions to arrive at a working definition of civilization from a hygienic perspective. If the depths of human depravity could be measured by dark, filthy bodies, the (inherently sexualized) crowding and commingling of bodies, and excretion in public, then by implication, civilization lay in the direction of clean white bodies, surrounded by circulating air and sunlight, evacuating all substances in private through carefully contained channels. This heuristic exercise sketches the outlines of the agenda, widely shared but rarely explicitly formulated as such, that runs throughout most of the literature of the French sanitarians between 1820 and 1880: a *hygiene of bodily separation and aeration* that diagnosed problems in the scientifically observed and investigated world, prescribed remedies both immediate and long-term by charting a course of reform, and held out the vision of a morally and physically healthier society in a more or less distant future.

What Villermé and his fellow hygienists seem to have been calling for was nothing less than a fundamental spatial reordering of the urban environment. (A similar project would presumably be appropriate for the countryside someday, though most reformers before 1880 focused on the city as the most urgent object of concern.) The imperative underlying many sanitary projects, proposals, and polemics was to reorder public and private space by separating and cleansing buildings and bodies. The basic individual elements of this agenda were neither especially innovative nor controversial. Popular hygiene manuals perennially recommended better domestic ventilation, and had railed against the widespread fear of drafts (*courants d'air*), or more generally of exposure to the elements: "In an apartment, you must be careful to open doors and windows and [thereby] sweep away vapors"; "respiration is effective only as long as a pure air, free in its course, odorless, sufficiently circulated and renewed, surrounds the human body"; "it is essential to renew the air, to make the quantity proportional to the number of inhabitants . . . [and] to make it circulate through ventilations."[87] Villermé himself was fanatical about ventilation, as the hospital broken-window story recounted earlier in this chapter shows.[88]

Bodily separation went hand in hand with ventilation, and addressed the same constellation of ills—especially overcrowding and "promiscuity," the indiscriminate intermingling of bodies in various contexts. When a wave of plans began to emerge for the construction of large, sanitary *cités ouvrières* or workers' housing complexes, Villermé was not the only hygienist to weigh in, though he was one of the most vocal and opinionated. In general, he looked upon the new *cités ouvrières* as a step in the right direction, but feared that they would repeat some of the same fatal design mistakes apparent in existing workers' housing blocks, in which the "indecently maintained" toilets were "placed no less indecently in the view of all those who went up or down the staircase [or] entered or left" the building. Commenting on a proposed *cité ouvrière* in Paris, Villermé expressed his fear that families could not be sufficiently isolated from one another: "It is doubtful, moreover, that everything has been calculated to avoid . . . even fortuitous communications among residents of a single block, especially between the two sexes. . . . Has the plan been set up so that one cannot hear what is being said in the adjacent room of the neighboring family's apartment? or so that if a door is open, one cannot see from another apartment what is happening there?" The hygienist was especially disturbed by the public visibility of that which should be most private and least visible, the excretory functions: "How to prevent those unfortunate encounters of a large number of individuals going up and down the same stairway every day, walking through the same corridors, or even noticing one another at the door of the facilities unfortunately common to several unrelated families, and where on the contrary one ought to be most hidden from all glances?"[89]

The solution to these ever-present dangers was an even more careful design of such housing projects on a smaller scale and according to moral and hygienic principles, with the goal of separating families as much as possible from one another, and surrounding each one with the essential health-giving influences:

> Each dwelling should be composed of two or three habitable rooms . . . and have its own separate entrance.
>
> All of these rooms should be well enclosed, well lighted, well aerated, and sufficiently large.
>
> The windows and doors would be arranged in such a way that when they are open, one can neither be seen by one's closest neighbors nor see what is happening in their apartments. . . .
>
> It is of course almost superfluous to note here how useful such dwellings could be for family life, and consequently for work, for savings, for good habits and for improved well-being, [which benefits one could not get] in the large cités ouvrières . . . [with] hundreds of people, [where] forced contact at every moment would be a continual and intolerable nuisance.[90]

Decades before microbes became the contagious health menace par excellence, human contact was dangerous here not because of the possible direct transmission of a specific disease, but in an even more frightening sense: because it could eventually break down the boundaries and inhibitions that ultimately constitute the basis of humanity.

The hygiene of bodily separation and aeration was by no means a uniquely French phenomenon. Sanitarians in Britain and elsewhere shared an obsession with overcrowded working-class housing, corrupted air, and bodily separation. As in France, these conditions did not merely present a physical threat to the population, though they were widely known to facilitate the spread of epidemic fevers; they were acute moral dangers as well, as Felix Driver has noted: "Cities (described as 'swamps' by one writer, and 'forests' by another) were said to provide countless 'places of darkness and conceal-ment' for the fermentation of moral disease. . . . The poor were repeatedly said to be housed *en masse* in countless courts and back-alleys, without re-gard for distinctions of age or sex, and with little differentiation between rooms according to their function." The only remedy for such alarming conditions, in Driver's rendering of the British sanitarians' "moral geog-raphy," was a thorough agenda of "segregation, ventilation, and inspec-tion" in a wide variety of settings, from working-class housing to prisons to hospitals.[91]

The French hygienists of the second quarter of the nineteenth century laid the groundwork for much of the public health knowledge that co-alesced after 1880, in the bacteriological era. Their method, their preferred objects of study, their confidence, their moral sensibility, and their tone all influenced the discourse of public health and disease prevention long after their work had lost etiological currency. The hygiene of bodily separation and aeration also survived as a conceptual ideal and a guide to practical action. For example, on the eve of the Bacteriological Revolution, in 1876, when Léon Colin attempted to classify systematically the pathogenic effects of overcrowding, he struck many of the same notes as had Villermé decades earlier. Colin focused on typhus and on nosocomial infections (where the effects of crowding seemed especially obvious), rather than on generalized moral consequences, but he zeroed in on the same problem of corporeal geography that had preoccupied his predecessors. In the case of typhus, Colin's research convinced him of "the benefit for everyone of a more com-plete life in the open air"; when a military unit was struck by the disease, "the ventilation experienced during a march continuously removed a cer-tain quantity of the typhic miasma." For hospitals, Colin had an urgent message: do not gather typhus patients together in one room or wing. Ag-glomeration made each case worse and facilitated transmission; dissemi-nation, on the other hand, limited the danger of the disease's spread and hastened the recovery of existing patients. The goal was to "confront the scourge with the barrier of the void," and to "give to everyone . . . a healthful milieu in which they do not have to expose themselves to the influence of their own emanations, nor to the emanations of others."[92]

From the innumerable investigations of epidemics in overcrowded neighborhoods to Villermé to Colin and beyond, the ideal of bodily separa-tion and aeration continued to shape the questions asked and the answers found in the literature of public health. In a sanitary environment, clean and clear boundaries separated individualized bodies;[93] abundant sunlight and ventilation constantly combated disease influences, whatever their precise nature; and every man was an island, entire of itself. The humanity of the individual body was enhanced (every day, constantly) by its being surrounded and bathed by fresh air and sunlight. Healthy bodies were solid, differentiated bodies, defined by their boundaries, by their solidity, and by their differentiation around the edges from the surrounding elements.

Both before and after the emergence of microbes, the hygiene of bodily separation and ventilation could not help but run up against tenacious popular antipathy toward drafts and toward bathing. In popular milieux where winds brought only chills and layers of dirt and grime protected the body from malign influences, it could actually be dangerous to open windows or to bathe;[94] even huddling together in bed with family members might be felt to be protective in certain circumstances. What appeared to be the stubborn resistance of superstitious inertia to progress can also be viewed as the clash of two alternative and coherent hygienic regimes: bodily separation and aeration versus bodily clustering and envelopment. Even a revolution in etiology would not be enough to resolve this conflict without a broader shift in popular mores. Although the outcome of the struggle might at times have seemed in doubt, the most enduring legacy bequeathed by the early French hygienists to their successors in the bacteriological era was the dogged determination to combat filth wherever it was found, in an ongoing battle that was more cultural than specifically etiological in nature.

Taxonomies of Transmission

Local Etiologies and the Equivocal Triumph of Germ Theory

*T*yphoid fever is caused by a bacterium first identified by Karl Eberth in 1880 as *Bacillus typhosus*, and later renamed *Salmonella typhi*. The mere fact that a disease could be said to have a single cause (whether a microorganism or not) is the product of an epistemological sea change that took place between 1875 and 1900, in the slipstream of the Bacteriological Revolution. But three years after Eberth's discovery, typhoid fever was caused by overcrowding, miasmatic emanations, and direct contagion in Quesnoy (Nord) and in the villages around St.-Malo (Ille-et-Vilaine).[1] This is a historical fact—relatively speaking. This is not to say that its victims were not infected by *Salmonella typhi*, nor that other factors such as contaminated water could not have been involved (although in the case of Quesnoy, the epidemic doctor believed he had demonstrated that the water supply was not to blame). Rather, it means that representative observers, weighing all evidence and considering all explanations reasonably available at the time to authorities in their position, concluded based on criteria prevailing in the time and place in question that these factors explained a particular outbreak of typhoid fever better (more persuasively, more usefully) than other possible explanations. Judged by the standards of other times or places, such claims might be patently false, even ridiculous; at this time and in these places, however, they were true.[2]

During the last quarter of the nineteenth century, just as monocausal bacteriological explanations of disease were beginning to gain currency in medical circles throughout the industrializing world, a host of infectious disease etiologies continued to proliferate. French health authorities attempted to impose some order on the chaos and to classify all reported epidemics nationwide by causal category. If standardized information concerning the causes of epidemics could be gathered, the reasoning went, more rational and more effective public health policies could be devised. "Epidemic doctors"—local physicians appointed to investigate disease outbreaks in their jurisdiction—were asked to fill out a form to accompany each report. The 1890 version of the form included the following question:

> 8. Presumed origin of the epidemic and causes of its development:
>   (a) Importation
>   (b) Poor water quality due to excessive organic matter
>   (c) Contagion
>   (d) Unsanitary conditions
>   (e) Defective waste disposal[3]

A century after the fact, the categories themselves seem oddly incommensurable and overlapping. But even at the time, when it was reasonable to conceive of such a taxonomy, the multiplicity and diversity of disease causes could not be contained by these categories, no matter how capacious they were.

EPIDEMIC DOCTORS, FROM THE OLD REGIME TO THE BACTERIOLOGICAL REVOLUTION

Beginning under Louis XIV in the late seventeenth century, the Royal Society of Medicine appointed provincial physicians to investigate rural epidemics. The doctors were to provide emergency medical care, distribute remedies, circulate the society's official therapeutic and prophylactic instructions, and report back to Paris on the causes, course, and lessons of each epidemic.

The system survived the demise of the monarchy, and an 1805 ministerial circular called for the appointment of a *médecin des épidémies* (epidemic doctor) in every arrondissement, to be paid on the basis of services performed. (Judging from the correspondence that survives in the archives, however, many epidemic doctors in the late nineteenth century had trouble getting reimbursed even for minimal travel expenses.) In 1848, departmental health councils (*conseils d'hygiène*) were established; although their responsibilities extended beyond epidemic diseases, the councils' investigative and advisory functions overlapped with those of the epidemic doctors. The inevitable conflicts did not take long to appear, and in 1851 a new directive made epidemic doctors ex officio members of the health councils, and required their reports to be sent to the councils as well as to the prefects.

Reimbursement for travel expenses was not the only problem facing the epidemic doctors in the late nineteenth century. Villagers, who tended to view all outsiders—and government representatives in particular—with suspicion, reacted to physicians' denunciations of their entire way of life with indifference at best, and outright hostility at worst. The epidemic doctor appeared as "a foreigner who has come to perform an inquisition," in the words of an 1882 report.

According to many critics of the system, most epidemics were never declared, and many of those that were declared were never investigated. When they did investigate, epidemic doctors were limited to advisory recommendations without the force of law or any power of sanction. It is easy to ridicule the whole system as an exercise in futility if not outright hypocrisy. But even the small percentage of reports that have been preserved testify to the remarkable zeal with which the epidemic doctors approached their task. As intermediaries between the medical world and the impoverished populations that furnished most of the victims of epidemic disease, they worked on the front lines of the negotiations that resulted in the sanitary-bacteriological synthesis, a workaday framework for understanding and combating infectious disease that proved both powerful and enduring.

In fulfilling the duties of official positions such as epidemic doctor, through the regular meetings of departmental and arrondissement health councils, and in the pages of specialized journals such as the *Annales d'hygiène publique* (est. 1829) and the *Revue d'hygiène et de police sanitaire* (1879), physicians (and some non-physicians) who worked extensively on public health–related matters established a distinct professional niche for themselves: that of *hygiéniste*—hygienist or public health expert. They established their own professional association, the Société de médecine publique, in 1878. Theirs was a niche both within and distinct from the world of medical practice, as it often demanded clinical expertise—treating patients and distributing medications were among the epidemic doctors' duties, for example—but its practitioners always had their sights set less on the patient's recovery than on the community's.

Sources: Camille Bloch, *L'Assistance et l'état en France à la veille de la Révolution* (1908; repr., Geneva: Slatkine-Megariotis Reprints, 1974), 244–45; Matthew Ramsey, *Professional and Popular Medicine in France, 1770–1830* (Cambridge: Cambridge University Press, 1988), 113, 121; Lion Murard and Patrick Zylberman, *L'Hygiène dans la république: La Santé publique en France, ou l'utopie contrariée, 1870–1918* (Paris: Fayard, 1996), esp. 17–18, 28, 76, 125–26, 140, 210.

The history of etiology is deceptively, maddeningly unstraightforward. From a bird's-eye view, the story seems simple enough: the ancient Hippocratic and Galenic hodgepodge of geography, climate, emanations, and humors finally gave way in the late nineteenth century to the specific, provable etiology of "one disease, one cause," a model that has only undergone further refinement since. But pinning that great shift down in time and space is surprisingly difficult. It is not that bacteriological advances had no resonance in the case of specific epidemics; rather, each local instance had its unique local causes. In most cases, locality trumped universality. Yet even as they frustrate those in search of simple historical narratives, the perplexing etiologies of the past reveal in remarkable depth and detail the cultural landscapes out of which they emerged. In these local contexts, politics, folklore, science, and shifting configurations of individual and collective identities fundamentally shaped knowledge about the causes of disease.

Etiology operates at many levels simultaneously, from the universal and theoretical to the practical and individual. The diverse modes of causal explanation can be illustrated by distinguishing four of these levels, heuristically designated "academic," "individual," "folk," and "local." Academic etiologies tend to be framed in terms of current research agendas, and (even when they are equivocal or uncertain) aspire to universality, as in these two 1884 explanations of typhoid fever:

> The disease develops around local focal points of infection, such as sewers, cesspits, [and] stagnant water, [which] spread putrid emanations; it is transmitted by contagion; the poison that engenders it appears to have as its principal vehicle the victims' fecal matter.[4]

> Typhoid fever is a *specific disease* and it has a *specific cause:* the action of an *infectious principle,* coming from outside [the victim's body]. . . . The infectious principle is, in the majority of cases (if not all cases), a contagion [that] emanates from the body of others with typhoid fever and is contained above all in their excretions.[5]

Individual etiologies, on the other hand, explain the origins of single cases within a framework dictated by the life circumstances of the individual patient. Different cases within the same epidemic could (and did) have completely different causes, discernible only through an examination of each individual patient's life history and illness narrative.[6] This report of an 1878 typhoid epidemic in a southern French mountain village gives a brief example, blaming the outbreak's origin on the extraordinary work habits and fatigue of the first patient to fall ill: "On July 9, the disease appeared in a house in the lower village. The first case was that of a M. Peynet, 33 years old, who had [recently] returned from two months of reserve military service. As he was more or less solely responsible for a small farm, he had since his return thrown himself into his work to an unusual degree; he was at that point essentially overworked. The illness took an insidious form in him, . . . ending . . . in delirium, coma, [and] death."[7]

It is important to note that in this case, if contagion or other patients' excretions were involved, they were not worth mentioning alongside Peynet's overwork. This individual etiology did not necessarily exclude all others; it could conceivably operate on a parallel track, explaining a different order of phenomena. Universal etiologies might help orient medical research or treatment, but they rarely did well at the culturally vital task of explaining why a specific person fell ill at a specific time. Individual etiologies offered the flexibility needed for this kind of explanation.

Similarly elastic but of wider utility, folk etiologies served either to reinforce behavioral and cultural strictures or to rationalize regional or seasonal health disparities, rather than to orient public policy or aid disease prevention per se. Rarely disease-specific, these etiologies featured a high level of flexibility and generality, as these French proverbs show:

Whatever you earn on Sunday will be spent at the pharmacy. [Excessive work will harm your health.]
Milk before wine is wisdom; milk after wine is poison.
It is better to sweat than to shiver. Heat is life, cold is death.
Circulating air is bad for you.
Wherever the sun does not enter, the doctor does enter.[8]

While their lack of specificity made them ill suited to the demands of medical science and public policy, folk etiologies managed persistently to link various kinds of transgressions with physical disease. This cultural patrol duty was (and is) a critical function of etiology in general.

The final category of disease causality to be examined here is the one that offers the greatest potential insight into the power of etiology to influence—as it is being influenced by—the currents and eddies of political and social change. Local etiologies reveal scientific knowledge in daily tension and dialogue with the social transformations, political agendas, and cultural norms I have already mentioned. Rather than being static, or changing only in sequential phases alongside major shifts in medical knowledge, the causes of any given disease differed from town to town, year to year, outbreak to outbreak. This extreme flexibility gave local etiologies greater potential applicability and utility than other ways of explaining illness. Not to be confused with "popular" etiologies, local etiologies were generated and negotiated by medical and lay observers alike, and included elements of bacteriology, miasmatism, folk wisdom, gossip, and prejudice. Regardless of the disease and the context, etiology always fulfilled one or more of several functions. It could reinforce moral strictures, cast blame and stigma, justify research programs, mobilize political forces, and dictate specific public health policies. Their flexibility made local etiologies uniquely well suited to all of these tasks—even, on occasion, all at the same time. The two primary distinguishing features of local etiologies are their continual mediation between the realm of medical knowledge and that of everyday life and their deep engagement with local social worlds.

THE WANING OF MEDICAL GEOGRAPHY

If the story of etiology and public health policy in the age of the Bacteriological Revolution could be divided into distinct "before" and "after" phases, it would be hard to find a better snapshot of the "before" phase than the 1873 epidemic of "intermittent fever"—malaria—in Bain-de-Bretagne (Ille-et-Vilaine). (Fig. 6.) The eastern Breton town endured the attacks of such fevers on a regular basis, but the outbreak of 1873 struck all observers as unprecedented. Residents went so far as to submit a petition to the prefect of Ille-et-Vilaine demanding that action be taken against the disease. They attributed the problem to the large pond that adjoined the town, and they asked the authorities to analyze its water, mud, and plant life in order to identify the culprit.[9]

Instructed by the prefect to investigate the outbreak, the departmental health council blamed the weather: after five years of relatively dry weather, a hot and wet autumn gave way to a mild winter, creating "vast" temporary marshes out of normally dry land. Each of these accidental wetlands in turn acted as a potential "hotbed of infection"; the council's report admitted that "the fever reign[ed] permanently" in Bain-de-Bretagne, but suggested that the unusual weather conditions "intensified the poison." The report dismissed the local residents' demand for laboratory analysis of the pond adjoining Bain, claiming such tests would be "useless" in determining the epidemic's cause: "The gases, solids, and liquids found in marshlands have been analyzed time and time again, but we know perfectly well that the fever cannot be attributed to any chemically defined principle, and that chemistry is absolutely powerless to show us the poison that spreads it." Likewise,

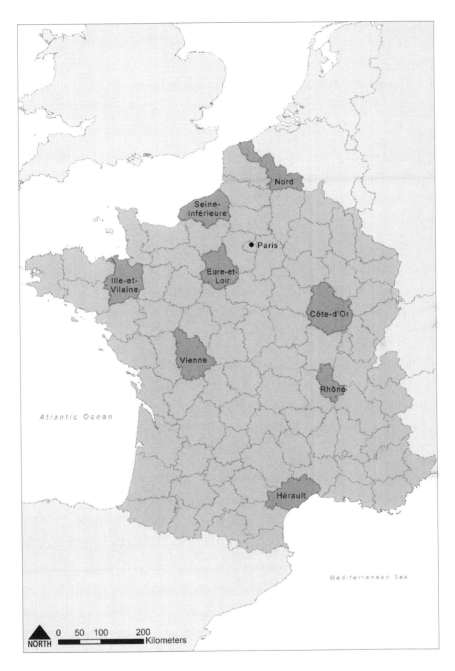

Fig. 6. Map of France, showing departments mentioned frequently in the text. Map courtesy of Cartographic Modeling Laboratory, University of Pennsylvania.

microbiological analysis was unlikely to help, according to the health council: "Of the numerous microscopic animals and plants whose presence in the pond's water or mud [the microscope] would certainly reveal, there is not a single one that we can indicate as constituting the precise cause of the fever. We know nothing about the nature of the material principle; we must limit ourselves to affirming . . . that it is an organic substance, poorly understood in its essence, [which] results from the decomposition of plant matter stagnating in a damp environment."[10] Not only was the existence of a specific organic cause not denied here, it was explicitly proclaimed. However, miasmatic reasoning called greater attention to the circumstances that gave rise to the specific principle (dampness, decomposition) than to the nature of the principle itself.

The health council's detailed investigation of the local circumstances in Bain revealed the pond as the almost certain source of the recurring fevers. They struck the hamlets and neighborhoods immediately adjoining the pond year after year with "a terrible tenacity," while areas just 500 meters away escaped the "paludal miasma" almost entirely. The shape of the pond itself explained its noxious influence, in the council's view: covering thirty-eight hectares, it was so shallow that at all times of year, one could cross it at its widest point without having to swim. In the dry season, the pond shrank to just over half its full size; the area left uncovered turned into "a veritable swamp, where decomposing plant matter produced the pernicious miasma in abundance." What was left of the pond at low water was dirty and clogged with plants and other organic matter. Its "unpleasant odor" was noticeable even at a distance.[11]

Who could have asked for clearer proof of the epidemic's cause? Even if laboratory analysis could have identified a specific microscopic culprit (which it could not), it was unlikely to have led to realistic preventive measures of the sort that were suggested by this kind of simple on-site observation. The health council acknowledged that the pond was too vital to the town's economic activity to be drained completely—among other uses, it supplied many local factories with water, and it constituted Bain's only watering hole. The report recommended instead that the pond's edges be modified to prevent the periodic uncovering and re-inundation that appeared to generate the deadly miasmas. An engineer from Bain and an architect from Rennes had proposed two competing plans for accomplishing this goal. One would have drained most of the pond's water through deep circular trenches, leaving only a small reservoir. The other plan would have built a very tall, nearly vertical embankment around the pond near its low-water mark, so that the water level could rise or fall along its edge without changing the surface area of the pond at all. This plan earned the endorsement of local notables and the health council alike, the latter urging the prefect to send it to Paris for review on an urgent basis.[12]

The departmental health council's report on the intermittent fevers of Bain-de-Bretagne in 1873 betrays a hint of impatience with the pretensions of chemical and microscopic analysis. It acknowledges the near certainty of a specific biological cause—here a miasma is an organic substance of as-yet-undetermined nature resulting from decomposition—but it regards this fact as of little practical relevance. This brand of miasmatism is neither unscientific nor fatalistic. It is capable of depicting the origins and the effects of the pathogenic influence, if not its essence. Like bacteriology fifteen years later, it is systematically empirical in its analysis and animated by a positivistic sense of mission and duty to the nation. It differs from bacteriology chiefly in its approach to causality and prevention, which is flexibly localistic rather than rigidly universal.

It is worth keeping in mind that this whole affair—investigation, report, and recommendations—began with a petition submitted by residents of Bain (whose identities are otherwise unspecified) to the prefect of Ille-et-Vilaine. The petitioners asserted that the pond was to blame for the unique vulnerability of Bain to intermittent fevers (which the health council's report confirmed), and argued that laboratory analysis of the pond water held the key to a solution (which the report denied). Although the petition may hint vaguely of a popular desire to find specifically identifiable causes of disease in the laboratory, there is no evidence of any kind of incipient lay consciousness of bacteriology running up against the scientific conservatism of authorities. What the petition does reveal is a background level of awareness of and engagement with public health problems among the general population, and a ready willingness to seek remedial action from the alliance of science and state.

These are the sorts of responses that one might expect to find in the heyday of germ theory in the 1880s and 1890s, not in the early 1870s. What was new after the rise of bacteriology was not public interest in or awareness of the causes of infectious disease per se, but rather the nature of the causes and remedies that took center stage. As a "before" snapshot, the intermittent fevers of Bain-de-Bretagne in 1873 testify to the local contingency of pre-Pasteurian etiology: even if there were a single specific cause of a single specific disease (say, intermittent fever), it manifested itself differently in different geographic contexts, and could only be understood and dealt with locally. Less than a decade later, the still-pervasive local frame of analysis would have to be reconciled with an increasingly universalizing agenda of etiology and prevention, in which local particularities began to matter less than did standardized responses such as laboratory testing, isolation, and disinfection.

The chronology of this shift can be discerned only in its broadest outlines. Although it is impossible to track specific etiological changes through the gross aggregation of reports on individual outbreaks, recognizable shifts do emerge in the Academy of Medicine's annual epidemic reviews and in other medical texts. Each year, the academy's Epidemics Committee digested all reports from prefects, subprefects, and epidemic doctors in an attempt to discern the state of the nation's health. The committee's annual reports are in effect hybrid etiologies—*academic* syntheses of dozens or hundreds of *local* etiologies. Like aerial photographs showing alterations in land use, a comparison of the sages' annual commentaries between 1875 and 1900 reveals a set of parallel changes that are not as readily legible in the epidemic doctors' individual reports.

SHIFTING LOCAL ETIOLOGIES: TYPHOID FEVER

A capsule chronology of causes singled out as primarily responsible for local typhoid fever epidemics during the late nineteenth century:

1869, Rouen (Seine-Inférieure): A prolonged epidemic at a boarding school prompted a debate in the departmental health council between those who blamed a mysterious "epidemic influence" combined with contagion and those who denounced the "disgusting filth" that prevailed on the school's grounds.[1]

1874, Laval (Mayenne): Residents complained about foul-smelling and -tasting well water they claimed was contaminated from latrines, but the epidemic doctor attributed the outbreak to overcrowding per se, especially in the courtyard of one residential building, which he identified as the epidemic's epicenter.[2]

1878, Fougères (Ille-et-Vilaine): In an annual epidemic chart for the arrondissement, causes are listed for three typhoid fever epidemics, as follows: "lack of cleanliness," "dampness of the soil," and "touched off by a young girl."[3]

1879, Langey (Eure-et-Loir): "Putrid miasmas" generated by evaporating runoff from manure piles.[4]

The Great Stink of Paris

1880, Academy of Medicine epidemics report: Typhoid fever is a "filth disease" (in English) "par excellence." Uncleanliness creates favorable conditions for the "seeds" (*germes*) of the disease to grow and multiply, but the presence or arrival of typhoid patients (i.e., contagion) is necessary in order for an outbreak to occur.[5]

1881, Academy of Medicine epidemics report: "As in previous years, the causes invoked vary according to [location]; but the preponderant influence seems to be that of putrid emanations."[6]

1883, Quesnoy (Nord): not caused by drinking water "in this instance"; primary cause importation and subsequent contagion; secondary causes overcrowding and fecal "emanations."[7]

1885, Academy of Medicine epidemics report: *Bacillus typhosus* is by now well known and well described. If some disagree about whether it can be transmitted through the air, "everybody agrees" that water contaminated by typhoid patients' excretions "is the most usual and most certain mode" of transmission.[8]

1887, Maconge (Côte-d'Or): Meticulous local investigation and mapping by epidemic doctor shows village's public fountain to have been likely contaminated by leaks and runoff from cesspits and manure piles situated close by and uphill from the fountain.[9]

1888, Houplines (Nord): Overcrowding caused the disease to spread by contagion.[10]

1893, Academy of Medicine epidemics report: In rural Brittany, typhoid fever is often caused by soldiers or other grown children returning home sick to be cared for by their families. Family members who care for the patients are forced by poverty to share the same room and breathe the same air; with the uncleanliness so common in those places, anything can "transport the morbid germs, without incriminating the drinking water supply."[11]

1893, Nogent-le-Roi (Eure-et-Loir): Water supply contaminated by leaks from latrines and other organic waste in river and wells.[12]

1895, Lille: Well water contaminated from surface runoff or leaks from cesspits.[13]

1896, St. Thibault (Côte-d'Or): Patients' family washed laundry in public *lavoir.*[14]

1899, Puligny-Montrachet (Côte-d'Or): Two wells located in the affected area, with a water table very close to the surface, are highly susceptible to contamination by surface runoff. A prolonged dry spell allowed accumulation of "organic debris," then abundant rains swept everything into the wells, contaminating the water supply.[15]

1. Conseil central d'hygiène publique, Seine-Inférieure, December 4, 1869, ADSM, 5 M 141.

2. Dr. Courcelle, epidemic doctor for arrondissement of Laval, to prefect, July 21, 1874, ADM, 5 M 56.

3. ADIV, 5 M 70.

4. Dr. Lancereaux, "Rapport général sur les épidémies de 1879," *Mémoires de l'Académie de médecine* 34 (1884): lix.

5. Henri Guéneau de Mussy, "Rapport général sur les épidémies pendant l'année 1880," *Mémoires de l'Académie de médecine* 34 (1884): clxvi.

6. Léon Colin, *RGE*, 1881 (Paris: G. Masson, 1883), 5.

7. Charlemagne Pilat, *Rapport général sur les épidémies qui ont régné dans le département du Nord pendant l'année 1883* (Lille: L. Danel, 1884), 12–13.

8. Georges Dujardin-Beaumetz, *RGE*, 1885 (Paris: G. Masson, 1887), 7–8.

9. ADCdO, M7 f I: 17.

10. Charlemagne Pilat, *Rapport général sur les épidémies qui ont régné dans le département du Nord pendant l'année 1888* (Lille: L. Danel, 1889), 28–29.

11. Jules Chauvel, *RGE*, 1891 (Melun: Imprimerie administrative, 1893), 28.

12. ADEL, 5 M 50.

13. Dr. Gorez, epidemic doctor, to prefect, October 1, 1895, ADN, M 303: 74.

14. Subprefect of Semur to prefect, January 17, 1896, ADCdO, M7 f I: 19.

15. E. Affre, epidemic doctor for Beaune, to subprefect, January 24, 1899, ADCdo, M7fl: 20.

One of the most striking etiological changes that took place during this period was the waning of geographical knowledge. For centuries the study of geology, climate, and what physicians called "medical constitution"—the prevailing disease profile of a specific place at a specific time—had served as a pillar of medical science. Before 1875, no self-respecting physician or hygienist would presume to say anything authoritative about public health without first specifying the geographical region under discussion and then cataloguing the particular geological and meteorological features that predisposed that region to particular diseases. Moreover, each season and year exhibited its own individual "constitution" of morbidity and mortality, as conjunctural causes both obvious and mysterious shaped the overall health of the population and resulted in the unusual prevalence of certain diseases at certain times. The Academy of Medicine's epidemic report for 1875 began as follows:

MEDICAL CONSTITUTION OF THE YEAR 1875.

The study of the medical constitution of each of the localities of France, that is, researching the pathological states that dominated there during the course of the year, is perhaps the best way to make known the sanitary status of the various localities.

The Great Stink of Paris

Each of the four seasons was discussed in turn, with a region-by-region accounting of prevailing weather patterns and dominant diseases. The report concluded that "cold and humidity" had predominated in France in 1875, resulting in a higher than usual overall mortality and an uncommon frequency of acute respiratory diseases.[13]

Even the increasing prevalence of terms such as "germ" and "virus" (in the sense of a poison specific to a particular disease) in etiological discussions did not banish medical constitution from the realm of scientific orthodoxy. There were simply some epidemiological peculiarities that could be explained persuasively only by climate and geography. For example, the academy's 1881 epidemics report considered why typhoid fever seemed to strike in many distant locations at once, when a contagious microbial disease might be expected to spread sequentially from place to place. Léon Colin, the report's author, speculated that some kind of "obscure" atmospheric influence or variation must have been at work, "thanks to which the germs of the affection [become] more or less active." Colin found support for this "atmospheric influence" on epidemiology in recent scientific research showing "viruses" modified by exposure to oxygen—a reference to Pasteur's experimentation with an anthrax vaccine at Pouilly-le-Fort.[14]

Blaming epidemics on the weather carried a faint whiff of resignation. If geological or meteorological circumstance were the primary or predominant cause of epidemics, what could possibly be done about it? It would be a mistake to trace the dawn of medical activism to the Bacteriological Revolution, and to associate all that came before with benighted fatalism; in prophylaxis just as in therapeutics and other branches of medicine, dedicated physicians and public officials were as likely to undertake heroic measures in 1800 as in 1900. Swamp drainage, to take just one example, grew out of the study of "medical constitution," and it is difficult to imagine a more activist enterprise than attempting to reshape the natural environment itself! Nevertheless, as long as climate could be adduced as an ultimate cause of disease, remedial inaction could be justified.

In 1880, when the prefect of Côte-d'Or inquired about a report of an epidemic among young children in certain neighborhoods of Dijon, the district's epidemic doctor reassured him that there was no cause for alarm:

It was not an actual epidemic, but rather a phenomenon that occurs every year, everywhere, at the end of summer: an increase in mortality among infants.

This increase in mortality, which is entirely unrelated to any kind of contagion, occurs regularly in August, September, and October, under the influence of [causes] unknown to us. What we know is that it is directly related to the temperature of the preceding months—so much so that one can predict it and even arrive at its approximate number based on the average summer temperature.[15]

Showing no concern for measures that might prevent or alleviate the problem, the epidemic doctor was content to attribute the deaths with confidence to the weather, without any further discussion or recommendation. What good would remedial measures be, if the true cause of the problem were the climate? The study of place- and time-specific disease profiles may not necessarily have encouraged fatalism, but it did provide a ready-made explanatory framework for those inclined to reassure and classify rather than intervene. The notion of targeting a specific disease for control would have been unthinkable within this framework. Fighting the weather was quixotic at best; reducing etiology to discretely identifiable entities like microbes encouraged grandiose ambitions.

Eighteen eighty-two witnessed a hidden landmark in French etiological history: in that year, "Medical Constitution" appeared as a separate heading in the Academy of Medicine's annual report for the last time. The academy's reporter, Jules Bucquoy, noted that the year's medical constitution had been "eminently catarrhal": "The year 1882 greatly resembled 1879. Like the latter, it was extremely rainy and humid; average temperatures were low. The cold and humid weather necessarily had a major influence on the medical constitution; we saw the seasonal illnesses rise and fall in parallel, so to speak, with the variations of the barometer and the thermometer." Although the peak period of summer heat caused an upsurge in gastrointestinal illnesses, the prevailing weather throughout most of the year endangered the respiratory tract above all. Even epidemic diseases such as measles and whooping cough, the report claimed, "despite the specificity of their cause, develop[ed] principally in cold and humid seasons." This is an important claim, with an equally important qualifier. Bucquoy neither denied nor ignored the new wave in etiology; he simply stood up for the old-fashioned knowledge and argued for its preservation alongside the new. He implicitly recognized the triumph of the new order, attributing specific causes to measles and whooping cough, whose microbial agents had yet to be identified at the time. Nevertheless, Bucquoy complained that fewer and fewer epidemic doctors included meteorological observations in their reports: "For whoever is concerned with epidemiology, it is scarcely necessary to insist on the importance of meteorological studies in establishing the influence of the atmospheric state on public health."[16] This energetic defense of medical constitution was doomed to failure, however, if the Epidemics Committee's reports and other etiological literature are any indication. After 1882, "medical constitution" never regained the status of a category unto itself in the annual reports, and future invocations of meteorological elements in etiology became increasingly defensive in tone.

After the final downfall of medical constitution in the 1880s, remnants of the old orthodoxy reappeared in new contexts to help explain outbreaks of infectious disease. By the end of the decade, most physicians and hygienists recognized microbes as the fundamental causes of most transmissible diseases and as the ideal objects of prophylactic intervention. Weather, instead of causing epidemics directly (or simply correlating with them in an implicitly direct manner), began to contribute to other more specific causes, which could be tied to disease outbreaks in a way that may have been less direct but fit better into a more instrumental and more utilitarian vision of etiology and prevention.

The 1889 typhoid fever epidemic in Givors (Rhône), near Lyon, presents a case in point. Out of twenty-five cases, there were three deaths—all in a single small dead-end street. The investigating physician, Dr. Pomme (also the town's deputy mayor), found several clues in this part of town: first, the cesspit serving the homes of the fatalities was not fully sealed, and its leaks may have infiltrated the drinking well water; second, a carpenter who fell ill late in the outbreak said that he drank water at the home of two early victims whom he helped lay to rest; and third, mapping cases of the disease in the town showed all of them to be within the areas of the two recent floods of the Rhône River. Further research concerning past epidemics revealed a regular correlation between Rhône floods and epidemics of both typhoid and diphtheria. The departure from traditional "medical constitution" came here: the deputy mayor added that "to fight effectively against an enemy as infinitesimal but also as dangerous as the bacilli of typhoid fever and diphtheria, one must know their habits and combat [them] before they have even entered our bodies." The combination of the town's geology and the recurring floods, Pomme argued, made contact between cesspits and well water all but inevitable. "We know that it is almost always by drinking, and especially by water, that the [typhoid and diphtheria] microbes are transmitted," he added, recommending that the town draw its water supply from a point farther upstream.[17] Medical constitution had survived, in a sense, but in a form that was scarcely recognizable. Local geology and climate persisted as etiological factors, but only in minor supporting roles—the scenic background, in effect, against which the leading players (germs) acted out their drama. Henceforth, it was left to nostalgic old-timers to mourn the passing of medical constitution as a prominent subfield of medical knowledge.[18]

It is important to note that the waning prominence of geographical knowledge did not mean the end of spatialized etiologies. The impulse to understand and categorize disease by linking it to particular places survived the Bacteriological Revolution intact. However, the meso-local knowledge of regional and annual medical constitutions gave way to a more easily measurable microgeography of disease, which also lent itself more readily to intervention and regulation. Instead of climate, it was the topography of wells, cesspits, manure piles, wash houses, and other sanitary nuisances— along with the microgeography of the contagious patient's deadly everyday travels—that dominated local etiologies after 1880. Etiological knowledge was fundamentally spatial throughout the nineteenth century—even after the triumph of microbial causation, which seemed to have reduced disease to a set of unitary and universal causes. Gradually, almost imperceptibly, however, the scale and meanings of space changed. Around 1800, one studied regional climatic and geological variation (that is, medical geography); around 1840, in addition to medical geography, one investigated the disposition of amenities and nuisances in (especially urban) public spaces; in 1900, medical geography was no longer on the agenda, as etiological attention was devoted to the regulation of both public space and domestic space.

OVERCROWDING AND SANITATION

Filth and crowding served as central pillars of many etiologies before the arrival of microbes on the scene. The sanitarian perspective that pervaded the research of Villermé, Parent-Duchâtelet, and their colleagues in the first half of the nineteenth century proved just as serviceable to epidemic doctors and academy members in the 1870s and 1880s. In the Norman port city of Le Havre, excessive population density caused both typhus and diphtheria, according to an 1878 report. The "poor hygienic conditions" prevailing in "certain neighborhoods," which went hand in hand with over-crowding, facilitated the spread of such diseases. The same report struck an equivocal note concerning typhoid fever, which it considered capable of spreading through contaminated water and sewers as well as contagiously

The Great Stink of Paris

from person to person. The typically pragmatic, sanitarian agnosticism regarding specific etiologies—virtually untenable a decade later—seemed the only responsible stance in 1878: "We do not know the exact nature of the typhus miasma"; diphtheria "appears to be" caused by overcrowding. But such ignorance was no barrier to remedial action.[19]

Four years later, in the midst of the initial excitement over the role of germs in disease, hygienist Jules Rochard defended the same pragmatic approach to etiology when faced with a serious typhoid fever epidemic in Paris. In a debate at the Academy of Medicine, Rochard took the floor to argue against complicating a simple practical matter with "theory and doctrines": "What are we really talking about here? About finding the causes that provoked the epidemic . . . [and] finding the means to make it stop. . . . It is thus a question of etiology and prophylaxis—a pure question of hygiene. When I speak of the etiology of typhoid fever, everyone understands that I'm not talking about its primordial causes, but rather about those causes that everyone can see, which are tangible and therefore suppressible." Overcrowding and uncleanliness were the tangible causes of the disease, Rochard continued, and they ought to be the targets of preventive efforts. Anyone familiar with the army or navy knew, he contended, that one only needed to "pile up too many young people in too small a place" to start a typhoid epidemic; likewise, one only needed to evacuate, clean, and disinfect the barracks to stop it. Germs, real or not, had no place in this straightforward equation: "I don't want to get dragged into matters of theory and doctrines. I will simply say in passing: if typhoid fever is due to a living being, to a microbe, the germs must exist all the time; they are everywhere, but these germs only develop, only become harmful, when they encounter a suitable milieu [or] atmosphere; well then, it is this milieu, this terrain, this atmospheric manure pile that is created by overcrowding, that is fertilized by the foul emanations that come from . . . negligence and disregard for the laws of hygiene."[20]

This is a crucial point. Especially in the early years of the Bacteriological Revolution, resistance and skepticism to the new paradigm arose from doubts not so much about the reality of germs, but about their relevance. Sanitarians like Rochard feared a focus on microbes might divert attention and energy from fighting the "tangible" and "suppressible" causes of disease. Their efforts to minimize the importance of germs were doomed to failure, but their defense of old-fashioned values—in essence, cleanliness and the ideal of bodily separation and aeration—proved too strong to ignore. Future etiologies would somehow have to continue to incorporate tangible causes, even as they turned toward the laboratory for the identification of new culprits.

CONTAGION WITHOUT GERMS

One important element of prebacteriological etiologies is easy to overlook: contagion. Contagion and microbes have become so intertwined in the scientific and public consciousness since the end of the nineteenth century that they seem to be inseparable. It bears repeating that the two are entirely distinct and historically independent. Contagion—the transmission of disease from person to person by direct contact—has been observed, described, and analyzed for centuries. Although microscopic organisms were observed before their role in disease processes was hypothesized (much less demonstrated), the identification of specific microbes as causes of specific diseases is a relatively recent phenomenon. Before germs, contagion often overlapped considerably with miasmatism, the spread of disease through emanations from decaying organic matter. Sick bodies and their excretions could also produce miasmas (as could swamps), and prebacteriological discussions of contagion often relied more on the language of emanation than on that of direct person-to-person transmission.

When Henri Guéneau de Mussy presented the Epidemic Committee's report for 1880 to the Academy of Medicine, the status of microbes was uncertain, but the fact of contagion was unquestioned. Despite the fact that the origins of epidemics were "mysterious," Guéneau de Mussy insisted that their spread could often be controlled by sensible policies:

> We see on every page [of the epidemic doctors' reports] smallpox, scarlet fever, diphtheria, and measles circulating freely and spreading as they go. This time, it's a child coming from a large city where her mother was living as a wet nurse, who brings the disease into the village; the next time, it's an itinerant salesman who camps out on the public square after having stayed in an infected locality, sometimes bringing with him in his caravan some family members who are already ill. Fairly often, it's soldiers who have recovered but have been sent home to their families on leave still covered with smallpox lesions. So it's the same story over and over again.

Guéneau de Mussy advocated more widespread provisions for the isolation of potentially contagious patients. He praised efforts that had been made in schools to provide such facilities, as "schools are the principal focal points from which [these diseases] irradiate."[21]

Prevention does not depend on etiology, and it never has. Specific etiological knowledge has never been a prerequisite for effective disease control measures. The U.S. Surgeon General knew no more in 1964 about the specific biochemical means by which smoking caused lung cancer than Edward Jenner knew in 1798 about the smallpox virus. Similarly, policies aimed at breaking the chain of contagion—from quarantine to enforced isolation, sometimes futile, sometimes effective—predated the science of germs by centuries. When they came, etiological breakthroughs certainly influenced disease control to a considerable degree; but in some cases they ratified existing policies rather than inspiring new ones. In 1880, making no reference at all to microbes (and admitting that the seeds or "germs" of disease were "mysterious"), Guéneau de Mussy proposed an expanded contagionist program of isolation for certain diseases. During the next two decades, as bacteriology fundamentally recast etiology, the core of the contagionist program remained largely unchanged. But if the triumph of germ theory did not give birth to these policies, it certainly gave them enhanced momentum, justification, and credibility; by the same token, the long history of belief, epidemiological observation, and advocacy regarding contagionism prepared the ground for the reception of microbial etiologies.

Even at the peak of the Bacteriological Revolution, the conviction persisted that contagion was possible (even common) in the absence of germs. In 1896, for example, the academy's epidemics report pointed out the large number of typhoid outbreaks in which Eberth's bacillus could not be found. Without taking sides, the report noted that "a certain number of observers" took this fact as evidence supporting the notion of "miasmatic contagion via dust." One epidemic was attributed to the mud in the harbor of the Breton port city of Vannes, exposed to the sun and wind at low tide, while others were blamed on construction work that had dug up "contaminated soil."[22] The fact that such explanations remained credible in respected medical circles in 1896 testifies both to the durability of long-held beliefs and to the limits of what could be discovered and explained with bacteriological techniques. Nevertheless, instances of "miasmatic contagion" in 1896 were anomalous even to those who believed in them; the default explanation for epidemics at the time, whatever the particular circumstances, involved germs.

The insinuation of germs into etiology began in the late 1870s, and gained irreversible momentum in the 1880s. The road to acceptance was not without bumps, however. One of the earliest manifestoes of the new agenda in the medical community can be found in the academy's epidemics report for 1877, written by Jean-Antoine Villemin, who had braved intense opposition when he claimed to have demonstrated the transmissibility of tuberculosis in the 1860s.[23] His review of epidemics in 1877 showed remarkable ingenuity and foresight, and also included the first mention of Louis Pasteur in the yearly academy reports. For example, Villemin wondered why, if filth caused typhoid fever, epidemics struck some filthy villages and not others. His answer suggested a creative and powerful analogy: "When we look at the wonderful experiments of our eminent colleague, M. Pasteur, we may find the answer to this question. This fecal matter, these sewers, these stagnant ponds, this water filled with organic matter, etc., seem to be the equivalent of the culture media in which M. Pasteur deposits an atom [sic] of infectious blood and which reproduce, in incommensurable proportions, the morbific principle they have received." Filth as biological culture medium: the comparison had the potential to reconcile the two seemingly incompatible etiological paradigms represented by the sanitarian perspective and the new science of germs. Villemin used the analogy as a lever to propose a bacteriological origin for typhoid fever, despite the absence of any specific laboratory findings to support such a hypothesis: "There is every reason to believe that the principle of typhoid fever, like that of anthrax, of chicken cholera, of septicemia, and perhaps of many other zymotic diseases, does not absolutely need the animal organism to survive and multiply. Culture liquids demonstrate this. These pathogenic agents exist independently of the diseases they provoke, in certain milieux that suit them, and their introduction into an organism is only a contingent phenomenon in their existence."[24]

Villemin's report, covering epidemics in 1877, was written in early 1878. (It was also around this time that the word "microbe" was coined. Retired physician Charles Sédillot devised it for use in a paper presented to the Academy of Sciences on the medical ramifications of Pasteur's work; Pasteur himself liked the word, and it achieved currency fairly rapidly.)[25] Research connecting relatively obscure diseases (at least among humans) such as anthrax and chicken cholera to specific microbes was dramatic and pathbreaking, but hardly comprehensive enough to justify a new model to explain all diseases. That Villemin invoked these scientific precedents in a discussion of typhoid fever—a very serious scourge among humans—was remarkable, even daring, at the time. His presumption that most diseases would eventually be found to fit the bacteriological mold did not take root right away in the late 1870s, but it ultimately took its place as the keystone of the sanitary-bacteriological synthesis, a new way of conceptualizing the place of disease in society at century's end.

Six years after Villemin's report, the etiological revolution was well underway at the academy and in the published medical literature, but it is unclear how drastically this intellectual change had affected *local* etiologies. The 1883 epidemics report also devoted considerable attention to typhoid fever, and contrasted the bacteriological reductionism of "the scientific movement" with the etiological pluralism of the local epidemic doctors. Its author, Félix Féréol, complained that his colleagues had been seduced by a doctrine that was "so eminently seductive in its simplicity," but incapable of accounting for the diversity of circumstances associated with a disease like typhoid: "Dominated by the idea of specificity and the parasitical doctrines, a whole school, I could almost say the whole modern school, is trying hard to reduce [typhoid's] causes to a single one. For them, there is no typhoid fever unless the specific germ of the disease has been brought into the organism from the outside by one way or another." Féréol even invoked Villemin's culture-medium analogy, albeit with a tone of mild mockery: "The other causes—putridity, overcrowding, uncleanliness, poverty, overwork, etc.—act only as adjuvant [causes]. . . . They are capable of promoting the blossoming of the seed, [but] incapable of giving birth to it. Sewers, latrines, slaughterhouse refuse, [and] *vidanges* can play no role other than that of M. Pasteur's culture broths; we need the seed to fertilize them. As for the human miasma, so much in favor just a few years ago, it is henceforth out of the question for this school."[26]

According to Féréol's report, the epidemic doctors were not quite so dogmatic, and clung to the explanatory arsenal that had served them so well for years. The majority of the academy's correspondents believed that typhoid could be caused by "numerous and varied" factors; in fact, they knew it for certain—they saw the evidence all around them every day. Most accepted that the disease was contagious, both directly and indirectly (through water, for example, or domestic objects), but could not accept such transmission as the sole possible origin of its outbreaks. There were simply too many cases in which a group of people placed in overcrowded conditions fell ill in the absence of any contact (direct or indirect) with a prior typhoid patient. The only possible explanation for such epidemics was the "human miasma" that resulted from overcrowding.[27]

Féréol's sympathetic stance toward the germ skeptics was nowhere to be found in the 1885 report. Its author, Georges Dujardin-Beaumetz, was positively enraptured by the promise of bacteriology, and had no reservations about proclaiming it as the future of medicine: "Thanks to the research of our illustrious colleague M. Pasteur, the history of epidemic and contagious diseases has taken a new turn." Gone were the qualifications and equivocations that characterized earlier discussions of microbes and disease: "Bacteriology allows us today to know the contagious agent of most [epidemic] diseases, and if all epidemic and contagious diseases have not yet yielded up their secrets, it is only a matter of time. We have every reason to believe that . . . all infectious and contagious diseases are [caused by] microbes."[28] Grandiose claims on behalf of bacteriology were nothing new in the mid-1880s. What makes this passage significant is its confident presumption that what had been learned about a few diseases—including anthrax, typhoid, tuberculosis, and most recently diphtheria (1884)—applied to all infectious diseases. It was one thing to predict great achievements for bacteriology in the future, but quite another to posit the microbial model as the standard, default etiology for disease in general.

This presumptive analogy—according to which diseases of unknown origin were presumed to follow the pattern established for other diseases, in which microbial pathogens had been identified—was already solidly in place by the time Dujardin-Beaumetz wrote his report in 1886.[29] By the turn of the century, the regularity with which germs were discovered for known diseases had almost become a running joke. The academy's epidemics report for 1898, having completed the review of diseases for which reports were filed, noted drily, "No doubt the list will continue to get longer, as we understand better the infectious character of many diseases that until now have not been classified [as such]."[30] It should be pointed out that one cannot trace the precise trajectory of germ theory based on the annual academy reports alone. The Epidemics Committee's membership turned over periodically, and members were assigned the writing of the report on a rotating basis; like the academy's membership as a whole, some of the authors were hostile to the germ theory of disease, while others were sympathetic.[31] However, the credibility, prestige, and authority of bacteriological etiologies roughly paralleled the chronology of the examples just mentioned: novel in the late 1870s, contested in the early 1880s, solidified in the mid-1880s, and taken for granted by the late 1890s.

The appeal of germs did not derive solely from the intellectual simplicity of reductionism. If it could not produce practical tools to advance the study of public health, the new science would have remained a sterile academic exercise—as it was, for example, after Robert Koch's mentor Jacob Henle proposed a new etiology based on microorganisms in 1840.[32] Actual therapeutic advances or vaccines were one thing; the disciples of Pasteur and Koch continually prophesied their imminent arrival, but with the notable

---

SHIFTING LOCAL ETIOLOGIES: DIPHTHERIA

A capsule chronology of causes singled out as primarily responsible for local diphtheria epidemics during the late nineteenth century:

- *1875,* Academy of Medicine epidemics report: primarily "atmospheric influences" beginning in autumn and lasting four to five months.[1]
- *1880,* Voulaines (Côte-d'Or): "intense" cold weather.[2]
- *1882,* Paris: contagion, assisted by miasmas from fermenting organic matter, which intensify individual susceptibility.[3]
- *1882,* Rennes (Ille-et-Vilaine): "The causes are unknown, outside of contagion."[4]
- *1883,* Hazebrouck (Nord): "spontaneous" origin during extremely humid weather.[5]
- *1883,* Ploërmel (Morbihan): humidity, filthy streets, and interior courtyards.[6]
- *1884,* Redon (Ille-et-Vilaine): "Even more than for smallpox . . . the propagation is due to contagion."[7]
- *1885,* Phalempin (Nord): "These children appear to have acquired the germ of their disease, which is essentially contagious, in the school itself."[8]
- *1888,* St. Broladre (Ille-et-Vilaine): contagion, failure to close the school.[9]
- *1888,* Nord (department-wide): "Cold weather and damp soil have as always played the principal role in the etiology of this terrible disease, which we nevertheless sometimes observe in warm and dry weather. Let us add that contagion sometimes played a part in the development and spread of the disease."[10]
- *1891,* Charente: cold and rainy weather.[11]
- *1897,* Academy of Medicine epidemics report: "direct contagion"; "it is almost always possible to follow the filiation of cases from the first patient stricken through all of those who contaminated one another secondarily"; "The discovery of Loeffler's bacillus has only pushed back the limits of the problem. We do not know which influences facilitate its expansion and

increase its virulence. . . . We are reduced to conjecture on the bacillus's mode of germination and penetration. It is almost certain that the air can serve as its vehicle; but precisely because of this, it is much more difficult to prevent its dissemination."[12]

1. Dr. Briquet, *RGE,* 1875 (Paris: G. Masson, 1878), 51–52.

2. Epidemic doctor of Châtillon-sur-Seine to subprefect, January 9, 1880, ADCdO, M7 f I: 16.

3. E. Vidal, discussion of report by Ulysse Trélat, Société de médecine publique, session of June 28, 1882, *RHPS* 4 (1882): 581.

4. Conseil d'hygiène, Ille-et-Vilaine, session of July 20, 1882, ADIV, 5 M 50.

5. Alexandre Decool, epidemic doctor of arrondissement of Hazebrouck, cited in Charlemagne Pilat, *Rapport général sur les épidémies qui ont régné dans le département du Nord pendant l'année 1883* (Lille: L. Danel, 1884), 20–21.

6. Alphonse Mauricet, *Compte-rendu des épidémies, des épizooties et des travaux des conseils d'hygiène du Morbihan en 1882* (Vannes: Imprimerie Galles, 1883), 23.

7. Dr. Gascon, annual epidemics report for arrondissement of Redon, 1884, session of April 9, 1885, ADIV, 5 M 71.

8. Charlemagne Pilat, *Rapport général sur les épidémies qui ont régné dans le département du Nord pendant l'année 1885* (Lille: L. Danel, 1886), 22.

9. Annual epidemics report, Ille-et-Vilaine, 1888, ADIV 5 M 71.

10. Charlemagne Pilat, *Rapport général sur les épidémies qui ont régné dans le département du Nord pendant l'année 1888* (Lille: L. Danel, 1889), 18.

11. Epidemic doctor to prefect dated November 1891, ADC, 5 M 29.

12. Ambroise Rendu, *RGE,* 1897 (Melun: Imprimerie administrative, 1899), 38–40.

exception of diphtheria antitoxin in 1894, progress was made only for diseases such as anthrax and rabies, which may have enjoyed relatively high profiles but were rare among human beings. Even in the absence of such dramatic breakthroughs, the new paradigm could earn its stripes with incremental technical innovations that promised new ways of approaching and measuring the problem of disease.

Initially, what the new science of germs offered above all was an identifiable and *measurable* entity that could stand in for the differential threat of disease in particular places and times. The incidence of various diseases could be measured in mortality figures based on cause-of-death certificates, and could be compared year to year and area to area. But a measurement of exactly where (in which substances, in which streets) germs tended to congregate might be able to focus preventive efforts more effectively than could, for example, the mere fact that diphtheria was common in certain neighborhoods. By revealing which spaces and substances were most dangerous, it could also lend scientific confirmation to the informal urban social geographies that ranked neighborhoods, streets, and buildings by the security and comfort—or fear and repulsion—associated with them.

Not long after the Great Stink of 1880, it was possible not just to find but to count microbes in the air, water, and soil, thereby substituting precision for the vagueness of dangers such as potentially pathogenic emanations.[33] In 1882, a commission studying sanitary problems in Le Havre heard a frightening yet exciting report in this regard. Doctor Jules Chauvel lamented the ignorance that had led legislators, government officials, and the general population to neglect both public and private measures to combat the causes of disease: "Whatever the agents of our diseases might be, they are material beings, and nature, which has given us over to their attacks, has also given us means of defense against them. . . . Already we have counted, measured, even cultivated them, and it is precisely this cultivation that [can] furnish us with precious information and dictate practical conclusions for us." Chauvel proceeded to describe the procedure by which air, liquid, or dust could be introduced into sterilized broth, blood serum, or other liquid culture medium, then left to "alter" or "putrefy" the medium. "When this work is completed," he continued, a certain quantity of the altered liquid is removed and examined under a microscope. The observer then had only to count the visible "microgerms" (*microgermes*) in the sample.[34]

The results could be unsettling. In Paris, researchers found 1,000 microgerms per cubic meter in the air of the Montsouris Park on the southern edge of the city, but 10,000 per cubic meter on rue de Rivoli in the city center, and 100,000 per cubic meter in the air inside the city's hospitals. Paris air contained ten to twelve times more microgerms per cubic meter than the air outside the city; the air of the capital's streets even exceeded four- to fivefold in "microgermic impurity" the air inside the sewers and at the Montparnasse Cemetery. (It is significant that these last two locations corresponded to the classic anxieties of the miasmatic era, when preoccupations focused on decaying bodies and bodily waste. These findings were less likely to alleviate concerns about sewers and cemeteries than to intensify fears about the urban environment as a whole.) Similar comparisons were performed on soil, water, and samples from different locations in and around the city; water samples from the Seine were more heavily germ-laden downstream from Paris than upstream, and dust taken from apartments in outlying arrondissements contained more microgerms than dust taken from apartments closer to the city center.[35]

Although he did not report how, by whom, and under what circumstances these findings were arrived at, Chauvel did not hesitate to add a few conclusions to these findings.[36] One-tenth of these microgerms found in Paris came "from the countryside," nine-tenths from dust arising from Parisian apartments and "especially from refuse in the streets"; their number always increased as one moved "from the periphery to the center" of the city. "Sinks, pipes, toilets, cesspits, street gutters, puddles in the roadway, the spaces between paving stones, sewers—these are the many laboratories of these infinitely tiny beings; food waste, miscellaneous detritus, refuse, and filth of every description in private lodgings or in the streets—these are the substances upon which they develop and multiply. This is where the air takes them and spreads them far and wide, sowing them in our drinking water, in our food, and in our lungs." There are echoes of the Great Stink of 1880 in these dire warnings: the enemy was lurking everywhere, insidious and prolific. It attacked us from within, thriving in our midst, gaining strength from our numbers. In 1882 perhaps even more urgently than in 1880, the time had come for spreading the news, sounding the alarm. The danger was clear to those who had taken the trouble to investigate; these were the sentinels who needed to warn their countrymen, in a voice as loud and insistent as the threat was imminent.[37]

One final finding reported by Chauvel added an ominous note to his warning, even if it was heavily foreshadowed by the rest of the report: rates of diseases such as typhoid fever, infantile diarrhea, smallpox, scarlet fever, measles, and puerperal fever "follow[ed] almost exactly with one week's lag" the relative numbers of bacteria observed, "so that a rise in the latter announces an increase in these diseases, just as the falling barometer announces bad weather."[38] (Here again, Chauvel did not report the source of these findings nor the methods by which they were derived.) Science could now identify, count, and grow bacteria; it could also induce disease with them in the laboratory. The missing link in the great bacteriological equation germs = disease was a direct correlation between the two elements *outside* of the laboratory, and it was imperative for Chauvel and others to address this gap if they wished to cement this relationship in medical science and in the public consciousness.

The precedent of measuring the concentration of germs—any germs, all germs—in various locations as a means of assessing degrees of danger persisted through the 1880s, before tests for specific microbes in specific substances became widespread. A public lecture in Lyon in 1886 reported 224,000 microbes in a liter of Parisian rainwater, compared to 80 million per liter in the city's sewer water; the corresponding figures for the Seine were 4.8 million on the upstream side and 12.8 million downstream.

The same speaker presented a chart showing airborne concentrations of microbes in locations ranging from the Atlantic Ocean to the high Swiss Alps to old and newly built houses and hospitals in Paris. Not surprisingly, ocean and mountain air proved microscopically cleanest, with one microbe per cubic meter or less. The old Pitié hospital's air ranked foulest with 79,000 microbes per cubic meter, ahead of the new Hôtel-Dieu hospital (40,000) and old residential buildings (36,000). Lest the audience get the message that only the immediate vicinity of such buildings was dangerous, they were told that in fact, it was windblown dust that carried microbes into the air and transported them long (but as yet undetermined) distances.[39] In this instance, measuring airborne germs again performed the work of ratifying nonscientific commonsense judgments regarding the disgusting and dangerous quality of various kinds of air and water. The supplementary commentary regarding dust in the wind added, in effect, a warning against complacency. A "safe" location provided no guarantee of security, as germs lurking elsewhere awaited only the next breeze to pay a deadly visit.

The shift from the indiscriminate measurement of microbes in air and water to the targeted testing of substances for specific pathogens took some time. In the 1890s, local bacteriological laboratories began to proliferate around the country as an integral part of the battle against infectious disease. The laboratory attached to Le Havre's municipal board of health (*bureau d'hygiène*) limited itself to tests for the chemical adulteration of foods and beverages from its creation in 1885 to 1896, when it was divided into a chemical section and a bacteriological section. In its early years, the latter analyzed primarily sputum samples (for the presence of the tubercle bacillus) and the "false membranes" of the throat characteristic of diphtheria (for the Klebs bacillus).[40] Around the same time, when the Le Havre health board looked to the Paris medical school in its search for a new director, it added some new qualifications to the job description. The board considered requiring a certificate attesting to the candidate's knowledge of bacteriology (in addition to a solid knowledge of chemistry "as it applies to public health"), but opted instead for a hands-on examination in bacteriological techniques in the laboratory of comparative pathology professor Isidore Straus, a key ally of Pasteur in the medical faculty.[41]

By 1900, the novelty of bacteriological laboratories functioning as an arm of municipal or departmental government had become a norm—not universally implemented by any means, but an established standard for the appropriate use of science in the exercise of public authority. Beginning in 1896, the Pasteur Institute of Lille provided laboratory services free of charge for the city of Lille and for the Nord and Pas-de-Calais departments. The institute analyzed 150 to 700 water samples per year, finding a large majority of them either "unfit for consumption" or "suspect/easily pollutable." In 1901, the institute reported, "these analyses were requested for the most part by government authorities, following epidemics of typhoid fever." Private interests, including brewers, distillers, and mineral water merchants, submitted their raw material for analysis on a paying basis, seeking to avoid spoilage and hoping for the scientific imprimatur that would validate their product's quality.[42] The routinization of bacteriological testing as a function of governments and scientific institutions signaled (while at the same time contributing to) the remarkable degree to which the germ theory of disease had passed from controversial to taken for granted.

LINGERING SKEPTICISM

The relatively rapid ascension of microbes to dominance in etiology did not take place without resistance. Many physicians trained in and intellectually anchored to an older causal paradigm refused to join Pasteur's revolution. Still more accepted bacteriological explanations of disease haltingly, grudgingly, and incompletely. There were "medical mandarins" such as Hermann Pidoux and Michel Peter in the Academy of Medicine who staked their reputations on a frontal combat against the Pasteurians, and found historical ignominy when they lost.[43] There were many ordinary practitioners who simply ignored the new science and went about their business as they always had (that is, unless a patient demanded access to a highly publicized innovation such as rabies vaccine or diphtheria antitoxin). There were also guerrilla warriors in the style of Achille Kelsch, France's leading military doctor and longtime member of the academy, who accepted the scientific validity of the germ theory but criticized its application in the realm of public health.[44] Kelsch used the Epidemics Committee's annual report (which he wrote in both 1892 and 1893) as a weapon in a rearguard, oblique attack on a doctrine that he thought was guilty of overreaching.

Epidemic diseases, Kelsch argued, were divided "naturally" into two categories: highly specific, "virulent" diseases and "irregular," seemingly spontaneous ones. Smallpox, syphilis, rabies, measles, and other eruptive fevers belonged in the first category; each case clearly resulted from a previous case, and the links of contagion were usually easily discernible. Typhoid, diphtheria, cholera, and pneumonia belonged in the second group; their origins were "obscure," their transmission "surrounded by mystery."

"How many times," Kelsch asked rhetorically, "have we seen them arise in conditions that exclude [the possibility of contagion] and that inevitably suggest the notion of spontaneity?"[45] To even refer to spontaneous generation in the 1890s outside the context of utter ridicule took some nerve, but Kelsch had it. "The old observations about spontaneous generation—now we say 'indigenous' [generation]—are still standing," he proclaimed, with this qualification: thanks to the new science of germs, the old theory, which had been "so mysterious," was "enlightened, understood, and situated within the general laws of pathogenesis."[46]

In fact, Kelsch prepared quite an elaborate scientific makeover of the hoary framework of spontaneous generation. The identification of what he called "saprophytic" organisms served as its keystone: "Bacteriology . . . teaches us that the germs of most contagious diseases live normally as saprophytes, in the ambient atmosphere or in our natural cavities, and that they can temporarily acquire their respective virulent functions under the influence of various circumstances—cosmic, telluric, hygienic, etc."[47] Saprophytes allowed a germ skeptic like Kelsch to acknowledge the scientific evidence in favor of bacteriological etiologies without abandoning the deep-rooted empirical knowledge that a variety of environmental factors could "cause" disease. "Etiology can never be exclusively microbial, because you need more than just a seed to make an epidemic," he argued. "Hygienic infractions" such as the fouling of soil or lodgings, poor diet, or excessive fatigue could "open the door to external germs" or "awaken to pathogenic activity" the saprophytic microorganisms that were previously living harmlessly in the body. In this etiology, germs were incidental—perhaps necessary, but far from sufficient, and certainly not candidates for becoming public enemy number one. Public hygiene, Kelsch insisted, could not afford to ignore the crucial "secondary" causes of disease in favor of an exclusive focus on the "primary" causes, "at the risk of ending up with an incomplete prophylaxis."[48] His plea was a pragmatic one, oriented toward the removal of multiple factors that contributed to the spread of many diseases, rather than the single specific causes of individual diseases.

A SYNTHESIS OF OLD AND NEW ETIOLOGIES

Viewed from a great distance in time, the conquest of etiology by germs was swift and thorough; the objections of Kelsch and others sound in retrospect like the carping of the defeated. The apparent clash of miasmatic/ spontaneous and microbial etiologies, however, concealed a deeper, subtler series of negotiations in progress throughout the 1880s and 1890s. Kelsch and his fellow skeptics were not the only ones unwilling to discard decades of sanitary wisdom, according to which filth caused epidemic diseases as surely as marshes gave rise to malaria—the evidence was overwhelming, no matter what happened in a laboratory. There is a fundamental difference between the spontaneous generation of disease from the sheer accumulation of bodies and bodily substances on the one hand and the transmission of specific diseases only through the ingestion or absorption of a substance containing the living essence of that same specific disease on the other. In practice, however, the gulf was bridged. What the new science of germs offered above all was a combination of epistemological simplicity and new techniques of assessment, measurement, and (in theory) control. These vital elements eventually proved reconcilable with the bedrock sensory certainty that overcrowding and filth made people sick. Exactly how these conflicting ideas were modified to accommodate one another is the story of the building of the sanitary-bacteriological synthesis.

A composite example of the sanitary-bacteriological synthesis in action: an epidemic doctor investigates an outbreak of typhoid fever in a small town. He establishes links among the various cases either through direct contact (between family members or neighbors, for example) or indirectly through contact with excretions or laundry. He denounces the unsanitary condition of the patients' lodgings, including the improper disposal of bodily waste and the careless handling of clothing and linens. He finds laundry being washed near wells or other sources of drinking water, which may also be contaminated by nearby manure piles or leaking cesspits. He sends water samples to the nearest bacteriological laboratory for testing, and recommends disinfection of patients' homes along with a stricter surveillance of the town's water supply (or the construction of an entirely new water supply or sewer system). Filth and germs are inseparable, not dichotomous etiological categories. Other scholars will doubtless recognize what I have called the sanitary-bacteriological synthsis. Without naming it as such, several historians—most notably Nancy Tomes[49]—have described analogous phenomena. By giving it a name and focusing explicitly on its development, I hope to empahsize its centrality in the development of new ways of understanding disease.

The constitution of the SBS cannot be dated with any precision; it took decades to accomplish, and in a sense it is still being renegotiated, continually, to this day. However, one can find signposts in the medical literature on etiology in general and on individual diseases, as well as in the epidemic doctors' encounters with disease outbreaks in the field. The first signs of

THE SANITARY-BACTERIOLOGICAL SYNTHESIS

- A new way of understanding, explaining, and combating the problem of disease in modern society . . .
- negotiated gradually over a period of decades among scientists, physicians, public health experts, government officials, and the general public . . .
- in which the overriding concerns of the early and mid-nineteenth-century sanitary movement (filth and contamination, cleanliness and morality) . . .
- were integrated *through the language of bacteriology*, with a persistent overlay of moralizing disgust, into a new set of meanings and practices . . .
- alongside a new germ-centered focus on (1) the danger of contact with sick or suspect bodies and bodily substances, (2) tests for the presence of potentially pathogenic microbes, and (3) the promise of their control through laboratory science.

---

a practical marriage of old and new etiologies began to appear in the early 1880s; by the mid-1890s, blending the two had become commonplace; eventually, it would be second nature.

An early attempt to synthesize filth and germs can be seen in a meeting of the Société de médecine publique in 1882. Dr. Hippolyte Marié-Davy warned city dwellers returning from vacations in the countryside that even the best-kept homes could become refuges for deadly microbes, especially when left uninhabited for long periods of time: "No house is so tightly sealed that dust from outside cannot penetrate it. These dusts contain microbes that come either from the street or from other . . . houses in the city. They can be counted by the millions in every gram of [dust] on the furniture, the rugs, the floors, the tapestries, the curtains. These microbes do not need to come from the sewer to be noxious; the streets, the gutters, [and] certain poorly kept houses are rich in putrefying organic matter, and people disacclimated by a long stay in the countryside are more sensitive to the city's miasmas than are [their] more sedentary [neighbors]." Marié-Davy urged returning urbanites to ventilate their apartments thoroughly, to wipe surfaces with a damp cloth wherever possible, and to "rigorously" dust everywhere else.[50] Urban "miasmas" here are utterly synonymous with germs; the undertone of foul emanations the term carried may have compensated for its increasingly old-fashioned flavor. The insistence on "large and prolonged ventilation" recalls the older sanitarian hygiene of bodily separation and aeration, henceforth invoked as a means to evacuate microbes.

Having established the mobility of germs, Marié-Davy went on to discuss the contagious threat posed by unsanitary working-class housing—a threat to the health of the bourgeoisie, that is, as "every day, rich houses . . . exchange their rare and harmless microbes in the street with the more suspect microbes that proliferate in poorly kept houses." For one thing, the lack of water in working-class toilets (located in tenement stairways and shared by many households) caused waste to overflow even to the doorways of apartments: "Even outside of these unspeakable toilets, the lodgings of the poor are impregnated from top to bottom with putrid or putrescent matter of all kinds . . . ; the floor is sometimes covered with a thick layer, which is incessantly beaten or stirred up by the inhabitants' feet or brooms. We also find in some of these houses 50 to 60 times more microbes than in the air of the foulest sewer." The juxtaposition in this passage of the lurid, disgusted description and the quantified scientific measurement is jarring. (No evidence is adduced here for the figures.) In a slightly subtler form, it would become a hallmark of the SBS.[51]

Of course, microbes in this instance are an undifferentiated mass, and even in 1882 not all microbes were considered equally dangerous. Marié-Davy addressed this problem not by distinguishing the causal germs of specific diseases from the rest of the germs (a task that was not feasible at the time), but by simply suggesting a calculus of probability. "By what special grace," he asked, "would these microbes all be harmless to us?": "If these microbes were all inoffensive, why would we see, every season, variations in mortality by [infectious] diseases follow in such a . . . regular manner the variations of the total number of microbes contained in the air that we breathe?" (Again, no evidence accompanied this assertion.) It is significant that already, in 1882, the burden of proof in etiology had shifted to such an extent that in the absence of direct evidence in either direction, it could be assumed that at least a large number of the microbes in question caused disease. Marié-Davy added that even the newest hospitals, scrupulously designed and maintained to prevent disease transmission, "abounded" at certain times with "the most suspect" germs. One could only imagine the magnitude of the danger in "these hovels swarming with human beings, where illness too often comes along to aggravate poverty, and where ignorance and inertia make [the residents] disdain the most elementary hygienic prescriptions." From this disgusted perspective, the "swarming," "ignoran[t]" poor were little better than microbes themselves.[52]

Marié-Davy concluded with a call for instilling "habits of . . . cleanliness . . . in the poorer classes" and for protecting the healthy from "air [that was] vitiated by sick people and . . . from food or drink that may have been contaminated by objects emanating from or . . . touched by a sick person."[53] In this remarkable intervention (apparently spontaneous, not based on a prepared text) before a meeting of fellow physicians and hygienists, Marié-Davy traced the contours of an agenda at which others were also hinting and that would dominate public health for decades to come. At the same time, he preserved the central elements of an older paradigm that had developed in response to the urbanization and social change of the early nineteenth century: contamination or "vitiation" of the air or of any part of the material environment represented a serious threat to the stability of both the individual organism and of the collective social body—regardless of the presence, amount, or nature of microbes that might be present. It simply stood to reason that filth and germs went hand in hand.

In the ensuing years, the SBS took shape primarily through the aggregation of local responses to particular diseases. However, a few important signposts at a more general level of abstraction also point to the gradual reconciliation of the sanitarian and bacteriological perspectives. As early as 1884, the underlying message of the SBS had been heard among rural officials outside of the medical profession. In July of that year, the mayor of the small town of Buffon in Côte-d'Or complained to the department's prefect that residents had been ignoring municipal ordinances indicating sanitary measures to be taken to prevent epidemics. He had posted notices requiring all piles of garbage, manure, and other waste to be taken out to the fields and buried, and also mandating the burial of animal cadavers at least 100 meters from the village and at least one meter deep in the ground. "But the difficulty of convincing country people," the mayor grumbled to the prefect, was such that instructions of this sort ought to be posted "in an *official* manner—that is, above *your* signature." He went on to request that the prefect direct each municipality to set aside a remote area for the burial of animals that had died of contagious diseases. The area should be securely enclosed, he urged, "so that live animals cannot get inside and contract certain germs—microbes, bacteria, bacilli, and others—as the immortal Pasteur's work on anthrax proves."[54]

Buffon was just one among thousands of battlegrounds large and small in the campaign to use the latest science to improve the nation's health. The mayor's appeal to the prefect reveals several crucial tendencies underway—at least haltingly—in 1884. Policing human/animal separation and fear of contamination by bodily waste represent an extension of earlier sanitary imperatives. The new elements of the hygienic agenda included, of course, disease-causing microbes, but also the spread of (at least partial) bacteriological awareness beyond the circle of scientists and physicians; the need to educate and civilize the hidebound populace; the acknowledgment of state responsibility for acting on scientific advances; and nationalistic pride in the glory of French science—including the ritualistic invocation of its brightest star. (Even in 1884, before the rabies vaccine, references to "the immortal Pasteur" already had something of the tone of a catechism to them.) These elements constituted some of the key building blocks of the sanitary-bacteriological synthesis. Ultimately, it matters little whether the mayor of Buffon sincerely believed what he wrote or simply rehearsed lines designed to elicit a favorable reaction from higher authorities. The bottom line was the same: even if words often outpaced deeds, the rules had changed, and the terms of debate in health policy had shifted at the local as well as the national level.

As a coda to this overview of etiology in the late nineteenth century, it is worth emphasizing that change happened unevenly and sometimes unpredictably. For example, how was it possible that the academy's epidemics report for 1901 referred to a disease caused not by specific bacteria, micrococci, or bacilli, but rather by "putrid germs"? Emile Troisier used that picturesque characterization in his discussion of an outbreak of gastroenteritis in a military barracks in Auxonne. The town and the barracks received their drinking water from a source that was "easily polluted after heavy rains"; the water "turned ocherous" after a snowfall in late January 1901, and the epidemic began the next day. "Various samples taken on February 5 caused [the water] to be declared impure [and found the presence of] putrid germs."[55] This etiology recalls the heyday of "medical constitution" and meteorological etiologies, but it also points to a critical factor in the gradual negotiation of the SBS. Brouardel and other hard-line Pasteurians had insisted in the early 1880s that "tout ce qui pue ne tue pas, et tout ce qui tue ne pue pas"—not everything that stinks kills, and not everything that kills stinks. Sensory evidence, in other words, could tell the observer nothing about a substance's potential pathogenic properties; only the evidence of the laboratory counted. But that dictum, to put it simply, failed the test of everyday experience and common sense. A durable and flexible etiological system could not be built on such a foundation. Water that looked, smelled, and tasted foul simply could not be bacteriologically innocent. (It is characteristic of the SBS that a corroborating verdict from under a microscope was a necessary component of the final explanation.) Troisier's report serves as a reminder of the failure of "tout ce qui pue . . . ," and although it lent credibility to the weather as a cause of epidemics, this endorsement could not have had the same impact in 1901 that it might have fifteen or twenty years earlier. With germ theory thoroughly triumphant and integrated into the SBS, Troisier's colleagues would likely have read his account of the Auxonne epidemic as yet another (perhaps quaintly framed) warning about the danger of contaminated water supplies.

Between 1875 and 1900, etiology was radically transformed—and remained largely unchanged. Miasmas and geology no longer caused disease at century's end; microbes and their contagious transmission had taken their place. But contamination by unclean bodily or organic substances still lay at the root of most epidemics, and transgressions against cultural norms remained highly pathogenic. The conundrum of continuity amid change lies in the reconciliation of old threats (both physical and moral) with a revolutionary new vocabulary and toolbox through which they could be explained and confronted. Old truths were true for new reasons, and new discoveries were adapted to fit old explanations.

4

Putting Germ Theory into Practice

*R*evolutionary etiological breakthroughs and the assimilation of time-honored sanitarian knowledge into the new language and new scientific paradigm of bacteriology were only the first steps in the establishment of a new public health regime in France. The new knowledge would prove barren if it did not produce practical strategies and policies to combat disease. Pasteur's 1881 anthrax vaccine demonstration at Pouilly-le-Fort (and his rabies vaccine four years later) promised miracle cures and vaccines for many other diseases, but promise was not enough. Epidemic doctors and others confronting devastating outbreaks and lamentable sanitary conditions on a daily basis needed new weapons immediately.

Their options were limited, but they seized them with remarkable zeal and conviction. By century's end, a guiding template for responding to infectious disease outbreaks at the local level had firmly taken hold. It rested on the twin pillars of isolation and disinfection, and joined to these immediate material interventions a long-term auxiliary strategy of popular education in the principles of the sanitary-bacteriological synthesis. Among scores of examples, the report on a 1900 scarlet fever outbreak in the Burgundy wine-making towns of Chassagne-Montrachet and Santenay (Côte-d'Or) demonstrates the extent to which short-term responses became formulaic, even automatic. The local epidemic doctor's investigation and report consisted of the following observations: the origin and cause of the outbreak were "unknown"; the sanitary condition of the towns was "good."

Chassagne-Montrachet:
> *Measures taken:* isolation of the patients
> *Measures proposed:* disinfection of linens, clothing, bedding, rooms.

Santenay:

> *Measures taken:* isolation of the patient
> *Measures proposed:* disinfection.[1]

Laconic in the extreme, this report represents the default option for busy epidemic doctors: when in doubt, recommend isolation and disinfection. By 1900, this strategy had become routinized to such an extent that an actual visit to the site of the outbreak was scarcely necessary. Along the way, however, the policy of isolation and disinfection in the short term accompanied by popular hygienic education in the long term, encountered resistance and contestation from various quarters before eventually achieving an uneasy and incomplete success.

The Pedigree and Theory of Disinfection

From setting fires in the streets to burning incense or sulfur indoors, communities have attempted to neutralize disease-causing influences by chemical and other means since ancient times.[2] By the mid-nineteenth century, the favored forms of disinfection—defined by the Larousse dictionary in 1870 as the destruction of "certain gases or certain exhalations produced by living matter, and called miasmas"—included the application of liquid chemicals, the burning of materials such as sulfur, and mechanical devices producing artificial ventilation through the forced circulation of air. Larousse's definition also complained about the popularity of so-called disinfections that "left much to be desired," merely masking unpleasant odors with stronger odors rather than truly "removing the harmful and stinking substances from the air." Such a definition both undermined and reinforced the equation of foul odors with disease, cautioning against superficial deodorization while at the same time suggesting that harmful substances did in fact stink and that genuine disinfection rendered dangerous substances "odorless and trouble-free," as if the two naturally went hand in hand.[3]

Meanwhile, beginning in the late 1860s, Joseph Lister began publishing accounts of his new "antiseptic" surgical practice, in which carbolic acid sprays seemed to drastically reduce the incidence of sepsis. Initially controversial among surgeons, Listerian antisepsis eventually gained converts in Britain and abroad. (Lister claimed Pasteur as a chief influence and inspiration, and maintained warm relations with the Frenchman.)[4] The benefits claimed for surgical patients both enhanced the status of chemical disinfection and accelerated the process by which it became linked with the germ theory of disease. An age-old practice was about to be reborn.

It took a combination of technical potential, scientific justification, and the mobilization of local authorities, however, in order for disinfection to become a central element of public health practice. For many years, disinfection meant little more than deodorization—literally, "dis-infection," when "infection" meant any foul stench. In 1877, for example, the district public health council in the Breton town of Montfort (Ille-et-Vilaine) responded to complaints of "ammoniac odors" produced by the town's newly installed public urinals by recommending their "disinfection" with a solution of chloride of lime; the council made no reference to any potential threat of disease.[5] Two years later, in Le Havre, the city council voted to fund the purchase of carbolic acid, ferrous sulfate, and chloride of lime for the newly established municipal health bureau. The chemicals were to be used to disinfect the lodgings of indigent Havrais after every case of a "contagious or infectious disease."[6] No specific mention was made of microbes or of these disinfectants' germicidal properties, but city officials clearly believed they could help limit the spread of disease. In 1880, the bureau added a detailed set of instructions for local physicians, who would often be initiating and overseeing the interventions of this first public disinfection program in France. The instructions defined disinfection somewhat equivocally as "the destruction or at least the neutralization of germs, miasmas, or dangerous principles that . . . can propagate epidemic or transmissible diseases." The booklet recommended particular chemicals for various applications (clothing, gutters, toilets, excretions, etc.), and warned that "substances that mask . . . odors are not always disinfectants, and disinfectants are not necessarily strong-smelling." Burning sugar in an apartment, for example, could remove odors but did not disinfect, whereas the bureau recommended the use of ferrous sulfate, which had virtually no odor.[7]

It did not take long for the link between disinfection and germs to become more explicit. In June 1880, the public health council of the Seine department delivered to the prefect of police a report written by no less an authority than Louis Pasteur himself, along with prominent physician Léon Colin. The report advocated the establishment of a systematic and scientific departmental disinfection program, coordinated by the Prefecture of Police and widely publicized among the Parisian working classes. Neighborhood police stations would provide chemicals and instructions for residents to use themselves—on a paid basis for some, but free of charge for those who could not afford to pay. After the death or recovery of a smallpox patient, for example, Parisians were to be instructed to place a kilogram of chloride of lime in each of four pans in the four corners of the room occupied by the sick person; they were then to combine 25 grams of hydrochloric acid and one deciliter of water, pour this mixture into each pan, and seal the room for forty-eight hours. At the end of this time, the room was to be thoroughly washed with a carbolic acid solution. Meanwhile, infected clothing and linens could first be soaked in the carbolic acid solution, then placed or hung in the sickroom (along with any infected furniture) for exposure to the chlorine vapors for the same forty-eight-hour period.[8]

Although their report avoided saying so directly, Pasteur and Colin must have known that such elaborate and time-consuming procedures were feasible only for a tiny fraction of the capital's population. (How many working-class households could afford to give up an entire room for two days?) They did acknowledge that "very few" Parisians had taken advantage of the existing disinfection supplies provided and subsidized by the Prefecture of Police: "It appears obvious that the habits of the working-class population are impervious to such sanitary precautions. It is only through moral pressure and by expanding the means of hygiene that we shall overcome this stubborn lack of concern." The properties of chemical disinfectants themselves posed another obstacle to the popularization of disinfection. Many agents were effective only in doses likely to damage or destroy the articles to which they were applied. The solution to this problem, in the authors' view, lay in Pasteur's experiments concerning the exposure of germs to heat. Fire, of course, had been considered the great purifier throughout human history, but Pasteur had shown that most microbes could be killed by a sustained exposure to even relatively moderate heating—that is, at temperatures that would not damage clothing or other household effects. Pasteur and Colin proposed the establishment of municipal disinfection tanks at various locations in the capital, in which such objects could be safely and reliably disinfected under scientific supervision.[9]

The Paris health council's 1880 report appears in retrospect as a definitive turning point in the history of disinfection: on the face of it, when the father of germ theory himself bestowed the imprimatur of bacteriology on this age-old practice and called for its systematic extension throughout Paris, the die was cast. But if scientific approval at the highest level was a necessary precondition for the spread of public disinfection services in France, it was far from a sufficient one. Publicity, education, and (perhaps most crucially of all) local bureaucratic will would be needed before the practice of disinfection finally became routine.

Calls for public disinfection services rang out repeatedly throughout the 1880s and early 1890s. Particularly during times of actual or threatened epidemics, hygienists and local government officials pushed for targeted disinfections, with uneven results. Faced with an alarming upsurge in cases of diphtheria, Colin used the Academy of Medicine's annual epidemics report in 1881 to call for the disinfection (by fire, if necessary) of all lodgings visited by the fearsome disease. When cholera invaded Mediterranean ports in 1884, the city council in faraway Lille debated whether to calm popular fears or to take advantage of them in order to undertake a major sanitation and disinfection program. Local newspapers angrily blamed an 1889 outbreak of diphtheria in Lambersart (Nord) on a Parisian family who had sent the undisinfected clothing of their recently deceased child (a diphtheria victim) to their impoverished northern relatives. When typhus struck western and northern France in 1893, suspicion focused immediately on vagabonds and itinerants. The Ministry of the Interior's director of public health and public assistance, Henri Monod, instructed all prefects to ensure the surveillance of all such migrants in their jurisdictions. The shelters and refuges where they slept were to be washed with a carbolic acid solution and their straw mattresses burned and replaced every morning, their walls whitewashed every week. The prefect of Nord urged judges to spray their courtrooms with disinfectant solutions after each session, if possible; prison officials in Douai soaked the clothes of all newly arrived inmates in mercuric chloride (or "corrosive sublimate") while the prisoners' bodies were thoroughly washed from head to toe and furnished with prison-issued clothing.[10]

The most significant milestone in the expansion of public disinfection in France, however, may have occurred in 1889, when the city of Paris began establishing the system first called for by Pasteur and Colin nine years earlier. After it was reorganized and expanded in the early 1890s, the municipal disinfection service operated four stations throughout the city and performed thousands of operations in homes throughout the city every year. Dr. André-Justin Martin led the effort to create the service, oversaw its operations, and served as its most tireless promoter before sometimes skeptical audiences—including the city council, the medical community, and the population of the city as a whole. (Fig. 7.) In theory at least, it was the very model of a modern, scientific public health intervention, staking its reputation on a combination of responsiveness, mobility, and safety. Even according to its proponents, disinfection was of little value if not performed in a timely manner, as exposure of neighbors and family members to the (deceased or recovered) patient's germs would be more likely if the

The Great Stink of Paris

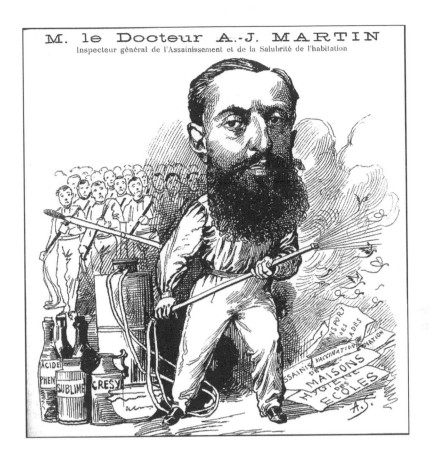

M. le Docteur A.-J. MARTIN
Inspecteur général de l'Assainissement et de la Salubrité de l'habitation

Fig. 7. André-Justin Martin, Paris disinfection chief, in an 1893 newspaper feature. *La Ville*, November 18, 1893.

operation was delayed; Martin took pride in his service's swift response to declarations and requests. The ability to send crews to apply disinfectants in apartments throughout the city and to bring infected belongings back to one of the stations for treatment was equally central to the program's reputation. A preoccupation with the scientific details of procedures designed to ensure efficacy and safety also distinguished the Paris disinfection service. Martin's description of the crews' safety precautions (see p. 147) may remind contemporary readers of the Level 4 biohazard crews of Richard Preston's medical thriller *The Hot Zone*. Of course, the degree to which such precautions were followed on a daily basis is an open question, but the fact that they figured so prominently in the service's self-presentation suggests, at minimum, that a scientific ideal of protection from germs had emerged as a common reference point in French culture by the turn of the century.

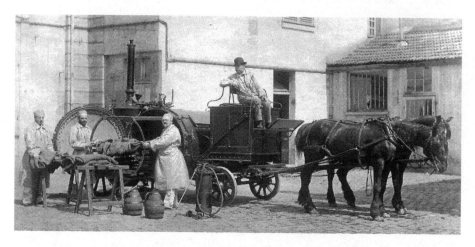

Fig. 8. A Paris disinfection crew, with mobile steam tank, at the time of the Universal Exposition of 1900. *La Préfecture de Police à l'Exposition universelle de 1900* (Paris: Imprimerie municipale, 1901), 217.

When Paris hosted the World's Fair in 1900, the Prefecture of Police featured the disinfection service as one of the centerpieces of its exhibits, touting its sophistication and efficiency. (Fig. 8.) At a time when surgical gowns and gloves were still new and controversial in hospitals, the pictured disinfectors wear protective robes and caps to prevent contamination from and of their clothing and hair; their facial expressions are more difficult to read, though it is possible to detect the hint of a smile suggesting professional pride on one or two faces. (Incipient smiles may also betray the strangeness of the circumstances of the photograph itself.) Disinfection had a long heritage, but its meaning was radically transformed by bacteriology. Laboratory science gave the old practice new momentum, prestige, and the credibility that came with putative precision. The case for disinfection could henceforth be made on specific scientific grounds rather than on vague intuitions of generalized contamination, infection, and contagion.

OBSTACLES TO DISINFECTION

Scientific reasoning alone, however, was not always enough to convince patients' families to entrust their belongings and lodgings to disinfection crews. Before the Paris municipal service was established, doctors despaired

The Great Stink of Paris

Each of the [four disinfection stations] is composed of two fully distinct parts. They are separated by a full wall and, in the disinfection rooms, by a metal partition at the level of the tanks. On one side is the arrival area for objects to be disinfected; on the other, that of the disinfected objects. No access is possible between the two parts of the establishment except by a hallway containing the locker rooms and a bathroom with shower. . . .

Personnel must keep their fingernails short, their beards trimmed, and their hair close-cropped. They have at their disposal soaps for washing their faces and hands, special brushes for their teeth, and toothpaste. Every evening before changing clothes to go home, they must take a shower, during and after which they are required to wash with antiseptic solutions. . . .

For residential disinfections, we follow the following rules: upon departing the station, each vehicle is accompanied by a coachman and two disinfectors. The wagons are enclosed, with smooth, impermeable interior surfaces. . . .

With the hose spraying disinfectant liquid, the agents begin by dampening one area, then they install in that area the packages, cloth covers, or baskets and place there (after folding them carefully) all objects capable of being taken to the disinfection tank. Packages must be hermetically sealed.

They then proceed to disinfect the rooms and the furniture by spraying the liquid [containing the] pulverized disinfectant on the walls, the ceilings, the paneling, the floors, any large carpets [not being taken to the station], the furniture, and especially the beds and all other objects left in the rooms. . . . If necessary, the large carpets and fabrics left at home because of their large size are detached from the walls and receive on both sides a prolonged spray of liquid disinfectant; the floors and the walls which they covered are also disinfected. The furniture, even the largest objects, must be moved and sprayed on all surfaces; the backs of paintings and the bottoms of bed frames must not be forgotten, and the same goes for the insides of cabinets and closets, and especially of bedside tables.

Disinfection with the spray hose must be methodical; on the walls, one must always direct the spray in the same direction from top to bottom, disinfecting section by section from a very close distance. After a certain amount of practice, disinfection can easily be done without subjecting the objects undergoing it to any deterioration, even when wetting them thoroughly; the disinfectors are trained in advance to acquire the necessary skill. . . .

When the various operations are finished, when every part of the residence . . . has been disinfected and cleaned, the agents themselves must be sprayed, in such a way as to have their shirts, their pants, their shoes—top and bottom—as well as their faces and hands, washed with the antiseptic solution; then they load the sacks containing the objects to be taken to the station into the wagon, and remove their work outfit to put into a special sack. After putting their uniforms back on, they submit the list of the objects they are taking with them.

Upon returning to the station, the agents ring the bell at the entry gate and give to an office employee their vehicle sheet. They enter the station only by the infected side.

. . .

The steam disinfection takes place as follows: the tank having been heated in advance, the orifice is opened by the infected side, whereas the opening on the disinfected side remains hermetically sealed. The carriage which goes inside the tank is steered onto the loading rails; its metallic parts are covered with a cloth sheet and each layer of objects . . . is also covered with a cloth sheet. Objects must not be folded nor crowded together, but rather spread out with care; those which are made of wool or feathers and might expand under the influence of the steam are always placed underneath. The carriage is then placed into the steam tank, which is solidly screwed shut, and the actual disinfection begins.

In the pressurized steam tanks, [disinfection] includes the following phases: five minutes of steam at a pressure of up to 7/10 atmosphere, one minute of rest, five minutes of steam as before, a second rest of one minute, [and a] third introduction of steam for five minutes under the same conditions as the two previous times.

Next the steam tank is opened, this time from the disinfected side, for five minutes; the carriage is rolled back on the rails and the objects unloaded. These are immediately spread out and shaken in the air for a few minutes; they are then stretched out—not piled up, not folded, not crumpled—to dry. Under these conditions, they dry rapidly. In one of our apparatuses, complete drying can happen even faster in the tank itself with the help of a draft caused by a ventilating mechanism and a powerful intake of air.

A. J. Martin, "Annexe: Note sur le service municipal de désinfection de la ville de Paris en 1901," *CMPR*, 1901, no. 184, 5–11.

of achieving appreciable results in the city's residential buildings. In 1885, the health council of the tenth arrondissement visited twenty-six apartments in which cases of smallpox, typhoid fever, diphtheria, or measles had been reported. When the council's representatives were not denied entry by concierges flatly denying that an illness had occurred in the building, they found that in most cases, not the slightest effort at disinfection had taken place. In several apartments, the council found that "disinfection" had consisted simply of washing some surfaces with carbolic acid solutions; in only a few instances was disinfection performed in a satisfactory way, by burning sulfur and by thoroughly washing all walls and floors.[11] When the newly established municipal service proposed opening its second disinfection station on rue des Récollets in the tenth arrondissement, the same council reacted with indignation when residents protested. A group of merchants and manufacturers near the proposed station signed a petition urging the city council to prevent its installation on the grounds that such a facility would "ruin" business by concentrating deadly infectious material in the neighborhood. The council met with a delegation of the petitioners, but rejected their worries as unfounded. In fact, its members made a point of affirming their pride in the installation of the city's second disinfection station in their arrondissement: as one member said, "It is an establishment that reassures the population" rather than endangering it.[12]

Hygienists complained incessantly about the popular tendency to misunderstand the scientific character of disinfection, and to associate it with simple cleaning or deodorization. The Paris daily *Le Temps* reported with wry amusement in 1892 on a physician's visit to the home of a child who had recently died of diphtheria. Asked whether the municipal service's crew had done its work properly, the victim's mother replied proudly, "I don't need the municipal service to take care of my house."

"I washed everything myself."

"That's not enough, Madam," the doctor answered. "You have to disinfect."

"I disinfected too, and your microbes are no longer here, sir."

Asked what disinfectant she had used, the mother replied, "Only the best": *papier d'Arménie,* an incense-like deodorizing paper that was folded on a plate and slowly burned. "We think the doctor began the operation all over again," the newspaper concluded dryly.[13] The anecdote may indeed be considered evidence of popular incomprehension, but the fact that a major daily newspaper considered its simple retelling humorous also points to a wide acceptance of the fundamental principles of disinfection (and perhaps, by extension, of germ theory on a basic level).

Occasional but memorable missteps bedeviled disinfection's advocates as well. In 1889, careless employees in central Lyon removed several straw mattresses from a home in order to perform the most reliable disinfection of all: incineration. When they began burning the mattresses in the street outside the building, an intolerable stench (of burnt corn husks, according to reports) suffocated the neighborhood. "The infection was such that the residents of neighboring houses had to close their windows immediately," according to a newspaper reporter. "Obviously, the disinfection of individual apartments is a very useful thing; but in doing it, you shouldn't infect an entire neighborhood."[14] (This incident illustrates the persistent double meaning of "infection" quite clearly: in 1889, it remained both foul odor and transmission of disease-causing influence.) After two deaths from diphtheria in January 1893, the mayor of the small town of Malaunay (Seine-Inférieure) wrote to the prefect to request that the departmental disinfection tank be sent right away; the victims' families had even agreed to hasten the funerals so that the operation could take place as soon as possible. The prefect sent the tank, but unfortunately, the technician who accompanied it arrived in Malaunay thoroughly drunk, and postponed the disinfection until the following day. When he finally began work, he found that the machinery needed repair, and he took it to Rouen, delaying the operation for the better part of another day and embarrassing those who had interceded to accelerate the victims' funerals.[15] Incidents like these could not help but tarnish the public image of disinfection.

Obstacles to disinfection were even greater in the countryside than in the city. The epidemic doctor of the arrondissement of Brest (Finistère) in Brittany claimed in 1897 that "the only way to disinfect a farmhouse in lower Brittany would be to burn it." Earthen floors and the absence of tiles made applications of liquid disinfectants problematic. Substances such as sulfur could still be burned, of course, but when a family lived in a single room, the prolonged evacuation of this room made even this measure impossible. Rural doctors nevertheless pleaded for the provision of mobile disinfection tanks to every arrondissement nationwide, preferring an imperfect system within which they could take some visible action to the alternative, which was the appearance of impotence.[16]

As disinfection gained in familiarity and popularity, the stigma and intrusiveness associated with it did not disappear; however, a countervailing influence emerged that seems to have succeeded (if not entirely, then at least to an appreciable extent) in subtly altering individual and collective expectations. In 1899, Le Temps bemoaned the fact that disinfection was still perceived by many as "a violation of a family's privacy" that caused disruptions comparable to the experience of a move, a burglary, or a fire. "Patients who have returned to health or families who have seen death visit their homes have no desire to prolong unpleasant images and upset-

The Great Stink of Paris

ting mental associations by imbuing their walls, their furniture, and their curtains with pharmaceutical odors, whose persistence will evoke painful memories." Such reluctance (along with the force of routine and inertia) could be overcome, the newspaper argued, by making public disinfection the equivalent of public school: mandatory and entirely free of charge. "Distributing health"—in this case, providing protection from germs—was a public service as essential as water supply, and ought to be acknowledged as such.[17]

It is impossible to know exactly how much impact prodisinfection propaganda of this sort had on popular attitudes in the 1880s and 1890s. What is clear is that both urban and rural disinfection services expanded considerably during this period. A combination of educational campaigns and increased visibility and familiarity not only weakened resistance to disinfection, but it also appears to have created a genuine demand for it, both in cities and (in time of epidemic) in the countryside. Disinfection became a routine feature of everyday life.

ACCEPTANCE AND DEMAND

Undaunted by public suspicion and the other obstacles they faced, the advocates of disinfection preached the merits of their cause tirelessly, both to the government officials holding the purse strings and to the general public. One official who scarcely needed to be convinced was Antoine Gailleton, mayor of Lyon from 1881 to 1900, physician, and holder of the chair in dermatology and venereology at that city's medical school. Gailleton considered it the municipality's duty to take all necessary steps to prevent the spread of disease, and every citizen's duty to participate in this effort. In 1889, he resolved to take action. The fact that many diseases had recently been shown to be microbial in nature gave the matter a new urgency, in the mayor's view: "They can be transmitted by numerous modes of contagion—not only by direct contact, but by laundry, clothing, bedding, domestic dust, toilets, cesspits, etc., etc." As a result, family members and neighbors were "exposed to a permanent danger by the failure to observe hygienic prescriptions." In recognition of this danger, Gailleton issued an executive order mandating that family members or others who cared for patients with smallpox, diphtheria, scarlet fever, typhoid fever, or other "contagious, epidemic, and infectious" disease make an official declaration of the case at the nearest police station or *mairie d'arrondissement,* so that the apartment could be disinfected. Neighbors or others with knowledge of such cases were encouraged to report them if the families failed to do so. Violators were subject to unspecified criminal penalties and civil liability, although there is no record of how intensively the order was enforced (if at all).[18]

Gailleton likely intended his order to make a strong statement rather than to actually punish those who failed to declare cases of infectious disease. Around the same time, the Rhône prefect Jules Cambon also issued guidelines to encourage disease reporting and disinfection, offering mayors throughout the department the use of the prefecture's mobile tank: "You should take care to recommend and propagate its usage, [as] nothing can offer greater safety, and there is no risk of damage to furniture, linens, or mattresses." Cambon cited Lyon as a leader in the popularization of disinfection, claiming that his departmental tank was in demand there nearly every day.[19] The actual number of disinfections in the city of Lyon was not reported until 1891, when it amounted to just under 800 operations per year; four years later, it had risen to 954.[20]

The public recognition achieved by disinfection in the late 1880s and early 1890s did not always come in the manner envisioned by its promoters—that is, by patients' families requesting the service. In Paris, the prefect of police noted in 1891 that the bulk of the municipal disinfection service's operations were requested by suspicious neighbors fearful of contagion rather than by concerned family members themselves.[21] In 1893, the epidemic doctor in Lille complained that a careless disinfection crew had left its carriage loaded with belongings from the household of several typhus victims unattended in the street for an extended period of time. Bystanders soon gathered, curious about the unfamiliar machinery and the accumulation of belongings: the load of "contaminated objects" was "surrounded by children . . . coming up as close as possible and playing with it like a toy."[22] This encounter can in fact be seen as emblematic of the challenge facing advocates of disinfection: the target population, which viewed this technology as a curious novelty, needed to be taught to respect and fear it as a potential vehicle of contagion, and at the same time to welcome disinfection into their homes as a routine and beneficent public service.

In the early 1890s, the combination of advocates' promotional efforts and specific local disease threats appears to have created a momentum in favor of disinfection that eased its eventual wider acceptance. The mayor of Le Tréport in Normandy (Seine-Inférieure) reported that prior to 1892, the typical family in his town rejected disinfection on the grounds that "my house is clean." After the cholera threat of 1892 triggered a major initiative to promote the service, residents' response to the offer of disinfection changed dramatically; increasingly, instead of waiting to be approached, they took the initiative and asked municipal officials what could be done to protect their homes and belongings. The mayor found himself so satisfied with the success of the disinfection campaign after the cholera scare that he could only lament that the town was unable to keep permanently the tank and machinery lent to it at the time.[23]

When diphtheria hit the town of Mons-en-Barœul (Nord) in 1894, doctors fighting the outbreak found an unexpected ally in the sensation-alistic newspapers of nearby Lille. Because the disease known as "croup" inspired a "terror" unmatched by any other disease, the slightest mention of it in the press (no matter how speculative or how flimsy the evidence) spread fear among the general population, thereby aiding those who were attempting to sound the alarm. According to local physician Georges Dumont, exaggerated stories in the press helped capture the public's attention, and laid the groundwork for the acceptance of disinfection and other preventive measures.[24] Doctors and local authorities in Mons-en-Barœul targeted the home of every diphtheria victim in town for thorough cleansing after the patient's death or recovery. Clothing and belongings touched by the patient were either incinerated or disinfected in boiling water before being left in a closed room while sulfur was burned. Walls, windows, and floors were washed with boiling water, then scrubbed with disinfectant. Many of the precautions recommended were redundant, Dumont admitted, "but in the country it is best to accumulate them, first to ensure that at least half of them are actually implemented, and second because stronger means (disinfection tanks, etc.) are often lacking." The municipality also made disinfectant substances available to the public free of charge, and had the town's schools disinfected after two children were stricken.[25] "All of these measures were implemented in a complete fashion . . . [and] they proved their efficacy by stopping the progress of the scourge; thus, the epidemic lasted only 25 days in the crowded rue du Bois, where deplorable hygiene was remedied by the careful disinfection of contaminated premises."[26]

Dumont's message was both encouraging and potentially unsettling. In Mons-en-Barœul, sensationalistic journalism and a deliberate policy of prophylactic overkill seemed to have enabled disinfection to defeat diphtheria. Fearmongering and heavy-handed tactics worked, in other words. But was it possible, as Dumont's report implied, that general hygienic improvement could be dispensed with as long as an adequate supply of disinfectants was available? This epidemic is one instance in which the bacteriological half of the SBS (that is, targeted disinfection) threatened to subvert the sanitary half (general cleanliness). Might targeted disinfection eventually obviate the urgency of public and private cleanliness? The possibility was raised by episodes such as the 1894 diphtheria outbreak in Mons-en-Barœul, but it would be left to many other epidemics over a sustained period of time to answer the question.

No locality in France had more experience with disinfection than Paris. Every malfunction that could disrupt a service's operation, every form of resistance that could be brought to bear against it, and every strategy that might be able to overcome such obstacles had been experienced in the capital. The raucous and volatile Parisian press reported with regularity on the municipal disinfection service as it progressed from curiosity to benefit to fixture in the everyday life of the capital. National dailies eventually proved a valuable ally in Martin's campaign to insinuate residential disinfection into the city's sanitary mores. *Le Temps* called attention in 1894 to the safety precautions it deemed vital to the success of the Paris disinfection program. The fact that disinfection procedures could sometimes cause significant damage to household goods and furnishings made the policy widely unpopular when it was first implemented. "We have seen grave popular movements—even riots, almost" when authorities urged disinfection on residents in time of epidemic, according to *Le Temps*. In response to such protests, Martin's department began to hold individual agents financially responsible for the damage they caused. The newspaper applauded this measure, and also praised the service's policy of disinfecting during the course of a patient's illness as well as after recovery or death. Other voices in the press echoed this sentiment, reporting that "the population, which appreciates the utility [of disinfection], cooperates with a laudable good will that we can only encourage."[27]

The district health councils in Paris (which, like their provincial counterparts, were composed of physicians, hygienists, and other neighborhood notables who regularly visited potential sites of disease spread) did not hesitate to criticize the local government when it came to public health policy. However, Martin's disinfection service began to enjoy consistent praise from the district councils in the mid-1890s. Disinfection in Paris was "well done," pronounced the fourteenth arrondissement health council in 1895: "The service functions to the general satisfaction [of all concerned], as there are never any claims [for damages] and our investigators could scarcely find three cases out of perhaps a thousand in which disinfection was requested but not performed."[28] Not all assessments were so sanguine, but the belief had become increasingly prevalent among hygienists not only that disinfection was an essential weapon in the arsenal of public health, but also that Martin's service in Paris effectively translated the ideal of disinfection into practice.

Even more important, lay minds had changed. As many observers pointed out, disinfection had many obstacles to overcome when the Paris program began. Aside from questions of efficacy and damage to property, Parisians were forced to confront the stigma of the disinfection crew's visit, which broadcast the presence of a dangerous infection to neighbors, customers, and passersby alike. When the city council met to discuss the municipal disinfection policy in 1898, councilman Adrien Veber proposed that merchants be spared bad publicity by having operations conducted at night. Martin shot back that cases of contagious disease tended to be widely known among neighbors anyway, and that the visibility of disinfection provided a vital public reassurance that the danger was being remedied. Most council members agreed with him that the operation ought to be publicized as much as possible, rather than hidden; one concluded with satisfaction, "The prejudices against disinfection that used to reign are disappearing day by day."[29]

Both Martin and the city council claimed, in effect, that a kind of "tipping point" had been reached, when for the first time the perceived benefits of disinfection outweighed its stigma. One must certainly take the self-serving claims of functionaries and elected officials with a grain of salt. Nevertheless, the statistical evidence regarding the total number of disinfections (and especially the number of demands for disinfection coming from private individuals) support the contention that during the 1890s, the practice definitively "enter[ed] into the mores of the population." In 1898, the council proposed adding thirty-six new agents to the staff of the disinfection service, noting that the existing manpower could not keep up with demand.[30] The following year, Martin congratulated himself on the success of his service, pointing with pride to the rapid escalation in numbers of disinfections performed in the capital. (Table 1.)

Especially remarkable (as Martin noted in a presentation to the city council) was the dramatic rise in requests for disinfections from private individuals—that is, people requesting that their own lodgings be disinfected, as opposed to doctors or civil servants reporting cases of contagious diseases that had come to their attention in the course of their professional duties. After fluctuating between 8,000 and 11,000 for five years, requests from individuals shot up to near 13,000 in 1898 and near 20,000 in 1899;

Table 1. Disinfection in Paris, 1893–1899

	1893	1894	1895	1896	1897	1898	1899*
	Disinfections requested at stations						
Requesters							
Private individuals	7,904	10,899	10,467	10,283	8,371	12,727	19,910
Doctors	3,340	3,069	1,770	1,814	1,903	1,859	2,787
Subtotal	11,244	13,968	12,237	12,097	10,274	14,586	22,697
	Disinfections transmitted to the service by official request						
Office							
Police	3,366	4,260	4,938	8,219	6,329	8,211	12,736
District administrative offices	11,465	7,015	7,229	5,161	5,662	6,016	6,141
Hospitals	4,166	2,880	3,128	3,156	3,866	3,416	3,343
Municipal Affairs Department	2,168	7,681	8,819	5,709	7,974	15,068	16,966
Schools	2,250	2,121	2,295	2,205	2,004	2,718	1,910
Subtotal	23,415	23,957	26,409	24,450	25,835	35,429	41,096
Total disinfections	34,659	37,925	38,646	36,547	36,109	50,015	63,793

Sources: "Rapport sur l'extension du service de la désinfection," CMPR, 1899, no. 83; figures for 1899 from "Rapport sur le service municipal de désinfection," CMPR, 1899, no. 183.

*Partial-year figures.

similarly, total disinfections in Paris suddenly rose from around 36,000 in 1897 to 50,000 in 1898 and nearly 64,000 in 1899.

Sooner or later, even the most successfully promoted policy would have to show some kind of results, and disinfection's advocates understood this fact. In addition to predicting routinely that disinfection would cause rates of infectious disease to decline, they periodically claimed that disinfection actually had reduced mortality. For example, Georges Dujardin-Beaumetz told the Academy of Medicine as early as 1894 that thanks to this relatively new program, "epidemics due to transmissible diseases are now stopped in a short period of time." "House epidemics, previously so frequent," he continued, "are coming to a halt, and those diseases that are thought to be the most contagious no longer claim more than a few victims."[31] An enthusiastic

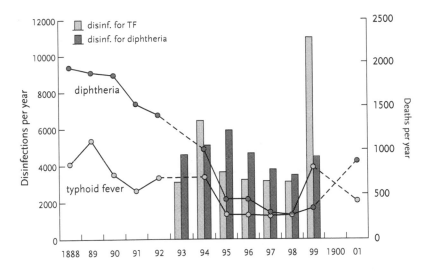

Fig. 9. Disinfection and mortality from diphtheria and typhoid fever in Paris, 1888–1901.

city council member echoed this claim in 1898: "Disinfection has brought about unquestionable results in the markedly improved sanitary state of Paris. Mortality has declined, and especially transmissible diseases have become relatively rare. . . . Epidemics are coming to a halt, and now have only a brief duration, for all diseases subject to [disinfection]."[32] Government statistics on this point are equivocal. As disinfections rapidly became a common feature of everyday life in Paris in the 1890s, mortality from the major contagious diseases fluctuated monthly and yearly according to rhythms that fail to fit an obvious pattern. (Fig. 9.) It is not inconceivable that the disinfection program could have favorably influenced infectious disease rates. Partisans of the program could certainly point to an apparent general downward trend in mortality between 1893 and 1899, but skeptics could find countervailing evidence in the same statistics, with some diseases seeming to increase dramatically after the popularization of disinfection. Diphtheria and typhoid fever—the two most prevalent diseases subject to disinfection—seemed to be in slight decline before Martin's service began operation, then declined more precipitously between 1893 and 1898. However, even this apparent triumph was equivocal, as both diphtheria and typhoid showed at least momentary increases after 1898, as disinfections remained high or continued to increase.[33]

It would be rash to reach any conclusive judgment about the effect of disinfection based on such a limited time period, particularly when the diseases involved tended to wax and wane in epidemic waves, rather than according to straightforward linear patterns. However, the fact of disinfection's increasing popularity and the apparently widespread belief in its efficacy stand in and of themselves as landmarks in the history of French public health, regardless of mortality rates. By the late 1890s, the tide had turned in the battle to win hearts and minds over to the microbial view of health and disease. Disinfection was both a weapon in this battle and a means of measuring its success. The sanitary-bacteriological synthesis took shape precisely through the kinds of practices that characterized the breakthrough of disinfection in Paris: medical advocacy, meticulous technical planning, debates in city council, reporting by official bodies and private citizens, resistance from tenants, persuasion by crew chiefs, word of mouth, and gradual habituation through increasingly frequent observation of disinfection crews at work in the city.

Even if they could be determined with precision, the actual rates of increase or decrease in infectious disease could not explain the increasing popularity of disinfection in Paris during the 1890s. Advocates of disinfection within the medical profession understood that the problem was a cultural one even more than a scientific or epidemiological one. Changing standards of cleanliness, the care taken by disinfectors with residents' property, neighbors' attitudes, and publicity about germs and infectious disease—in addition to perceived efficacy—all contributed to the increasing desirability of disinfection. Increasing demand, however, did not always mean more sanitary housing in the city, and many physicians complained that disinfection was too often being done poorly and for the wrong reasons. In 1892, shortly before the reorganization that expanded Martin's municipal service, Dr. Eugène Deschamps was torn between enthusiasm and caution as he delivered a report to the Paris health council on the state of disinfection in the capital. At the time, private companies competed aggressively for business in the new marketplace, and bacteriology was not always the disinfectors' ultimate guide. Deschamps hailed the growing popularity of disinfection, and bragged that its "utility and necessity . . . [had] rapidly become, for a significant part of the population, an obvious truth."[34]

The report warned, however, that the hard work of physicians, hygienists, and bacteriologists would go for naught if private companies continued to be allowed to cater to the caprices of an undereducated public. According to Deschamps, when customers submitted their belongings to be disinfected, what they really wanted most often was not so much a verifiable destruction of bacteria as a thorough cleaning. Success was measured by the absence of dirt and odors; if these were gone, the germs must have gone with them. Because the municipal disinfection service occasionally returned articles with stains still visible—whereas "for the majority of the population, a bedsheet or mattress cover . . . is only disinfected if it is perfectly whitened"—Parisians were turning increasingly to (unregulated) private companies to perform the service. Deschamps's report alleged that these firms' advertising sought deliberately to foster the equation in potential customers' minds between a thorough cleaning and disinfection. The fact that they had neither the training nor the equipment to perform actual disinfections did not deter these companies: "The important thing is to attract customers, and since disinfection is much discussed these days, they must appear to be doing it."[35]

Private "disinfectors" were not the only ones targeted for blame by Deschamps in his report to the health council. Far too many Parisians, he claimed, treated their lodgings and belongings with culpable recklessness after a case of a contagious illness. Linens and clothing were simply washed or sent to the cleaners; rugs were beaten in the courtyard (as if to share one's misfortune with the neighbors); and windows were opened to ventilate the apartment. "Those who fancied themselves scientifically minded" hired the phony, profitmongering disinfectors, who made a show of treating every room with a barrage of chemicals. Those determined to disinfect their lodgings for themselves chose from several options: "[For some,] burning a few pinches of sulfur . . . is enough, without taking into account the volume of the room or its openings . . . ; others burn *papier d'Arménie* or some other so-called 'antimiasmatic' paper invented by some entrepreneur always ready in time of epidemic to exploit the public's credulity and fear; for still others, the vapors of aromatic plants are a powerful and safe antiseptic; others, finally, apply on the floor (and only on the floor) a great variety of solutions (phenic acid, Bobeuf phenol, tar, *crésonaphte Faucon*, etc.)."[36] To an expert observer such as Deschamps, the offense was all the more grievous because disinfection was not a distant, hypothetical ideal, but rather a real practical achievement, lacking only sufficient awareness and resources to be adequately implemented on the ground.

In retrospect, this Paris health council report, issued shortly before a major expansion of the municipal disinfection service, signals more than just medical protest at abuses of science. It represents a rare insight into the reasons for disinfection's very success—and by extension, for the success of the bacteriological project as a whole. Deschamps is in fact telling the attentive reader (perhaps without realizing it) that disinfection could and would gain a significant foothold in society only to the extent that it reconciled new scientific advances with old cultural imperatives. The need to make bodies and their surroundings look and smell clean proved every bit as powerful as the demonstrated ability to neutralize the causes of deadly diseases. The impossibility of civilized living in dirty surroundings was not a perception born in the nineteenth century, although it did gain urgency as a social problem when urbanization accelerated after 1830, and (as shown in chapter 2) it expressed itself poignantly in the work of Villermé, Parent-Duchâtelet, and the other early sanitarians. When the cultural imperative of filth-fighting was harnessed by a scientific program promising concrete results in public health, the momentum was established for an unprecedented medical success story—not necessarily in the defeat of disease per se, but in the remaking of public perceptions concerning bodies and health. The fact that the enlistment of cleanliness and disgust in the service of germ theory was not (for the most part) deliberately planned did not make its effects any less dramatic.

ISOLATION, OR THE TIES THAT BIND

Hygienists and epidemic doctors recommended disinfection and isolation together so often that the two words seem almost to merge into one in the public health literature: *"isolement, désinfection"*; *"désinfection, isolement."* Like disinfection, the isolation of patients who were thought to be contagious had been practiced for centuries. Also like disinfection, isolation gained new justification and new momentum from the science of germs. (Bacteriology did not create the danger of contagion ex nihilo, of course; several diseases, including smallpox, had been widely perceived as contagious for centuries. However, the triumph of germ theory did spawn what I have called the "presumptive analogy" according to which *most diseases* were or *disease in general* was presumed to be microbial and therefore potentially contagious.) Unlike the partner with which it was so often paired, however, isolation encountered considerable resistance that did not appear to wane with the increasing popular awareness of bacteriology.

The fear that caused houses to be placarded and patients forcibly shut up in lazarettos when plague struck between the fourteenth and seventeenth centuries had not necessarily abated by the late nineteenth century. Placarding, for example, remained a central element in cutting-edge public health movements such as New York's antidiphtheria campaign in the 1890s, and in France around the same time even patients with a chronic, endemic illness such as tuberculosis found themselves shunned and worse in their neighborhoods.[37] However, when it came to what might be called domestic or "everyday" epidemics—typhoid, diphtheria, measles, and the like—most French hygienists and policymakers favored education and persuasion over police powers. Surely the discoveries of bacteriology could eventually convince family members of the wisdom of keeping patients in a separate room with a bare minimum of contact with other people. (If nothing else, self-preservation alone would seem to be a powerful argument in favor of isolation.)

There were times, certainly, when officials felt the need for education to become more persuasive. When diphtheria broke out in Lyon in 1890, the city government began disinfecting the lodgings where cases had been reported. As the outbreak continued and showed no signs of letting up, the departmental epidemic doctor called the prefect's attention to the alarming situation. "It is urgent," wrote Dr. Louis Bard, "that we concentrate on isolating the patients and convalescents, and on monitoring the patients' contacts." He even called the prefect's attention to a single address in Lyon, at which at least five cases of diphtheria had been reported. During another diphtheria epidemic, when parents took two still-contagious children home from the hospital against doctors' wishes, Dr. Bard took an even tougher line in a letter to the Rhône prefect: "The only useful precaution would be to have the local police investigate the habits of the children involved, to notify their neighbors about the danger that could result from their presence, and to find out if any new cases of diphtheria have been caused by them; and given that their parents were warned of the existing danger, to examine whether they might be subject to prosecution for damages caused by negligence."[38] The implied threat may have been an idle one; there is no definitive evidence even that the police warned the children's neighbors about the danger they faced. Nevertheless, the fact that the prefect was personally involved in a discussion of such enforcement options in response to two cases of a common epidemic disease shows that by the end of the 1880s, isolation had been placed near the top of the public health policy agenda at the local level.

Promotion of isolation continued throughout the 1880s and 1890s at every level, from epidemic doctors castigating negligent parents to elite Paris physicians advising cabinet officials. Listening for tone, one notices a persistent frustration with the public's apparent imperviousness to the obvious necessity of isolation. The Academy of Medicine's 1898 epidemics report, for example, insisted that this measure alone would neutralize the effects of whooping cough: "We must spread among mothers the conviction that a prolonged stay in the bedroom, and even in the bed, is the best way to shorten the duration of the illness and to avoid [complications] . . . ; isolation must be imposed upon whooping cough patients until the complete cessation of the illness, in other words for six weeks, two months, and often even longer. Isolation and absolute confinement to the bedroom would have the advantage above all of almost always [preventing] bronchial pneumonia, which is the principal cause of death."[39] Mothers stubbornly (and wrongly) insisted on the value of the patient "changing air" regularly, the academy report noted. Even at this late date, the task of educating people to treat not only their neighbors but also their loved ones as potentially dangerous remained to be accomplished.

Scattered signs suggest that the hygienists' message was not always ignored. Perhaps the most familiar dynamic in the machinery of late nineteenth-century French public health was that which saw prefects harangue mayors over insufficiently active responses to epidemics, while mayors claimed they were doing the best they could under the circumstances. It was not often, though, that a mayor's report to the prefect toed the hygienic line as diligently as did the one concerning a case of diphtheria in Vaux-sur-Somme (Somme) in the spring of 1900. Following the formula laid down in the centralized national system of reporting and response that (in theory) flowed from town to prefecture to Paris and back (at times stopping in the subprefecture along the way), the Somme prefect had directed the mayor of Vaux-sur-Somme to ensure that all necessary precautions were taken to prevent the spread of diphtheria. Among other things, the parents of the stricken child were to receive a copy of the Comité consultatif d'hygiène publique's official instructions prescribing strict isolation as well as disinfection in cases of diphtheria.[40]

According to the mayor, the parents and their family doctor acted aggressively, implementing all applicable precautions even before receiving the government's instructions. "The child was immediately isolated, and the other children of the house were moved to friends' houses," the mayor assured the prefect. The child recovered, and no further cases of diphtheria appeared in the town.[41] The nonepidemic of Vaux-sur-Somme in 1900 stands as testimony less to the actual prevalence of isolation as to the mayoral self-defense reflex in response to prefectural demands for action. Nevertheless, it is significant that when faced with such pressure from above, the mayor chose to emphasize thorough isolation as proof of his vigilance in combating disease. At century's end, isolation had joined disinfection as a central pillar of the public health edifice at the local level.

RESISTANCE TO ISOLATION

Isolation's path to acceptance seems to have been even rougher than that of disinfection, however. Just as many had resisted the intrusion of disinfecting crews into their homes, patients' families were not always willing—or able—to isolate their loved ones from relatives and neighbors. Even as they tirelessly preached the necessity of isolation, hygienists acknowledged that the small and overcrowded dwellings that housed the populations most at risk from infectious disease made this measure all but impossible to implement. The Academy of Medicine's Achille Kelsch called isolation in rural lodgings "easier to prescribe than to achieve."[42] Jacques Botrel, epidemic doctor for the arrondissement of St.-Malo (Ille-et-Vilaine), confronted this fact in 1881 when investigating a typhoid fever outbreak in the village of Roz-sur-Couesnon. (Fig. 10.) No stranger to this disease, Botrel saw a new and troubling element in this epidemic: typhoid fever seemed to be spreading through contagion—that is, directly from person to person: "The surest way to stop the disease would be to isolate patients in [rooms] where it would be easy to expel the miasmas with ventilation; this method is extremely difficult—often impossible—to achieve in rural houses." Less stringent measures were still possible and advisable in such cases, Botrel argued. In addition to rigorous disinfection and cleanliness, he recommended patients' movements be strictly limited, and the care of patients confided to a small number of relatives selected from low-risk populations, including the elderly.[43]

As the new bacteriological contagionism gained currency during the 1880s, this limited "isolationist" agenda began to seem almost quaintly lenient. Epidemic doctors promoted an increasingly strict doctrine of patient isolation, and railed against the folk customs and sheer carelessness that stood in the way of its realization. For example, when diphtheria broke out in the arrondissement of Redon (Ille-et-Vilaine) in 1884, the local epidemic doctor blamed the spread of the disease at least in part on the ritual visits paid to the sick and dying: "Nothing equals the imprudence of insouciant mothers who, carrying a young child in their arms and dragging others behind them, enter out of curiosity a house where someone has [diphtheria]. Unfortunately, it is not only peasants [and] ignorant people who commit these grievous misdeeds." In this case, the report continued, the violation

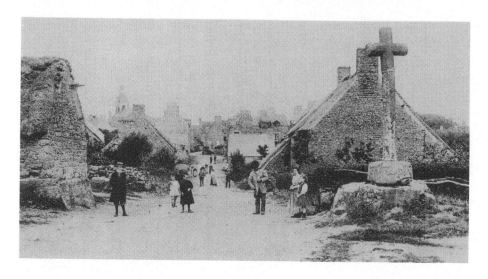

Fig. 10. Roz-sur-Couesnon, a village in the arrondissement of St.-Malo (Ille-et-Vilaine), ca. 1900. Photo courtesy of Musée de Bretagne, Rennes, France.

of hygienic norms was especially flagrant, and came from an unexpected source: "During the course of [one] epidemic . . . a six- or seven-year-old girl died of croup; she had barely expired when the teacher brought three other young girls in to kiss for the last time the face of their playmate. Out of the three, two were taken with croup and succumbed. This fact needs no further comment."[44] The scandal here was the commission of such a severe transgression by a *teacher,* of all people—the very personification within the village of the secular, positivist republic. The same act committed by a peasant mother would be taken for granted, and likely escape mention altogether in the investigating doctor's report. That hygienic progress was subverted here by the person upon whom progress depended above all only added insult to injury. That "no further comment" was needed indicates a lack of interest on the part of hygienists in the cultural importance of rituals such as the schoolgirls' final goodbye. Here Botrel's flexibility in the enforcement of isolation, taking into account extenuating local circumstances, had given way to a more dogmatic approach that brooked no compromise.

Small acts of kindness and charity loomed as potentially deadly sins against public health in the new regime of microbial contagion. Two diphtheria epidemics in the department of Seine-et-Marne in 1887 illustrate the point: in Bray-sur-Seine, the outbreak began in a Catholic school "irreproachable from a hygienic point of view," in which a teacher insisted

The Great Stink of Paris

on visiting and caring for her students when they fell ill. "The next day she would teach her class in the same clothes as the day before, and every day a new case broke out." In Nangis, another nun guilty of the same "generous imprudence" caused the same result. "The affection of a school director for her students [and] the devotion that she shows when they are stricken with a fearsome disease, doubtless result from a noble sentiment, *but they are in no way to be proposed as a model.*"[45] When Auguste Ollivier reported these epidemics in the annual Academy of Medicine report, he went out of his way to advise teachers and other nonfamily members of their "moral responsibility" *not* to visit sick children: "It is certainly painful to not be able to say a word of consolation to a child fighting against a terrible illness, but duty trumps all, and one of the first duties of a teacher is not to . . . bring to school the germs of diphtheria. The care of parents and nurses is enough; no visits other than those of the doctor should be allowed."[46] Ollivier seemed to be drawing a reasonable circle around the patient, allowing parents, physicians, and other caregivers, but excluding friends and other outsiders. Even this stance betrayed too much permissiveness for many hygienists, however. Anything less than complete isolation (ideally in a hospital, or at home attended by only one family member) threatened contagion.

Popular customs continually undermined hygienists' efforts at reform and progress. For example, they complained about the funerary practice of children visiting the body of a deceased friend and accompanying it to its gravesite. In 1889, the prefect of the Rhône department issued an order prohibiting this ritual, and directing schoolteachers to ensure that it was carried out: "Teachers will see to it that their students never enter into infected houses and never carry flowers, crowns, or shrouds to which morbid germs might become attached." The prefect noted that his order was motivated by didactic as much as practical concerns, explaining that reforms had to be enacted in times of relative good health in order to take root in popular habits: "Populations have a tendency in time of epidemic either to become excessively frightened or to neglect all precautions; it is the duty of the [governmental] authorities to care for the public health, and to take account of this [psychological] tendency. Policies intended to prevent epidemics must penetrate, little by little, into popular mores. To this end, they must above all be instituted when the sanitary status is satisfactory, as it is now."[47] Mayors were instructed to post the order prominently in their towns.

The prefect's practical commentary on the challenges of public health reform can also shed light on the problem of popular resistance to isolation. As a modern, progressive administrator, he was frustrated both by the archaic custom of maintaining contact with the bodies of deceased loved ones and by the seemingly irrational popular oscillation between panic and apparent indifference. But he did not draw the implicit connection between the two: might it not have been the family and friends of the potentially contagious victim who "neglect[ed] all precautions," while others panicked? This inference has the advantage of helping to explain some of the seemingly contradictory evidence regarding popular behavior in the face of infectious disease. Where officials saw patients sowing infection all around them, those most closely involved saw sons, daughters, and neighbors in need. To abandon them, or to deprive them of the everyday care and contact that constituted social life in their community, might risk something worse than diphtheria: a breakdown of the relationships on which both healthy and sick alike depended for sustenance. In short, the resistance to isolation that seemed backward and irrational to hygienists might in fact simply have grown out of a different logic than that of bacteriological contagionism.

Once laboratory science had linked contagion (and other mechanisms of infection) to microbes, and established a presumptive analogy according to which most diseases were regarded as likely caused by germs and therefore contagious, any unnecessary movement of a sick person became dangerous. (Once again, it should be emphasized that concern about contagion predated germs by centuries, but the Bacteriological Revolution greatly expanded and intensified that concern.) Hygienists continually warned patients against travel of any kind, and presented as cautionary tales local epidemics putatively started by patients arriving in a particular area from out of town. But French people—city dwellers and peasants alike—had the stubborn habit when they fell ill of returning home to be cared for by family members. The Academy of Medicine's 1891 epidemics report cited a dysentery outbreak in Rambervillers (Vosges) as evidence of the threat posed by sick soldiers returning home to recuperate with their families: "The same danger can come from sick civilians who also rush back home or are sent home by their employers. To safeguard the public health, every individual with a contagious disease who cannot receive the care he needs at his home should be transported without consultation to the hospital and kept there as long as he is capable of spreading infectious germs."[48]

The following year's academy report sounded the same note with even greater insistence and frustration. The spread of a diphtheria epidemic in Feuquières (Oise) "appear[ed] to have been encouraged by the neglect of the most elementary prophylactic precautions." When the local epidemic doctor first visited Feuquières in early July, he saw a five-year-old girl with diphtheria roaming freely through the village, and he discovered that the same had been true of all affected children since the beginning of the outbreak. When school resumed at summer's end, the epidemic redoubled in intensity, killing six children in a single week. This turn of events finally forced the mayor to do what local physicians had long been clamoring for: he closed and thoroughly disinfected the schools, strictly prohibited all gatherings of children, and turned the town hall into a temporary hospital where diphtheria victims could be both treated and isolated from the rest of the population. (This epidemic occurred two years before Roux's and Behring's antitoxin treatment for diphtheria first became available.) "Unfortunately, part of these wise measures was thwarted by an unconquerable prejudice. Fathers, even when reduced to the most extreme poverty, refused to send their sick children to the hospital, considering it a dishonor to admit them to an establishment where they would receive all the care that they couldn't get at home."[49] The question of exactly what treatment for diphtheria the children might receive at the town hall / hospital is certainly relevant, and may help explain parents' decisions in a moment of anxiety and crisis.

Nevertheless, even if one assumes that patients would be well cared for in isolation, the incomprehension of the epidemic doctor (and his colleagues on the academy's Epidemics Committee) is striking. In the absence of proven specific treatments, physicians were asking parents to give up contact with their children (during what might be their last days of life) in order to prevent a hypothetical exposure of a third party to the disease. If the new scientifically oriented public health intended to stake its claim to authority on these grounds, pitting hygienic wisdom against the enduring bonds of family and community, it was doomed to failure.[50] What looks in hindsight like inevitable progress looked like an overweening and unjustified imposition more than a century ago.

At times, epidemic doctors seemed to recognize that there was more than just ignorance or indifference behind popular resistance to isolation, but they showed little inclination to do anything more than denounce those who failed to conform to their hygienic precepts. For example, when diphtheria broke out in the town of Ruffec (Indre) in 1884, attention focused on the first reported case, a child in an isolated farmhouse. After the child was brought to Ruffec to see a doctor, he died, but not before leaving behind a cluster of cases in the town's schools, as the epidemic doctor later reported: "[The schools] were closed, but the isolation of patients was not practiced. On the contrary, everyone came to see them, especially women, with small children in their arms. *This is the local custom.*" After a month, the outbreak seemed to have ended, and residents demanded that the schools be reopened. As soon as local officials gave in and authorized the reopening of the schools, six new cases of diphtheria appeared in Ruffec. At this point, the epidemic doctor was called in. Dr. Dion immediately re-closed the schools, and with great difficulty succeeded in preventing the patients from receiving visitors. He even requested in vain that a room in the town's girls' school be set aside as an isolation room for diphtheria patients. The epidemic lasted for six months and caused 60 deaths (including 44 children) among the 250 inhabitants of Ruffec.[51] It seemed a classic case of prevention thwarted, in which rigorous isolation in the early stages of the epidemic might have cut short what turned out to be a devastating outbreak. Authorities acknowledged that showing support for patients by visiting them was a local custom, but as was the case so often elsewhere, popular customs were treated as a baffling obstacle to progress rather than a sensible and deeply rooted response to adverse circumstances.

Nevertheless, optimism prevailed that such barriers would be overcome. At century's end, hygienists congratulated themselves on the progress they had made in a relatively short period of time. According to the Academy of Medicine's 1899 epidemics report, many epidemic doctors had noted a decreasing incidence of diphtheria in their jurisdictions. The academy attributed this trend to the combination of "serotherapy" (antitoxin) and the success of isolation and disinfection—both of which were accepted "fairly regularly" where diphtheria was concerned: "Whereas measles is generally regarded as a minor illness, diphtheria . . . inspires a justifiable terror[.] They call the doctor as soon as they suspect that a child has diphtheria, and they follow his recommendations."[52]

It is worth recalling that the academy's epidemics report represents a selective but revealing compilation of information supplied by epidemic doctors nationwide. The claim that isolation, for example, was widely accepted for diphtheria in 1899 contrasts sharply with the chorus of complaints from epidemic doctors and other local authorities in the 1880s and earlier in the 1890s. (The problem of healthy carriers in typhoid and diphtheria did not become a significant topic of discussion among French hygienists until after 1900.) However, the scope of this assertion has limits. It refers vaguely and collectively to both disinfection and isolation being implemented "fairly regularly" (*assez régulièrement*), and it applies only to diphtheria. It also gives no explanation of how the problem of dwellings with insufficient space to permit isolation might have been overcome. What this passage suggests more than anything else is that those who were the object of the epidemic doctors' attentions responded to different infectious diseases differently, and, more generally perhaps, responded to any illness on the basis of a pragmatic calculation of risk and benefit. They neither accepted nor rejected wholesale the measures urged upon them by doctors or subprefects. They chose to accept (even if only partially) those that reasonably promised a desirable result without threatening bedrock elements of family identity and community stability; they rejected those that they saw as excessively risky or unacceptable. Theirs was not a scientific or hygienic logic, certainly, but it seems to have been a coherent *cultural* logic; by dismissing it as simple backwardness, hygienists only made their job harder.

POPULAR EDUCATION

While most public health authorities agreed that isolation and disinfection were their best short-term weapons against infectious disease, they also feared that their best efforts would come to naught without education. The ignorance and heedlessness that the epidemic doctors witnessed all around them would surely undo even the most energetic interventions from physicians or the state. Only through the combination of aggressive short-term measures with a concerted effort to educate the population as a whole in the basic principles of hygiene could one hope to effect lasting improvements in public health.

Once again, the technique enlisted in the service of the hygienic project predated the germ theory of disease. While bacteriology gave new justification and urgency to disinfection and isolation, popular education in personal and family hygiene gained new importance in the eyes of health reformers as the microbes responsible for the major infectious diseases were identified. Even before Koch's work on tuberculosis and Pasteur's rabies vaccine, however, hygiene education received a great impetus from the humiliating French defeat in the Franco-Prussian War of 1870–71. On March 4, 1872, at 8:00 p.m. in an auditorium on rue Jean-Jacques Bel in Bordeaux, Dr. Arthur Armaingaud began a series of weekly lectures as part of a "Municipal Hygiene Course" that would become a local institution and a model for other cities throughout France.

Armaingaud's first lecture included an introduction to the study of hygiene, and covered such topics as "hygiene and patriotism," France's demographic decline, and "the validity of the French race," concluding with a discussion of the question, "Has the race degenerated?" Fear of degeneration—the putative racial decline of a population through the hereditary transmission of acquired vices and weaknesses—plagued Germans and Britons and other Europeans, but after military defeat and decades of declining fertility, it struck Frenchmen with all the foreboding of a recurring nightmare.[53] The principal effect was an intensification of the pronatalist drive to increase the birth rate, but the vitality of a population could be increased just as much by early deaths prevented as by additional births, and disease prevention assumed a higher priority in the early Third Republic than it had enjoyed previously. In other respects, Armaingaud's first hygiene course in 1872 could have been lifted from the pages of the *Annales d'hygiène publique* in the 1830s or from Diderot's and d'Alembert's *Encyclopédie* in the late eighteenth century. The lectures highlighted heredity, climate, and moderation in food, drink, and physical activity as the keys to health. Contagion was conspicuously absent from Armaingaud's course, while "vitiation of the domestic atmosphere by the respiration of men and animals," "the effects of overcrowding," and "ventilation" occupied one lecture. It was a standard pre–germ theory synopsis of sanitary/miasmatic wisdom, combined with a guide to clean and upright bourgeois living.[54]

During the 1870s, the Bordeaux hygiene course began to focus increasingly on specific diseases and their prevention. In 1876, for example, Armaingaud added a lecture on "contagious, infectious, and epidemic diseases," which covered plague, typhus, yellow fever, cholera, and smallpox. Another lecture covered "endemic diseases"— "swamp fevers . . . including goiter and cretinism"—and posited their increase over the past fifty years as an index of degeneration. This schema divided disease into two categories: exotic plagues imported from abroad and domestic afflictions caused by geology and heredity. No mention was made of germs.[55]

By the early 1880s, the Bordeaux hygiene course had not abandoned its roots in the domestic advice genre, but it had added a significant component that reflected the incipient bacteriological orientation of public health nationwide in those years. In 1883, an entire lecture dealt exclusively with typhoid fever, covering its causes, transmission, and statistical incidence, as well as a segment devoted to "Preventive Hygiene of Typhoid Fever: Applications to Hygiene of M. Pasteur's Discoveries." At the same time, Armaingaud began distributing printed summaries of each lecture's key points to everyone in attendance. He also wrote and published a special pamphlet intended for popular audiences on the causes and prevention of typhoid fever.[56]

One of the most noteworthy changes in Armaingaud's approach at this stage was his insistence that the bourgeoisie pay careful attention to "the extent to which [their] domestic servants *know how to, want to*, or *are able to* implement the hygienic measures" he recommended. With contagion once again near the top of the public health agenda, prevention and protection no longer involved only one's own behavior and way of life; the working class—the servants and neighbors of Armaingaud's audience—were now directly implicated in the health of everyone in the city. Moreover, given the still-prevalent vertical segregation of many urban neighborhoods (in which working-class and bourgeois families often lived in the same apartment buildings), an updated version of miasmatism made even indirect cross-class contact dangerous: "The diffusion of gases that are given off by poorly installed or poorly maintained toilets . . . carries morbid airborne germs into the farthest reaches of the building; and if the better-off tenants don't take an interest in the well-being of their humble neighbors out of humanity, then let them do it out of a sense of self-preservation."[57] This "socialism of the microbe"—in which the health of rich and poor were inextricably linked, for better or for worse—eventually became a widely preached chapter of what has been called the "gospel of germs" in many countries, including France.[58] Armaingaud was slightly ahead of the curve by emphasizing it in Bordeaux in 1883, just as he was a pioneer in French popular hygiene education more generally.

At this early date, Armaingaud was attempting to inculcate into his Bordeaux audiences the core elements of what would eventually become the dominant framework for confronting disease: the sanitary-bacteriological synthesis. On the one hand, cleanliness inside and outside the house was imperative in the prevention of infectious disease. (Typhoid fever served as Armaingaud's chief case study, and he published a separate pamphlet of "instructions" based on his typhoid lecture.) He called for "the distancing of all varieties of filth," which entailed the evacuation of waste through the sewers with an abundant supply of water; the "hermetic closure" of all sewer and toilet openings to prevent the spread of odors; street cleaning with regular and thorough sweeping and spraying with water; and the strict application of unsanitary housing laws so that nobody would have to live in "revolting slums." At the same time, the doctor taught his Bordeaux audiences that isolation of patients, ventilation, disinfection of lodgings as well as clothing and all bodily excretions, and "laboratory analysis" of potentially harmful substances were indispensable elements of a responsible preventive policy.[59]

The message differs only in its comprehensiveness, perhaps, from that spread by legions of epidemic doctors and other hygienists through-out France during the first two decades of the Bacteriological Revolution: the core of the civilizing agenda of sanitarian hygiene must be integrated alongside new (and newly refurbished) scientific techniques into a multi-faceted strategy aimed at protecting society from filth and germs. What is remarkable about Armaingaud's curriculum is that it gathered all of these elements together in a succinct form so early and brought them all to bear on a single disease—typhoid fever. The mixture of breadth and specificity that would make the SBS so powerful and so durable were already on dis-play in the auditorium on the rue Jean-Jacques Bel in 1883. The struggles of epidemic doctors and local officials over the next fifteen years remind us that it was not always easy to put the agenda into practice.

No attendance figures exist for Armaingaud's municipal hygiene courses. Judging the state of popular attitudes about disease prevention from the content of a series of public lectures would be a dubious affair even if the course was offered in every city and town in the country. Though hygiene courses were also taught in Limoges and Reims in the late 1860s,[60] there is no indication that they lasted into the bacteriological era. In 1887, the Conseil général (departmental council) of Pyrénées-Orientales consid-ered replicating Armaingaud's course in its department as a response to troublingly high infant and child mortality rates. The prefect endorsed the principle, but objected that establishing such courses in every town with high death rates—much less ensuring that those who needed to be reached would attend—would be utterly impractical. They settled on a resolution designed to reach as large an audience as possible: the prefecture would distribute copies of Armaingaud's printed instructions (which in Bordeaux were handed out at each lecture) to all schoolteachers in the department; the teachers would read the instructions aloud in class and give copies to all pupils, who would then take them home to their parents. The best way to reach the adults who seemed impervious to hygienic wisdom, the prefect reasoned, was through their children.[61]

Notwithstanding Armaingaud's ambitious agenda and the enthusi-asm of the officials in Pyrénées-Orientales, popular hygiene courses did not spring up across the nation before the turn of the century. Those who learned of the new infectious disease paradigm in the 1880s and 1890s did so for the most part by other means. Only around 1900 did it become commonplace to teach about microbes, cleanliness, and disease through courses and publications intended for a wide popular audience. By then, the marriage of filth and germs had been consummated, and the SBS governed most public and private disease-prevention initiatives.

Popular hygiene literature at century's end taught the new orthodoxy to lay audiences by highlighting the novelty and wonder of bacteriology, and by holding out the promise of immediate practical benefits. For example, Ernest Monier's 1897 book *Hygienic and Scientific Chats* announced that Pasteur's "tremendous revolution . . . which has shaken medical science to its foundations," had already vanquished puerperal fever and would soon (if its lessons were heeded) defeat the other infectious diseases. It would do so "because we know the microbe [that causes] the contagion, and we know how to keep it away through rigorous cleanliness."[62] Monier also grasped a fundamental truth that eluded the bacteriological apostles of "not everything that stinks kills," who rejected the sanitarians' straightforward association of the unpleasant with the pathogenic: no matter how dazzling the science, health-related knowledge and behavior could not be divorced from the senses, nor from powerful cultural norms.

While dramatizing the interplay of genius, persistence, and serendipity that produced scientific discoveries, Monier also sang the praises of the esthetic purity that bacteriology seemed to demand. Aseptic surgery provided the most elegant example. What had been a messy and unruly encounter of instruments and bodies had now become a supremely ordered and pristine intervention in which the bodily envelope was protected from microbial violation. Whereas the pioneer of antisepsis Joseph Lister sounded the rallying cry of "tout ce qui pue ne tue pas" by boasting that his patients' wounds were "esthetically dirty" but "surgically clean," the advocates of asepsis protested that a carbolic acid spray was no substitute for scrupulous, sterilized cleanliness.[63] Monier became positively enraptured when he described for his lay audiences the atmosphere of the aseptic operating room:

> Look at this simplicity, the nudity of the room, the walls, and the . . . operating table. . . . No cornices, no ornamentation, no corners—nothing, in a word, that could give asylum to dust. Everything is painted and varnished in light and clean colors, with a strict, surgical cleanliness; the instruments . . . shine in their metal containers through the antiseptic liquids in which they are constantly submerged. . . . No extraneous bystanders around the surgeon and the patient; air, sunlight, all of this sterilizes and renders antiseptic; it is even forbidden for the assistants to put their hands in their pockets during the entire duration of the operation, in order to avoid picking up microbes. Finally, it is forbidden to cough, to blow one's nose, almost even to talk. Silence is antiseptic.[64]

"Silence is antiseptic"? Of course talking could theoretically spread germs, but Monier is exaggerating for effect here, carried away on his own conceit of synesthetic purity and cleanliness. If one truly subscribed to the full program of synthesis between the old sanitary science and the new bacteriology, then simple cleanliness in public spaces and public services (e.g., water supply, sewage, street cleaning) was not enough. Everything that came out of bodies—even sounds—was potentially dangerous, and therefore suspect.

The Schoolhouse as Battleground

While they were attempting to popularize the fight against germs for adult audiences, hygienists in the 1880s and 1890s did not neglect the most obvious educational platform available to them: the nation's public schools. In 1881 and 1882, a pair of laws named after Jules Ferry (who occupied various cabinet positions, including that of prime minister, during the 1880s) established mandatory, universal, free, and secular public schooling in France for the first time. The public schools in every urban neighborhood and every remote village nationwide were more than just educational institutions; they became the most prominent symbols of the democratic and secular republic in the making. More than any other institution, the primary school was the republican regime's outpost in the village, and the teacher was often its most powerful local agent. Charged with inculcating citizenship and national identity in addition to reading and mathematics, schoolteachers came to embody the authority, prestige, and values of the republic, especially in the countryside.[65]

In the 1890s, primary school students were taught "hygiene" as part of both the "physical education" and "intellectual education" curricula. Children were inspected upon arrival at school and required to exhibit "absolute cleanliness." Their games were monitored "from a hygienic point of view." Beginning at age seven, they were given "practical advice" on diet, clothing, and bodily hygiene. On the "intellectual" side, students learned "very elementary notions" about the human body and hygiene from age five. For eleven- through thirteen-year-olds, the content had progressed to "digestion, circulation, respiration, the nervous system, the sensory organs" as well as tobacco and alcohol abuse and "practical advice on hygiene."[66] Beginning in 1890, twelve one-hour lectures on hygiene became a mandatory component of the secondary-school curriculum. Designed by Adrien Proust of the Paris medical faculty, the hygiene course emphasized germs, infectious diseases, and the various means by which they could be transmitted (including food and water), but both domestic and bodily cleanliness also figured prominently in the lectures.

Hygienists and educational administrators reminded teachers insistently that instruction in the principles of hygiene was not enough. Students, they were told, needed to learn clean and healthy living by example, every day in the classroom. Teachers themselves were expected to serve as role models in bodily cleanliness, including bathing, toothbrushing, hair combing, and fingernail cleaning. Classrooms and school buildings were to be kept scrupulously clean—especially the toilets. An 1884 report proposed a variety of possible toilet installations that would be relatively easy to keep clean, but it acknowledged that mechanical solutions could never fully address the underlying problem: inculcating habits of cleanliness. "We want to teach the child to sit [on the toilet seat] voluntarily, and not by force. The goal to be attained is less to have clean privies than it is to habituate people to not soil the toilet

---

SECONDARY SCHOOL HYGIENE CURRICULUM, 1890

Official curriculum of "Hygiene" course instituted as part of anatomy and physiology instruction in *classe de rhétorique* (sixteen-year-olds) beginning in 1890, and later moved to *classe de philosophie* (seventeen-year-olds):

Twelve one-hour lectures

1. (Two one-hour lectures)
   - *Water.*—The various kinds of potable water: spring water, river water, well water.—Only spring water is pure; all others can be contaminated; modes of contamination.
   - Means of purifying potable water: filtration, boiling.
2. (Two one-hour lectures)
   - *Air.*—The quantity of air necessary in dwellings, etc.—Dangers of confined air.—Circulation of air.—Ventilation.—Alteration of the air by dusts, gases.
   - Proximity of swamps.
3. (Two one-hour lectures)
   - *Foods.*—Principal adulterations of everyday foods, solids and liquids.
   - Dangerous meats: parasitism and infectious germs (trichinosis, cysticerosis, anthrax, tuberculosis); putrefied meats (poisoning by pork, sausages).
   - Alcoholic beverages.—Alcoholism.
4. (Two one-hour lectures)
   - *Contagious diseases.*—What is a contagious or transmissible disease?

Example: a typical disease which is experimentally easy to transmit. Anthrax, experiments of M. Pasteur.

- Rapid indication of the principal contagious diseases of man; avenues of transmission: air, water, the respiratory tract, the digestive tract.
- Ringworm, scabies, eruptive fevers, smallpox, measles, scarlet fever, tuberculosis.

5. (Two one-hour lectures)
- *Vaccination. Revaccination.*—Mortality from smallpox.
- Preventive measures.—Prophylaxis.—Disinfection.—Bodily cleanliness.
- Healthy housing conditions.—The sanitary house; the unsanitary house.
- Diseases transmitted by human excretions: typhoid fever, cholera.

6. (Two one-hour lectures)
- *Basics of sanitary control of animals.*—Diseases transmissible to man. Rabies, glanders, anthrax, tuberculosis.
- Slaughter, burial. (Law of July 21, 1881 on the sanitary control of animals.)

Sources: "Arrêté du ministre de l'instruction publique, fixant le nouveau programme de l'enseignement secondaire classique dans les classes de lettres (28 janvier 1890)," *Recueil des lois et actes de l'instruction publique,* année 1890, premier semestre, 105–106; "Circulaire relative à une nouvelle répartition des matières de l'enseignement scientifique dans les classes supérieures des lettres (12 août 1890)," *Circulaires et instructions officielles relatives à l'instruction publique,* vol. 11: June 1889–December 1893 (Paris: Delalain Frères, 1894), 280; Adrien Proust, *Douze conférences d'hygiène, rédigées conformément au plan d'études du 12 août 1890,* 2d ed. (Paris: G. Masson, 1895).

---

seats." "Where there is running water," the report continued, signs should encourage children to flush the toilet before as well as after each usage, in order to dampen the porcelain and minimize the chances of solid material sticking to the sides of the basin. The report discouraged the use of automatic flushing mechanisms, because they allowed children to avoid taking steps to ensure cleanliness, rather than inculcating good habits in them.[67]

For the hygienist, public schools were not just an arena for health education; they were also potential hotbeds of contagion, and they turned into battlegrounds where the state's interests in education and in disease prevention often came into conflict. The issue was fraught with uncertainty and the stakes were high: if schools were kept open too long after cases of contagious diseases had appeared, local authorities could be responsible for sparking an epidemic. If, on the other hand, schools were closed every time a child came down with sniffles or a rash, the vital purpose of universal secular education would be undermined. Authority for school closure rested with mayors, but teachers, epidemic doctors, subprefects, and prefects often had a say in the decision. When individual children were diagnosed with contagious diseases, they were kept out of school for forty days in cases of smallpox, scarlet fever, and diphtheria; twenty-five days for chicken pox, measles, and mumps; and thirty days after the disappearance of symptoms for whooping cough. Any sick child whose diagnosis was not registered with the school could return to school only with a doctor's certificate specifying the exact nature and duration of the illness.[68]

When several children were involved, however, the question of school closure inevitably raised itself. Teachers were always caught in the middle: they were the only adults who saw all children on a daily basis, and they were responsible for the day-to-day operations of the school. If they failed to notice or report an incipient outbreak in time, they could be blamed for failing to stop an epidemic. If they sounded the alarm unnecessarily, they incurred the wrath of parents, whose lives were disrupted by having to arrange for the care of their children for extended periods of time. Judging from the surviving reports and administrative correspondence, schoolteachers seem to have had a prejudice in favor of keeping schools open, while epidemic doctors frequently advocated closing schools when a nascent outbreak was possible but not proven. (In principle, all school facilities were to be chemically disinfected during a closure.) In order to soothe the worries of alarmists without "frightening the population," the health council of the Laval arrondissement (Mayenne) proposed during an 1894 diphtheria scare that school attendance be made optional rather than mandatory during the course of the putative "epidemic."[69] That proposal went nowhere, and if there is a lesson in the school-closure debates, it is that like etiologies, they were all profoundly local. Every decision was colored by the personal and political temperament of the parents, the teacher, the mayor, the epidemic doctor, and the prefect. Even in the midst of a revolution in universal etiologies and attempts to apply universal national policies for school closure, each potential epidemic could only be understood as a local phenomenon interpreted by local actors. The equivalent of an automatically flushing toilet for school-closing decisions had yet to be invented.[70]

"A MAYOR WHO DOESN'T WANT TO ACT, A PREFECT WHO DOESN'T DARE TO ACT, AND A HYGIENIST WHO IS UNABLE TO ACT"

The periodic disputes over school closings raise the vexed question of local officials' inertia in matters of public health. The recent historiography has not been kind to the early Third Republic's public health policy in general, and most of the blame has fallen upon paper-pushing prefects and those champions of smug inaction, small-town mayors. French officials have been accused of "political expediency," "legislative inertia," and general "pusillanimity" where public health and social welfare were concerned. Confronted with the apparently successful example of the no-nonsense Germans and their comprehensive state initiatives, the French dithered and ultimately failed to muster the political will necessary to take meaningful action.[71]

Members of the Academy of Medicine's Epidemics Committee and other Parisian observers never tired of scolding lazy prefects, subprefects, mayors, and epidemic doctors who submitted annual reports marked only with the single word "*néant*"—"nothing," i.e., nothing to report, as if all diseases had miraculously managed to bypass that department or arrondissement entirely. Even the public health reform law of 1902, one critic noted wryly, left all responsibility in the hands of "a mayor who doesn't want to act, a prefect who doesn't dare to act, and a hygienist who is unable to act." The result was what historians Lion Murard and Patrick Zylberman have called an "orthodoxy of nothingness" and a "thwarted utopia."[72]

France's public health achievements in the late nineteenth century indeed pale in comparison to those of its neighbors, especially Germany and Great Britain. The French found direct and heavy state investment in medical care politically unpalatable, and preferred exhortation to coercion or taxation. Focusing on government budgets and legislative weaponry risks ignoring slower-moving and less immediately visible changes in behaviors, knowledge, attitudes, and mores—culture, in a word. Health policy narrowly defined also cannot account for such ostensibly non-health-related phenomena as agitation for shorter workdays and workweeks, higher wages, and better working conditions, which may have had a significant effect on public health in the long run. When historians judge France by the Anglo-Saxon standard and find it wanting, they implicitly assume that government health programs (and only government health programs) actually improved the health status of populations. In fact, the jury is still out on this question.[73]

Nevertheless, it is true that judged according to the standards aggressively set forth by French hygienists themselves, France failed to build a modern administrative infrastructure in public health, and lagged far behind Germany and Britain in health-related spending and legislation. Health reformers called loudly and continually for laws and programs that never materialized. One can only call this aspect of the hygienic program a failure. But inertia in the legislative arena should not obscure extraordinary

The Great Stink of Paris

activity in realms less easily assessed by objective measurement. French hygienists worked to educate people about infectious disease and its prevention, to enlist medical science in the creation of a durably secular and republican citizenry, and to bring culturally backward segments of the population into a clean new world of civilization. During the last quarter of the nineteenth century, the everyday behaviors and mores of ordinary French people, the very definition of a healthy and civilized lifestyle, the place of medicine and science in French society, and the contours of national identity all underwent dramatic transformation in France. Here we are far from the realm of "nothingness," and far even from a "thwarted utopia." We are in the messy human world of experts and lay people with sometimes conflicting agendas, caught up in changes the magnitude of which they often did not fully understand, attempting to survive in and sometimes to improve the world around them.

Among those whose motives and performance are most difficult to evaluate are France's mayors. Damned if they did take any action that threatened entrenched interests, they were most certainly damned (by hygienists and, later, by historians) when they did not. "The point for a mayor," according to Murard and Zylberman, was "to stay mayor"—that is, "to not annoy his constituents." Typhoid fever killed around twenty people per year in the town of Lure (Haute-Saône), where all drinking water was drawn from the lowest point between the cemetery and the sewage farm. The water's quality was notorious, and the health council reported to the mayor that it putrefied after a few hours in a bottle. An expert laboratory analysis was commissioned, but the mayor refused to release its results to the city council. His only comment was to reaffirm the water's "excellence."[74] Similarly, an 1892 outbreak of typhoid in Bellefois (Vienne) gave the local epidemic doctor a strange sense of déjà vu: "Typhoid fever is endemic in Bellefois. Every three or four years it becomes epidemic. In my report on the epidemics of 1879–80, I warned . . . about the causes of insalubrity in the village of Bellefois and I demanded that the gutters of rural route 24 . . . be rebuilt, that the drainage ditches be cleaned every day, and that the stinking ponds they flow into be drained." The epidemic doctor concluded by recommending drily "that the mayor's attention be drawn to these facts, and that he be requested to attend to the sanitary cleanup of the village."[75] There is no shortage of examples that could be cited to the same effect. Abundant evidence shows that many mayors dragged their feet when deadly health hazards needed to be removed or when urgent reforms needed to be implemented. However, too few accounts exist of exactly how mayors made the decisions they did.

Careful examination of incidents in which mayors faced difficult choices with lives on the line allows a more nuanced picture to emerge.

Prefects and epidemic doctors occasionally found themselves in the unfamiliar position of praising mayors and of holding them up as examples for their less energetic brethren. The prefect of Rhône did as much to the mayor of Lyon in 1889, when he offered the municipality the use of the brand-new departmental mobile disinfection tank. (The city had ordered an identical model, but it had not yet arrived from the manufacturer.) The prefect commended the mayor's recent ordinance mandating the reporting of contagious diseases, and explained that the similar departmental measure he himself had ordered was intended only "to compensate for the often dangerous negligence and ignorance of rural towns and villages." Lyon had distinguished itself by "taking all measures necessary for the care of public health." Big-city mayors were not the only ones singled out as doing things right; prefects and epidemic doctors also called attention on occasion to the cooperation of small-town and rural mayors in the fight against outbreaks of epidemic disease. After departments acquired mobile disinfection tanks in the late 1880s and early 1890s, mayors (even of the smallest villages) developed the habit of requesting that they be sent when a disease outbreak occurred in their towns. For once (one can imagine mayors and prefects thinking), there was something material, specific, and targeted that could be undertaken by local governments to combat infectious disease.[76]

Mayors themselves did not hesitate to pat themselves on the back for the scrupulous care they gave to the protection of public health. When an epidemic was declared and the prefect demanded action, mayors could be counted on to respond as the mayor of Allaines (Eure-et-Loir) did in the midst of a typhoid outbreak in 1895:

> I have the honor of informing you that I have taken the essential measures prescribed by the Comité consultatif d'hygiène publique to prevent any new cases of typhoid fever . . . in this town.
>
> I have prescribed the strictest cleanliness in streets, courtyards, and residential buildings, the disposal of manure piles and all manner of refuse, the isolation of patients, and the disinfection with carbolic acid of infected lodgings. Thanks to these precautions, the epidemic is in decline; no new cases have been brought to my attention.[77]

Clearly, such a self-serving account must be read with considerable skepticism. However, for all that it may not be a transparently accurate record of the average mayor's actual behavior during an epidemic, it does display a clear awareness of what was *expected* of a mayor during an epidemic. The existence of an investigating official (the epidemic doctor) who could visit and file a report might also have been a check on some mayors' creative license. Change in France was taking place less at the level of policy than at the underlying level of expectations, norms, and perceptions. Faced with the conflicting and categorical testimony of Parisian authorities complaining about mayoral inaction on the one hand, and mayors proclaiming their hygienic zeal on the other, the historian can either choose to believe one party, reject both versions out of hand, or attempt to interpolate carefully between them.

In 1889, the municipality of Montlay (Côte-d'Or) notified the prefecture of "several" cases of typhoid fever, including two deaths. This notification was more than just a formality required by bureaucratic protocol; there was genuine alarm behind it. "In the presence of this situation, which is very worrisome for the townspeople, we ask you, M. le Préfet, to order an investigation." The prefect sent the epidemic doctor, who reported back that "the epidemic of typhoid fever, which motivated this investigation, does not exist." The investigation revealed that two young sisters had died several days apart from typhoid fever: "These two deaths, in the same house, within a short interval, vividly struck the imagination of the town's inhabitants. Every headache seemed to be the prelude to a grave fever; the doctors in Précy were called at the drop of a hat, and the request for an investigation came from this panic." No cases other than the two fatal ones had been found, and the epidemic doctor was unable to trace the origin of the first sister's infection. "I therefore have no protective measure to prescribe."[78] This was no cholera panic: there were no rumors of an exotic foreign plague invading the land with horrifying symptoms and sudden death. Two girls died of an unfortunately familiar infectious disease, and an apparently well-developed dynamic of alarm and demand for action was set into motion. No action was taken; the inertia thesis would incorporate this case as further evidence of "nothingness," but such an interpretation would miss the heightened state of awareness regarding the threat of infectious disease that pervaded towns like Montlay in the late 1880s and 1890s.

Whooping cough struck the town of Lanneray (Eure-et-Loir) in October 1895. The mayor wrote directly to Ernest Hiblot, the epidemic doctor of the arrondissement of Châteaudun, reporting forty-five cases: "I ask you therefore to come as soon as possible, so that we can discuss what measures to take, in the interest of the schools, which I have dismissed for the time being." Hiblot found that the epidemic had been brought to Lanneray by a child sent to a local wet nurse, that girls had been hit harder than boys, that a few adults had been stricken, and that "in general, the cases are benign, but fairly persistent." There was no need to keep the schools closed any longer, he maintained, though isolation should be encouraged and teachers should be careful not to allow any afflicted child back to school until a full month after the disappearance of symptoms.[79] Here again, the municipality treated the epidemic with more urgency than did the epidemic doctor or departmental officials, who were left to reassure the anxious mayor that he could safely relax his precautions.

Not far away and just two months later, in December of 1895, it was diphtheria that alarmed the mayor and residents of Gallardon (Eure-et-Loir). The successful introduction of Roux's serum less than a year earlier had not diminished the fear attached to this disease. "Five or six cases"—all of them successfully cured—"caused a very legitimate emotion among the population," according to the mayor: "They are of a nature to make people believe that the town is in the grips of an epidemic of croup—a grave one, if we are to judge by the number and frequency of cases reported by public rumor. The patients, thankfully, are well . . . but if they were stricken with diphtheria, measures must be taken in order to avoid the spread of this dreadful disease." The mayor added that no official declaration of cases had been made at the town hall, and asked the prefect for instructions regarding "the conduct appropriate to such circumstances." The prefect then sent the epidemic doctor to investigate, even though (as he felt compelled to remark to the mayor), "contrary to the prescriptions of the law, no declaration of epidemic illness in your locality has been transmitted to me." The investigation found only five suspicious cases in Gallardon, all of which had been treated with Roux's serum, and all of which had shown signs of full recovery. All five lived on the same street, and "all indispensable precautions" had been taken to prevent the further spread of the disease, including rigorous isolation and disinfection. The prefect could only reply to the mayor that all necessary measures having been taken, no further action was called for.[80] In the case of Gallardon, as in Lanneray two months earlier, the mayor and local population were attempting to rouse the administration and the medical profession to action, rather than vice versa. If there was indifference and inertia, it was not coming from the mayors.

Eighteen ninety-two was a trying year for a cluster of villages along the Dive River in the central-western department of Vienne. Successive epidemics of sweating sickness and typhoid fever taxed local government re-

The Great Stink of Paris

sources and residents' composure to the breaking point, and mayors found themselves on the front lines of what seemed at times a hopeless battle. Mayor D. Martin of Vouzailles first reported an unusual rise in mortality in a March 18 letter to the Vienne prefect in Poitiers. "We have seen people of all ages taken from us; those who seemed the most robust were cut down almost suddenly," Martin noted. The case of Auguste Suret, "a vigorous man" who died after an illness lasting only five or six days, prompted Martin to consult the treating physician. The doctor's diagnosis was sweating sickness (*suette miliaire*), an epidemic disease characterized by its sudden onset, rapid course, and fever accompanied by profuse sweating and extreme thirst. (The disease had most recently swept across Vienne and neighboring departments in 1887.) In the interests of his "justifiably worried" and "greatly distressed" constituents, Martin asked Prefect Mastier to "take the necessary measures to stop, if possible, the scourge that seems to be descending upon us." He followed up five days later with a handwritten chart listing all thirteen deaths in the village since November 1891 by name, date, age, and cause.[81]

If Mastier took any action, it had little long-term effect, as the epidemic flared up again in September 1892. The mayor of Cuhon complained to the prefect that women from Massognes were washing laundry that might have belonged to *suette* patients in the Roche Bonneau creek, thereby threatening the health of Cuhon's residents. At the same time, Mayor Valet of Massognes pleaded with Mastier to send help to his village:

> The sweating sickness is claiming new victims every day in Massognes. Many are dying for lack of care or of everyday necessities. Entire families have been stricken, leaving nobody to care for them; others lack everything: meat, linens, etc., and are languishing in filth; it is a dire squalor.
>
> M. le Préfet [is asked to] have some consideration for this situation and to allocate to our village three hundred francs of emergency relief, in order to meet the most pressing needs: remedies, disinfectants, aid, etc.

The only response on record is the prefect's order that Mayor Valet put a stop to the washing of Massognes's dirty laundry in public waterways.[82]

Meanwhile, the arrondissement's epidemic doctor, Dr. Jablonski had visited the affected areas and had found cases of sweating sickness in Mazeuil and Verger-sur-Dive as well as in Massognes and Cuhon. Mastier had earlier proposed a joint tour of the region in order to ascertain the true state of affairs on the ground, and Jablonski suggested that the time had come to

—a.k.a. sweating sickness, miliary fever, *sudor anglicus* (English sweat)

Symptoms: sudden onset of acute fever and profuse sweating; severe headache; stomach pains; sensation of chest constriction; anxiety; and skin rash marked by a large number of very small "miliary" lesions (i.e., the size of a millet seed); in severe cases, coma and death can ensue within forty-eight hours of first symptoms' appearance.

Suette miliaire, or "sweating sickness," may be the only significant infectious disease familiar during the Bacteriological Revolution whose etiology remains a mystery to this day. Although it is best remembered for a series of deadly sixteenth-century epidemics in Britain, sweating sickness persisted into the early twentieth century, and periodically plagued several French departments in the west-central regions of Berry, Poitou, and Charentes. In 1880, for example, 1,200 inhabitants of the small island of Oléron off the coast of Charente-Inférieure were stricken with *suette miliaire,* and 150 died. The departmental archives of Vienne contain reports of several devastating outbreaks in the countryside around Poitiers in the late 1880s and early 1890s. The mayor of Massognes (Vienne) pleaded in desperation to the prefect for help during the 1892 epidemic:

> Sweating sickness is claiming new victims almost every day in Massognes. Many are succumbing from a lack of medical care or everyday necessities. Entire families are stricken, and have nobody to care for them; others lack everything: meat, linens, etc., and are left to wallow in filth; it is the most dire destitution [*c'est une misère oire*].
>
> In consideration of this situation, M. le Préfet will kindly accord to the town three hundred francs in emergency aid to deal with the most pressing necessities: medicines, disinfectants, financial assistance, etc.

France's last recorded outbreak of *suette miliaire* struck in the Indre department in 1947.

Nineteenth-century observers blamed the disease on geological factors, "fetid emanations," poorly maintained housing, contagion, and a variety of other factors. Over the years, physicians and scholars have periodically attempted to uncover the secrets of the mysterious sweating sickness. Most agree that it must have been a viral infection transmitted by an insect vector; several studies have hypothesized that the *campagnol* or field vole served as the animal reservoir for the virus (a member of the arbovirus family), and ticks or mosquitoes transmitted it to humans.

Sources: Ann G. Carmichael, "Sweating Sickness," in Kenneth F. Kiple, ed., *The Cambridge World History of Human Disease* (Cambridge: Cambridge University Press, 1993), 1023–25; John A. H. Wylie and Leslie H. Collier, "The English Sweating Sickness (*Sudor Anglicus*): A Reappraisal," *JHMAS* 36 (1981): 425–45; Jean Héritier, *La Suette miliaire: Une maladie mystérieuse* (unpublished thesis, Université de Paris VIII, 1948); Chantal Beauchamp, "La Crise salutaire: Stratégies de la guérison dans la suette miliaire, XVIIIe–XXe siècles," *RHMC* 45 (1998): 807–21; Academie of Medicine's reports, *RGE*, 1880, 1881, and 1891. Quotation: Mayor Valet of Massognes to Prefect (Vienne), ADV, M 5: 40.

put the plan into action: "If you are not available on Monday, we could postpone the trip until Tuesday, but I believe the sooner the better." The visit would comfort the terrified, uncertain patients, the doctor argued, while at the same time functioning as a fact-finding mission and an opportunity to spread knowledge about infectious diseases and their prevention. (Presumably at the suggestion of Mayor Valet, he mentioned the names of three families in Massognes who were especially deserving of financial aid from the department.) Jablonski also reassured the prefect that he had seen the department's mobile disinfection tank at work in Massognes, that it was being used correctly, and that he had ordered it sent on to Cuhon and Mazeuil. The epidemic doctor also enclosed his own handwritten "Instructions for Mayors," with detailed directions for sanitary precautions, prompt burial of corpses, and disinfection of belongings and lodgings.[83]

Just four days after Jablonski's update (and presumably just after the joint fact-finding visit), Prefect Mastier received a report from Mazeuil's mayor that deserves to be quoted at length as a revealing glimpse into the state of mind of a rural mayor during a severe epidemic. The handwriting is extremely difficult to decipher, as if the writer had not slept in days, and the tone is equal parts desperate and fatalistic:

Those measures that could be implemented were prescribed today.

The streets have been cleaned and the material collected from them has been transported east of town. The washing of patients' laundry in the public washbasins has been prohibited. I have ordered that such laundry be boiled for at least a half hour in a solution of [illegible].

Tomorrow I will make available for those who can't afford it a supply of copper sulfate, chloride of lime, and [illegible].

Meanwhile, the health news was not good. The mayor seemed determined but exhausted, and there is little optimism in his report:

Around ten new cases occurred today. Among the four people gravely ill, one died yesterday at [illegible]. Another is much better and the other two are stable.

The doctors appear to me to be fairly indifferent to the patients, and are not prescribing any of the measures contained in the instructions that you sent me.

I will continue tomorrow to take other measures if necessary. This is the situation, M. le Préfet. Tomorrow I will keep you updated on what happens.[84]

Judged by standards of efficacy, this may not have been an exemplary public health program, but whatever its shortcomings were, they cannot be imputed to a lack of energy or commitment on the part of local officials.

Even when the sweating sickness subsided, there was no rest for the weary mayors of northwestern Vienne. Typhoid fever arrived in November, and after three cases in his town, Mayor Martin of Vouzailles was quick to ask the prefect's help yet again. In support of his request, Martin specifically evoked the devastating impact of the *suette* epidemic on "our poor population," who could not handle any "further ravages." An investigation to identify possible sources of drinking water contamination was ordered, and the departmental disinfection tank was once again dispatched. The 1892 experience was so traumatic, in fact, that a single death from sweating sickness in late June of 1893 caused Martin to appeal again to Prefect Mastier for guidance and resources, in the hopes of avoiding a repeat of the "terrible epidemic" of the previous year.[85]

The dedication and persistence shown by these rural mayors (and the epidemic doctor) in 1892 is impressive, and even moving. Although there is confusion, uncertainty, and even a hint of panic in their responses at times, there is never the slightest indication of complacency or inertia. It is possible but highly improbable that three or four exceptionally active and public health–conscious mayors coincidentally happened to be in office in neighboring villages in Vienne at the same time, and that most mayors were passive and negligent. Representativeness in such cases is impossible to determine. More likely, the accident of archival survival has provided a rare glimpse of a pattern of activity on the local level that was not altogether uncommon, even if it was not the general rule. Similar emergencies happened every year in hundreds if not thousands of towns and villages throughout France. A certain degree of responsiveness on the part of mayors and other government officials was expected by hygienists and constituents alike; many officials met the standard, and at least some exceeded it.

Evidence of popular imperviousness to the sanitary-bacteriological synthesis on the local level is everywhere, and it fills the correspondence of the epidemic doctors and their colleagues, who so often portrayed themselves as voices crying out in the wilderness. However, just as disinfection found favor where isolation failed because it seemed immediately and materially useful to families, there are indications that popular attitudes toward the hygienic movement moved toward a selective embrace during the last quarter of the nineteenth century. The fervor of the embrace and the means by which it expressed itself varied drastically depending on the context.

The residents of Nouméa outside Dijon (Côte-d'Or) clung desperately to a portion of the hygienic agenda when they submitted a petition to the prefect asking, in effect, for a new neighborhood. The Nouméa quarter had been built up haphazardly over the previous fifteen years along the outer edge of Dijon's customs wall, its streets neither aligned nor graded. Ninety-six of the quarter's working-class residents had had enough of their living conditions and felt entitled to something better when they signed the petition in May 1889: "M. le Préfet, the inhabitants of . . . the so-called Nouméa district have the honor of bringing to your attention, notifying you [sic] of the danger that an epidemic could break out any day, given the state of uncleanliness in the streets, the cause of which cannot be attributed to the residents." The petitioners certainly intended to grab the prefect's attention with the mention in the first sentence of a possible epidemic. They had also obviously become accustomed to being blamed for the filthy state of their neighborhood. "[Our] streets are not aligned and not graded[;] as a result of water not flowing out, refuse thrown into the streets, which are nothing more than a quagmire, ferment, rot, and stay there, as no city garbage collectors pass through the neighborhood. . . . Several requests have been made to the municipal administration about the sanitation of our quarter, all have been fruitless." The petition concluded by asking the prefect to submit "our justifiable complaints" to the departmental health council.[86]

The council sent two of its members to investigate the history and sanitary conditions of Nouméa. The investigation found dangers not even mentioned in the petition (such as a serious risk of flooding) while it substantiated and documented the residents' claims in unpleasant detail. Poor drainage caused rainwater to collect and stagnate in a foul mixture with household garbage. Trash heaps grew so big that they interfered with traffic. Drinking water was drawn from numerous shallow wells, and the close proximity of cesspits often facilitated contamination. The health council agreed that the state of affairs in Nouméa was "lamentable," and expressed the rueful belief that a little advance planning when the quarter first began to spring up could have avoided the situation entirely. Short of razing and rebuilding the entire neighborhood, the council could recommend only the distribution of clean drinking water and the removal of the garbage lining Nouméa's streets. The prefect passed the recommendations on to the mayor of Dijon with the injunction, "It is up to you . . . to prescribe the measures indicated." (As is so often the case, the surviving records are silent on the matter's ultimate resolution.)[87]

The Nouméa petitioners did not mention germs in their purely sanitarian brief, although the health council reformulated their complaint to refer specifically to the spread of typhoid and cholera through fecal contamination of the water supply. While it is possible to imagine similar complaints being made in earlier decades, the fact remains that the public discussion of health and disease in 1889, at the height of the Bacteriological Revolution, eclipsed in volume and alarmism anything that had come before. Motivated no doubt, like all participants in the sanitary-bacteriological synthesis, by a combination of cultural/esthetic and health concerns, the residents of Nouméa pleaded their case on the grounds of health.

How representative of wider working-class attitudes toward public health was this one petition? The vicissitudes of archival conservation present us with an idiosyncratic sample, and hold out the tantalizing prospect of an iceberg effect: what is visible above the surface represents a much bigger invisible mass below the surface. The careful historian will resist this dangerous interpretive temptation, while attempting to reconstruct the context and read the tone of the original source for clues suggesting its typical or exceptional character. Relatively few reports from epidemic doctors survive; direct testimonials regarding working-class or peasant perceptions of public health are even rarer. In the end, it is the conditions of possibility behind pieces of evidence that hold the key to their interpretation. Certain perceptions and realities become thinkable and knowable at certain times and under certain circumstances. The conditions of possibility that make things utterable—whether true or false, self-evident or controversial—define the landscape of debate and knowledge at that time in that cultural environment. This cultural reality does not determine the course or outcome of debates, but it makes some things possible (thinkable) while others are not.

That some rural mayors and epidemic doctors worked doggedly to fight disease does not mean that all mayors and epidemic doctors did so; rather, it means that an environment existed in which such a course of action had become a desirable norm or professional standard. It is not overstretching plausibility to infer that at least some other mayors and epidemic doctors acted similarly and that highly uneven archival preservation has hidden their activity from historical view.[88] Likewise, that workers outside Dijon used alarmist health claims to demand cleaner streets does not mean that all (or even most) French workers had learned and internalized the essence of the sanitary-bacteriological synthesis. It does mean that in 1889, certain realities prevailed—some of them old, and some new: health claims carried particular weight in the public arena; filth was associated with disease in general and certain kinds of filth with specific diseases, through a vivid language of disgust; and even the poorest Frenchmen claimed the right to live in at least minimally acceptable sanitary conditions, and expected public remediation when those standards were not met.

The Capstone of the Sanitary-Bacteriological Synthesis

In 1894, the bacteriologists' laboratories finally produced what many had been predicting for more than a decade: an effective treatment for a disease common among human beings. Pasteur's anthrax and rabies vaccines had achieved renown and provoked expectations transcending the actual magnitude of those diseases,[89] and it is remarkable that the absence of any other prophylactic or therapeutic breakthroughs had not damaged the credibility of bacteriology. In terms of practical disease-fighting strategies, the SBS had coalesced and achieved consensus based on little more than refurbished versions of the age-old practices of isolation and disinfection, and the unfulfilled promise of discoveries to come. There is little doubt, however, that the availability of diphtheria antitoxin significantly enhanced the profile of the new microbe-oriented public health agenda, and fueled expectations that further advances in the fight against disease would come from the laboratory. "Dr. Roux's serum" proved to be the capstone in the edifice of the SBS.[90]

The importance of Pasteur's work as a precedent—especially his rabies vaccine, introduced in 1885—cannot be exaggerated. Even though rabies did not rank as a major public health threat, it was a dramatic and fearsome disease that was 100 percent fatal. The news of a life-saving injection that instantly turned a doomed victim back into a happy-go-lucky child not only made a strong impression in the medical and scientific worlds, but also struck the popular imagination with a force far beyond the statistical incidence of the disease.[91] Hygienists realized that this therapeutic innovation had the potential to add popular credibility to the entire public health agenda. The

Academy of Medicine's annual epidemics report for 1890 expressed great optimism that the "vulgarization" of the new science of disease would lay the groundwork for public acceptance of a variety of preventive measures:

> If this presumption might encounter some incredulity, one has only to look back on the practical consequences of the discovery recently made by our illustrious colleague concerning the prevention of . . . rabies.
>
> Thanks to the immense impact of this scientific conquest, [almost] overnight all those haunted by the fear of a horrible . . . death rushed from the remotest hamlets, in France and across the entire world, to seek salvation. [There was] no delay, no hesitation in this impetus toward the remedy, [even though] its therapeutic mechanism was difficult for limited minds to grasp.

It would be far easier, the report reasoned, for the public to understand the preventive value of (and therefore accept the need for) measures such as the cleaning of wells and the disinfection of contaminated houses and personal effects.[92]

Pasteur's rabies vaccine could serve as the leading edge of the new science, opening minds to the benefits of public health. Moreover, unlike Jenner's smallpox vaccine, the rabies vaccine was the direct product of a bacteriological laboratory (even though the rabies virus would not be identified until 1962), and it carried with it the promise of even more dazzling breakthroughs to come.

When Emile Roux announced his new serum treatment for diphtheria to the International Congress of Hygiene and Demography in Budapest in September 1894, the effect was almost immediate. By October, physicians and local officials in France were already scrambling to get their hands on reliable supplies of antitoxin. Reports on diphtheria outbreaks henceforth routinely included updates on the treatment's availability and requests for replenishment of stocks. While urban patients were the first to be treated, departments and arrondissements quickly acquired supplies that could be sent anywhere in the event of a diphtheria outbreak. Soon epidemic doctors were reporting dramatically lower fatality rates even in village epidemics when Roux's serum was widely administered. Eventually, the treatment's success allowed physicians to enlist public cooperation in taking early symptoms seriously and reporting new cases right away. Not long after its introduction, antitoxin was also used prophylactically on asymptomatic contacts of diphtheritic patients, again with favorable results.[93]

Diphtheria antitoxin was no panacea: its efficacy was much lower when it was not administered early in the course of a patient's illness, quality control was not always reliable, and it was difficult to maintain adequate supplies in some localities. However, the new treatment quickly became part of the hygienist's routinized response to epidemics. In fact, its appeal was so great that it threatened to supplant the other standard tools of public health in the sanitary-bacteriological era. In late 1895, a little more than a year after Roux's Budapest announcement, Gabriel Maunoury, epidemic doctor for the arrondissement of Chartres (Eure-et-Loir), investigated a diphtheria outbreak in the town of Berchères-la-Maingot. His report differs strikingly from the typical preantitoxin responses to diphtheria. After an overview of the epidemic's course and a summary of each case, Maunoury listed five immediate practical recommendations:

1. Close the schools until January 10, and longer if necessary.
2. Request 20 tubes of 10 grams of antidiphtheritic serum from the Pasteur Institute and deposit these tubes at the Town Hall in Berchères. . . .
3. In the event of new cases, [prescribe] preventive injections of 5 grams for all persons living in the same building as the patient and for everyone with [symptoms] that could be confused with diphtheria.
4. In the event that the epidemic continues, it would be appropriate to give this preventive injection to all children in the area.

The last recommendation was more radical than Maunoury's matter-of-fact tone would suggest:

5. There is no reason at the present time for disinfection . . . which, as advisable as it was in the past, has lost much of its importance since [the introduction of] serum injections.[94]

The familiar, almost ritualistic litany of hygienic precautions—public and private cleanliness, waste disposal, isolation, disinfection—was gone, replaced by school closing and a blanket of antitoxin treatment covering all those potentially infected. Disinfection, a pillar of public health strategy, now appeared almost quaint compared to the specific, targeted injection that was both therapeutic and prophylactic. The epidemic doctor's job must have seemed suddenly easier.

"Not everything that stinks kills, and not everything that kills stinks." In the long run, as appealing as this doctrine was to many scientific-minded physicians and hygienists, the highly disease-specific bacteriological approach to public health that explicitly divorced itself from the perceptual "common sense" of sanitary moralism failed as a guiding structure for public health as a whole. In contrast, what I have called the sanitary-bacteriological synthesis promised practical benefits derived from science without sacrificing the cultural resonance and moral serviceability of the filth-disease connection. Similarly, Maunoury's proposed abandonment of disinfection for diphtheria failed to take hold even in his own department. Antitoxin treatment occupied a privileged position in the fight against diphtheria, but it continued to be advocated alongside—not instead of—disinfection, isolation, and cleanliness.

The terrible diphtheria epidemic of 1901 in Châteaudun (Eure-et-Loir) illustrates the full implementation of the SBS in its mature form. Authoritative, scientific, and moralistic, epidemic doctor Ernest Hiblot's report was both confident in its grasp of the problem and exasperated at its seeming intractability. The year-long outbreak sickened at least 175 people and killed 14 in Châteaudun, and Hiblot was certain that many nonfatal cases were never officially declared. The disease took root in the poor working-class neighborhoods of the lower town along the river, largely sparing the upper town. Hiblot lamented that repeated disinfections of the local schools had no effect on the epidemic, inasmuch as the working-class families lived most often in a single room each, and therefore could not possibly have their lodgings disinfected. They refused to send their loved ones to the hospital, and certainly could not manage to isolate patients within the home: "What's more, these poor people are often ignorant and fatalistic; they meet the doctor's recommendations with the force of inertia; they do not prevent the neighbors from coming into their contaminated house, and the [neighbors then] transport the germs . . . and enlarge the scope of the epidemic." "With the exception of a few enlightened people of a certain social condition," the families generally refused prophylactic injections of antitoxin, Hiblot found, but all accepted therapeutic injections, which were uniformly successful when administered early in the illness.[95]

In Hiblot's own hospital-based practice, the disorderly and unmanageable reality of the working-class neighborhoods gave way to a controlled and predictable universe. He treated fifty-three diphtheria patients in 1901, the majority of them between four and eight years old; six were diagnosed too late to be saved: "In the hospital, all rules relating to the isolation of diphtheria patients and staff members, as well as the disinfection of objects that came into contact with patients, were rigorously observed. . . . It goes without saying that I always took care to enforce the most scrupulous cleanliness in my ward." Hiblot treated every one of his fifty-three patients with serum provided by the Pasteur Institute in Paris. His report included a detailed description of the protocol he used to administer different doses to patients depending on their age and on the severity of their symptoms. The experience left him more convinced than ever of the value of the serum as a safe and "specific medication against diphtheria."[96]

Hiblot was clearly as frustrated at the difficulty of implementing disinfection and isolation effectively in Châteaudun as he was satisfied with the efficacy of Roux's serum. Nonetheless, like most hygienists and unlike Maunoury, he did not abandon the older tactics in favor of an exclusive use of the "specific medication." No matter how effective it was, treatment without cleanliness, isolation, and disinfection was unimaginable. The laboratory innovation was seamlessly integrated with the existing sanitary and bacteriological weapons. Meanwhile, the public accepted the hygienic program very selectively: like disinfection in many places, therapeutic injections appeared to offer immediate, practical benefits, while isolation, cleanliness, and prophylactic injections were either impractical or threatening. As the twentieth century began, the (partially) new regime of public health knowledge had definitively taken the shape that would govern responses to the threat of disease for decades to come.

5

Toward a Cleaner and Healthier Republic

When Jacques Botrel, epidemic doctor for the district of St.-Malo (Ille-et-Vilaine) in Brittany, reported to the departmental health board on the epidemics that had afflicted his district in 1882, one disease in particular preoccupied him: typhoid fever. This persistent scourge regularly devastated local towns, and Botrel found its ravages easy to explain: "The explanation is quite simple, and it comes not from theoretical reasoning, but from an examination of the state of affairs in the homes of those struck by the fever."[1] The most cursory glance inside the rural dwellings where typhoid reigned exposed the reasons for its prevalence: the proximate cause was "contagion," according to Botrel, but it was contagion of a very specific sort. His observation had convinced him that the ultimate cause of this disease was an insufficiently civilized way of life. (Fig. 11.) The fetid, promiscuously overcrowded housing that was all too common in the small towns and hamlets around St.-Malo, he explained, allowed typhoid fever to spread from person to person with relentless predictability: "A kitchen containing several box-beds, where sick and well lie together, cluttered with various furniture items, pierced only by a door and a small window, serves at the same time as dining room and bedroom; the residents spend all night there, and often the daytime as well, in a limited volume of air that circulates very little, so that the atmosphere is rapidly vitiated and exercises its deleterious action on anyone who breathes it and lives surrounded by it." The presence of a single sick person, Botrel continued, turned this vitiated atmosphere deadly: "A person with typhoid in such a place soon fills the air with the specific miasmas that are exhaled by his skin, by his respiration, and above all by the intestinal matter that he excretes frequently, and before long, these miasmas contaminate those who care for or sleep near the patient." In contrast, Botrel rarely saw typhoid

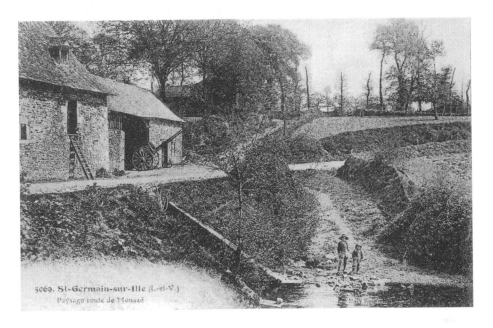

Fig. 11. St.-Germain-sur-Ille, a village in the arrondissement of St.-Malo (Ille-et-Vilaine), early twentieth century. Photo courtesy of Musée de Bretagne, Rennes, France.

spread contagiously in urban homes with several rooms, where patients could be isolated, and attended by family members who came and went from the sick room rather than effectively stewing in its vitiated air.[2]

The curious blend of miasmatic and contagionist language in Botrel's explanation of typhoid's causes is striking. His reference to the "specific miasmas" of the disease and his emphasis on the danger of the patient's excretions seem to grope haltingly toward a microbial etiology of typhoid fever. Indeed, three years before Botrel's report, the German bacteriologist Karl Eberth announced that he had identified the causal microbe of typhoid fever, baptized *Bacillus typhosus* at the time (and later renamed *Salmonella typhi*). It seems reasonable, therefore, to read Botrel's etiology of typhoid as a confused and slightly backward blend of old-fashioned miasmatism and dimly understood bacteriological contagionism. After all, a busy country doctor could be forgiven for not keeping up with the latest big-city scientific literature.

It is also possible, however, to see this particular local etiology not as a step on the scientific path from error (miasmatism) to truth (bacteriology), but rather as a salvo in the battle to move the French peasantry forward along the cultural path from backwardness to civilization. In their capacity as epidemic doctors in remote towns and villages, Botrel and his colleagues acted as front-line operatives in a political and cultural struggle to strengthen the foundations of French society. The 1882 report on typhoid in St.-Malo represents the fusion of the ongoing hygienic battle against filth with the incipient science of germs. It serves simultaneously to rationalize dramatic health disparities and to pursue the Kulturkampf aimed at transforming (in Eugen Weber's phrase) "peasants into Frenchmen."[3] Paradoxically, the doctor's abhorrence of the unconscionable and barely human disorder in which rural Bretons were living (and dying) served simultaneously to define this subset of the population *out* of the civilized world of Frenchmen and to call them urgently *into* that world.

The urgent need to civilize the savage elements in French society for the sake of the nation's physical health was felt not only in Brittany, and not only in rural environments. Around the time of Botrel's typhoid report, another epidemic doctor was asked to investigate the "constant . . . intensity" of typhoid fever in the industrial city of Hazebrouck (Nord) near the Belgian border. Just as Botrel saw a "specific miasma" of typhoid emanated or discharged by its victims, Alexandre Decool of Hazebrouck speculated about the existence of "a special principle, unknown element, germ or seed which . . . communicates and develops the typhoid-causing property."[4] However, this hypothetical "special principle" or "germ" of typhoid fever did not answer the most important questions posed by the disease. Like Botrel, Decool considered the existence of a specific causal agent of secondary importance. He found in the dwellings of Hazebrouck's industrial workers and day laborers the most repugnant filth and overcrowding, which combined with the residents' "unclean habits" and poor diet invariably resulted in typhoid fever—whatever its biological cause. How could one be surprised that this disease was endemic, Decool wondered, in a city where one could find living together in two small adjacent rooms . . . twelve rabbits, two cats, one magpie, and ten human beings?[5] After receiving Decool's report, the subprefect of Hazebrouck appealed to the prefect of the Nord department for intervention in order to help enforce the sanitary housing laws in cases of such blatant disregard for the most elementary standards of civilized and hygienic living. All of these officials seemed to realize, as the subprefect observed, that the root of the local typhoid problem lay in the people involved: "This population, held in mistrust of all physical or moral progress, and of all change in habits, bears no resemblance at all to those of towns growing in dignity, where each person improves his situation by taking intelligent care of himself." "This population" consisted of working-class Flemish families, whom the subprefect described as "impervious to progress and lacking any spirit of initiative." In the end, the mayor of Hazebrouck was prevailed upon to issue an order cracking down on the raising of rabbits, goats, and chickens inside apartments and houses.[6]

The reports of epidemic doctors such as Botrel and Decool in the early 1880s resound powerfully with forty-year-old echoes of Villermé's and Benoiston de Châteauneuf's voices. Not only did the latter two hygienists spend considerable time observing depravity and disease in the hovels of rural Brittany and urban Hazebrouck and its department, but they also took pains to ground a science of public health in the meticulous description of living conditions among the sickly poor. One key element is added in the early 1880s: an incipient attempt to link filth with disease by means of a "specific miasma" or "germ." In Botrel's and Decool's work, the notion is introduced as a secondary factor, a trigger of sorts, which activates the underlying causes and turns them into disease. Before long, these secondary factors would become full partners in the etiological equation: inseparable from the filth and depravity out of which they arose, they constituted a specifically measurable index of danger and an irresistible target for intervention. As such, germs opened a new front in the battle against infectious disease: by introducing the identifiability of disease-specific organisms in the laboratory, bacteriology first threatened to subvert, then proved to complement, the moralistic etiology of filth and transgression. By the mid-1890s, the association of microbes and uncleanliness provided mutual reinforcement: the linkage with already proscribed practices rooted germs in familiar dangers, while the thought that everyday substances might be teeming with pathogenic organisms added urgency to the battle against filth. As Georges Vigarello has shown, the imperative of cleanliness was the product of a "social code, not [of] science." The new bacteriologically driven public health adopted and ratified the cultural imperative, even in the face of laboratory advances (such as diphtheria antitoxin) that threatened to render cleanliness medically moot.[7] Swimming against such a powerful cultural current, the notion that disease could be fought exclusively with the weapons of the laboratory—in other words, the "not everything that stinks kills" school of thought—didn't stand a chance.

This chapter traces the contours of the mutually reinforcing relationship between filth and germs as it developed during the 1880s and 1890s. The everyday interpenetration of medical knowledge and behavioral mores played a central role in the formation of the sanitary-bacteriological synthesis. In fact, it is misleading even to speak of separate domains interpenetrating, inasmuch as medicine and culture have never been and can never be truly separate from each other. However, there are historical moments—including this one, the Bacteriological Revolution, which many consider the turning point in the maturation of modern scientific medicine—in which medical science staked its claim to authority so strongly on its objective, scientific nature and on its opposition to the old etiologies of supposition and superstition that it is worth emphasizing the extent to which the new science was grounded in preexisting cultural imperatives.

A Taxonomy of Disgust

The banishment of excrement and other substances that served as a reminder of human animality did not happen overnight. It expressed a disgust among respectable bourgeois observers that had been solidly entrenched for decades—certainly since the days of Villermé and Benoiston de Châteauneuf, and in partially recognizable form since the 1780 Cemetery of the Innocents calamity (see chapter 6) or even earlier. (This disgust was not the exclusive preserve of the bourgeoisie; reformers tried hard to spread it to workers and peasants throughout France—with at least some success, as some of the evidence discussed in this chapter suggests.) While no single historical starting point can be identified for the intense disgust focused on bodily substances, it is possible to identify its primary constitutive elements and to trace the gradual process by which they were associated with disease transmission in general and microbes in particular.

The investigation of a typhoid fever epidemic in the city of Rouen (Seine-Inférieure) in 1869 expresses in a nutshell the dilemma of hygienists worried about filth and disease on the eve of the Bacteriological Revolution. After the disease swept through a government-run boarding school, students and parents accused the school's administration of neglecting even minimal standards of cleanliness on school grounds and in preparation of students' meals. The departmental health council seemed inclined to agree: "the students' diet is bad, and this fact . . . combined with a disgusting uncleanliness in meal preparation and in the upkeep of students' rooms to cause this year's [epidemic]," claimed Achille Flaubert, member of the health council and brother of novelist Gustave. Other council members seconded Flaubert's accusations, adding their own regarding the school's physical education system, water supply, overcrowded dormitories, and poor ventilation. Still others on the council blamed the epidemic on contagion and an "epidemic influence whose essence escapes us." A rough consensus was reached on the need to improve physical conditions and food quality at the school, but the array of "causes" invoked to explain the typhoid epidemic diluted the strength of the council's conclusions.[8] Local causes of disease outbreaks were varied and nonspecific, just as they had been in the era of the early sanitarians. They would remain so several decades later, in the fullness of the Bacteriological Revolution, but with one crucial difference. The parallel recognition of specific, identifiable, and measurable causes—that is, germs—gave a qualitatively different kind of heft and specificity to the filth-disease nexus. When pathogenic microbes could (at least theoretically) be found in bodily excretions, drinking water, animal carcasses, and any number of other substances, the denunciation of various kinds of filth ceased to be merely one among many items in an etiological laundry list, and became a reliable and uniquely effective weapon in the hygienists' arsenal.

Overcrowded lodgings, the commingling of humans with animals, manure piles, and disorderly defecation: these transgressions were the most commonly recurring targets of disgusted hygienists' wrath in the early bacteriological era. Taken together, the reports of epidemic doctors and others charged with improving both urban and rural health articulate an acute concern with separation, containment, and boundary maintenance that resembles an updated version of the sanitarians' hygiene of bodily separation and aeration. (See chapter 2.)

Health reformers denounced overcrowding as consistently and vociferously in 1900 as they had in 1830. Here as in so many areas, if hygienists' reports are to be believed, the antithesis of civilization was to be found in rural Brittany. Typhoid outbreaks too often began there when a sick soldier was sent home on convalescent leave. "Then in the same house," wrote Jules Chauvel in the 1891 Academy of Medicine epidemic report, "we see fall ill in succession the parents, the brothers and sisters, those who care for the patient, those whom poverty forces to live in the same room, to breathe the same air." Given the lack of cleanliness "too common in such milieux," Chauvel elaborated, family members' hands, linens, and belongings could "transport the morbid germs" whether the water supply was contaminated or not.[9] In the academy's epidemic report ten years later, the problem and the region remained the same, even if the disease had changed. When scarlet fever sickened 191 residents of the Breton town of Audierne (Finistère) in 1901, killing four of them, the local epidemic doctor highlighted the sordid living conditions of the victims: "Cramped rooms sheltering up to ten people, overcrowding, insufficient windows, unbelievably dirty furniture, floors and walls that disappear under a layer of inveterate filth, accumulated garbage in the bedrooms, defective diet—here is the *modus vivendi* of the [Audierne] resident, no matter what his occupation."[10] Reformers frequently claimed that hygienic conditions had improved over the years (as Villermé had in his historical study of epidemics as early as 1833), but outrageous examples of atavism continued to figure prominently in their investigations throughout the nineteenth century and into the twentieth. As depicted by hygienists, the Breton peasant family remained as disgusting as it had been when Villermé and Benoiston had written their scathing report in the early 1840s. Overcrowding caused disease in 1901 just as surely as it did in the pregerm era, but microbes endowed the causal relationship with greater specificity and a new kind of certainty.

Just as disgusting and dangerous as the crowding together of human beings was their indiscriminate commingling with animals. The domestication and exploitation of animals may have been a distinguishing mark of human development in its upward progress from barbarism, but civilized nineteenth-century society demanded a strict separation of human and animal bodies in everyday life.[11] In the words of a local health board concerned about the presence of animal parts and blood on streets and inside markets, the failure to enforce appropriate separation and disposal was "as contrary to the most rudimentary [standard of] cleanliness as it [was] to public health."[12] As was the case with so many other perceived health hazards, the notion of disease-causing microbes did not itself make animal-human contact disgusting, nor did it make it dangerous, but it did refocus attention in a new, more specific, and potentially more alarming way on the danger posed by the disgusting. In 1879, for example, the newly created health board in Le Havre urged the mayor to enforce a cleanup of certain intersections in the city where particular kinds of refuse tended to accumulate. Particularly disturbing were the "residues of dead dogs" that "compromise[d] public health" by giving off "dangerous emanations."[13] Four years later, the Bordeaux physician Arthur Armaingaud warned in his "popular instructions" about typhoid fever that pets should be kept out of bedrooms "not only [because] they contribute to the vitiation of the air, but also [because] they can serve as vehicles for disease germs."[14]

At times, the animal-disease connection appeared as a simple empirical juxtaposition, as in the response to an incipient dysentery outbreak in Givors (Rhône) in 1889. Two cases occurred in the same house within a few weeks of each other; when the house's well was emptied, a dead dog

The Great Stink of Paris

was found at the bottom.[15] When a Lille city council member complained in 1893 about dog corpses lying in stagnant water near the general hospital, he posited a disease link with an ostensibly scientific justification: "During the hot weather, flies will throng to these cadavers and will then go deposit the virus on the meat at the slaughterhouse."[16] The same claim could have been made in nearly identical terms in the pregerm era, but the currency of bacteriology in the 1890s made the danger slightly more real and more immediate. Finally, elaborately bacteriological justifications were occasionally offered to support calls for animal separation and disposal. One doctor hypothesized that animal-human contact might have helped lay the groundwork for the serious diphtheria epidemic that swept across the Nord department in 1894 and 1895. Housecats and barnyard fowl in particular were capable of spreading the Loeffler bacillus, Lille physician Georges Dumont argued. "Gallinaceans go into houses, and I have seen some of them pecking at dust that might contain the dried sputum or vomit of diphtheria patients." Dumont reported that during the epidemic, birds in some patients' houses showed signs of illness, and were immediately killed. For their part, cats posed an even greater danger: "Cats, which climb onto beds and play with sick children, can serve as vehicles for infection; the microbe travels to the throat either directly or . . . from the animal's fur, which it licks; they then contaminate their fellow animals, and spread the epidemic far and wide. In one of the centers of the epidemic . . . two cats fell sick; one, which had been petted by [patient] number 12, began coughing and remained sad with no appetite for several days; the other died, after showing the same symptoms."[17] The animals' mobility and potential intimacy threatened the human body's separateness and self-containment; the Loeffler bacillus only enhanced the status of the threat.

Perhaps the ultimate statement of the danger represented by the everyday commingling of animals and humans can be found in the fourteenth arrondissement of Paris in 1895. The deliberations of the district health commissions in the capital consisted in large part of reports concerning visits to residential and industrial buildings that had been the object of neighbors' complaints or the site of deaths from infectious disease. The state of affairs discovered by the commission's investigators at 133 rue de l'Ouest simply defied civilized hygiene in nearly every way imaginable: "In a fairly small courtyard, chickens and pigeons confined in wire netting, spreading unhealthy odors. . . . Past this small courtyard, an extremely cramped room inhabited by a woman and her daughter, who have suffered from measles and typhoid fever: in this room there are, in addition, a dog, a cat and a guinea pig, [and they all] spread bad odors. On the second floor, a room where a three-year-old child has had [diphtheria], and across the way, a tiny room occupied by a woman and a large dog." One might imagine various remedies that could be proposed for this house, but for the district commission's reporter, there was one that imposed itself above all others: "The elimination of all of these useless animals is indispensable in order to avoid the return of contagious diseases."[18] The description recalls Dr. Decool's report on the lodgings of Flemish workers in Hazebrouck (without the ethnic stereotyping): the stench, disorder, and fundamental disregard for the civilized arrangement of bodies are so blatant that the reporter does not even need to draw a direct medical connection between the animals and the contagious diseases. The disgusting scenario speaks for itself.

In the countryside, of course, animals (especially of the larger sort) were far from useless, and nobody thought to propose their elimination. They did, however, tend to produce large amounts of waste—*fumier*, or manure—which could be both a source of agricultural prosperity and a health hazard. Like animal bodies, manure could be tolerated in a civilized society only if it were carefully contained and managed. Most often, *fumier* crises that threatened public health originated in individual farms, but occasionally entire towns seemed to be drowning under mountains of manure. Marcolez (Cantal), a village in the rugged Massif Central region, was a case in point in 1879, when typhoid fever "invaded" from two towns a short distance to the north. The 600 residents lived along a single street, in two-story dwellings described vividly by the local epidemic doctor in his report to the Academy of Medicine: "The lower story is occupied by animals, most often pigs; the family lives on the upper story. The inhabitants, all small farmers, consider manure their most precious source of wealth. They accumulate around their house all of the detritus they can gather, they collect stagnating rainwater, and they add—either by throwing out the window or by a hole connecting the [house's] two stories—all of their garbage and refuse."[19]

In Marcolez, the rural ethos of letting nothing go to waste and the embrace of animal excrement as a vital element in the organic cycle collided head on with the newer, urbane code of hygienic containment and separation. The village's drinking water was taken from two troughs whose edges were flush with ground level and encouraged the mixture of the drinking water with the runoff from the "layers of manure." Even before the typhoid epidemic, the population looked "sickly and debilitated," according to the report, their skin "discolored, or rather with a drab and grayish coloration":

"Mediocre physical development, slow movements, inactivity. Truly this whole poor etiolated population expresses something miserable and sickly. If one adds to these conditions the introduction of typhoidal elements, the rapid spread of the disease can be easily understood." The author of the academy's epidemic report, Dr. Henri Guéneau de Mussy, considered Marcolez's typhoid epidemic a typical scenario, combining the key elements and underlying chronology of the average French epidemic in 1879: "Before the arrival of two subjects afflicted with the illness, no fever, despite the most deplorable hygienic conditions; after the introduction, combination of circumstances most favorable to the dispersal of the germs [germes], and to their mixture with the drinking water."[20] Although the report was likely written in the early months of 1880, before Karl Eberth's claim to have identified what he called *Bacillus typhosus*, the typhoid bacterium, Guéneau de Mussy used "germ" in the older, more general sense—a seed of disease, of whatever nature, in some way particular or unique to a given disease.

This early case provides a clear and straightforward example of how the new germ theory was linked with and integrated into the old etiology of filth and transgression. As *germes* gave way to microbes and etiological links became more specific and more directly verifiable, the causal role of filth was refined, and bacteria could actually be found in certain disgusting substances. The core of the nascent sanitary-bacteriological synthesis, however, shows through even in the Marcolez typhoid report. Two years later, accumulated manure reportedly caused another typhoid epidemic in the Breton village of Lanhouarneau (Finistère), a place described by its local epidemic doctor in a tone recalling that of the Marcolez account: according to Léon Colin, author of the academy's 1881 epidemic report, "The endemicity of typhoid fever in . . . Lanhouarneau is tied to local conditions of uncleanliness so revolting that one could scarcely believe it; imagine dwellings [situated] below the stables, so that the liquid runoff [from the manure] floods down into them without being able to drain out; so much so that the only room of the dwelling is a stinking pool, in some places 20 centimeters deep, in the middle of which one must put large stones in order to ford it from one piece of furniture to another, [or] to get to the table, the bed, or the door." It was impossible to know whether the disease originated spontaneously in such filthy conditions or whether they merely presented fertile soil for the "reproduction of its germs [germes]." What was important to emphasize, in his view, was that observing "the precepts of public hygiene" could have prevented the epidemic.[21]

The same refrain sounded regularly through the 1880s and 1890s, particularly when typhoid fever struck rural communities. Favorable topographical and geological conditions and an ample supply of clear water, "which dissolves soap perfectly," did not save another Breton village, St.-Sulpice-des-Landes (Ille-et-Vilaine), from an epidemic in 1890. Filth trumped the town's natural advantages: nearly every house had a manure pile in front of it, which when washed by the rain gave rise to innumerable puddles of infection. One of the largest pools adjoined the town's only well. The epidemic doctor lamented this spoilage of nature's bounty, and denounced the "revolting dirtiness" of the area around the well; indignant disgust seems to have fueled even the most restrained and scientific interventions in the discussion of filth and infectious disease.[22]

Hygienists found themselves amazed at the variety of ways in which backward peasant mores could harm public health. Upon investigating a typhoid outbreak in Les Andelys (Eure) in 1901, the local epidemic doctor discovered a quaint local custom. There were three ponds around the town, each of which was fed by manure runoff and in each of which residents regularly washed their laundry. Water from these three ponds was rumored to make the best cider in the region.[23] Moreover, *fumier* did not only cause typhoid fever, according to contemporary accounts. When a particularly serious measles epidemic hit the town of Mèze (Hérault) in 1890, local authorities demanded that all manure piles be removed, in conjunction with street cleaning and the distribution of disinfectants.[24] A 1901 scarlet fever outbreak at the girls' primary school in Angerville-l'Orcher (Seine-Inférieure) was likewise blamed on a manure pile next to the school.[25]

Peasants' own thoughts about the possible danger of carelessly kept manure piles do not appear in the written record, for the most part. Hygienists assumed that a combination of apathy and economic self-interest drove most farmers to accumulate manure regardless of whatever health risk it might pose. There are scattered bits of evidence, however, suggesting that at least some peasants had become relatively less tolerant of potentially hazardous filth. Local authorities were occasionally called upon to intervene when rural neighbors accused one another of violating basic standards of cleanliness and public hygiene on their property. In 1898, for example, one resident of Courlon (Côte-d'Or) wrote to the prefect (in a halting script riddled with grammatical and spelling errors) urgently requesting help in enforcing the cleanup of a neighbor's manure pile that had been "flowing into the street" and was "very unclean." (The prefect managed to persuade the mayor to intervene, and the matter was apparently resolved.)[26]

Although it is impossible to know exactly how representative such attitudes were among the peasantry as a whole, the fragmentary evidence suggests at least that demands for increased cleanliness occasionally came from the bottom up, and were not the exclusive province of hygienists and government officials.

The final major category in this taxonomic review of disease-causing filth is the one that overshadows all the others: human excrement. No substance provoked as much hand-wringing, outrage, investigation, and reportage as did this most elemental and natural of human productions. The central dynamic of the sanitary-bacteriological synthesis played itself out in the case of this primal threat as it did with most of the others. First, before the Bacteriological Revolution, excrement was disgusting and caused disease in ways that were nonspecific and based on descriptive observation. Subsequently, references to the germ theory and analogies to recent medical discoveries suggested that it could carry and spread "germs" in conjunction with other disgusting substances and behaviors. Finally, when laboratory methods could identify and culture specific pathogenic microbes in samples of excrement, the demonstrable presence of these microbes took center stage, with the disgusting elements assuming a supporting role.

Thus, "old fecal matter" that had accumulated in the sewers beneath a secondary school in Lyon was denounced as "the source of infectious germs" in 1881.[27] In 1883, Armaingaud called attention to a danger that was both more specific and more wide-ranging:

> The *contagious principle* [of typhoid fever] is contained if not exclusively, then at least principally in the *intestinal excretions* of the patient. . . .
>
> As a consequence, these excretions play a preponderant role in the spread of the disease, and all objects that may have been in contact with this substance, all places where they have been deposited or may have penetrated—even if just in the form of an . . . imperceptible particle, dried up and mixed with dust—can serve as a support structure, a medium of preservation, and a vehicle for this contagious principle.

Here Armaingaud took a crucial step in the development of the SBS: the fact that the specific causal agent could be found in visible and palpable samples of excrement did not mean that hygienic efforts should be oriented only in that direction. He urged that preventive policies such as disinfection should target *all* of the places and objects that may have been contaminated even indirectly by excrement:

patients' clothing, linens, bedding, furniture, curtains, all objects in their sick rooms, the containers in which they have defecated and urinated, toilets, cesspits, sewers, the ground on which their excretions might have been emptied, the air in which they subsequently spread when dried, the particles of these substances deposited on furniture, clothing, between floorboards, the drinking water provided by wells, fountains, watercourses, gutterspouts . . . [and] finally the milk that we drink, into which these particles can be mixed either through the water that sellers often add or through the water in which containers are washed.[28]

Air, water, soil, indoors, outdoors, manmade objects, everyday living spaces: it seemed the "contagious principle" of typhoid fever, though it originated in excrement, could be lurking anywhere and everywhere! Indeed, the technical challenge for disinfectors and hygienists was daunting. However—and this dimension of the question ultimately lay at the heart of the SBS—individuals could and should protect themselves by regulating their own personal lifestyles. In the same pamphlet intended for popular audiences, Armaingaud insisted on the need for moderation in all things: "It is therefore necessary to be more sober, more regulated than ever in one's habits; to avoid excesses and fatigues of all sorts." Individuals should also make sure to avoid all contact with human excretions, and to make sure that toilet lids and all other openings connecting the air of the house with a sewer or cesspit be fully sealed to prevent contamination.[29] Three years after the Great Stink of 1880, a sophisticated preventive agenda focused on specific microbes was well under development, but the notion of germs spreading through fecal emanations remained credible and frightening.

The Lasnier family of Flamets-Frétils near Neufchâtel-en-Bray (Seine-Inférieure) represented both the zero point of civilized hygiene and a cautionary tale regarding the dangers of indiscriminate defecation. Around the first of August 1892, soldier Eugène Lasnier was sent home to Flamets-Frétils on convalescent leave from his unit's garrison in Africa. At the time, Lasnier was partially (but not fully) recovered from a serious attack of dysentery contracted in Africa. A week after his return, his mother fell ill; on August 15 it was his brother Ernest's turn, then a few days after that his other brother Emile became sick. On August 23 the widow Callot, who had washed the Lasnier family's laundry, took ill, followed a few days later by her nineteen-year-old daughter. All had the obvious symptoms of dysentery. The succession of cases did not stop there: a road construction worker named Séraphim Présumé, who had complained of foul odors when walking by the Lasnier house, but had never entered it, became sick on August 28, the same day that Eugène Lasnier's mother died. Two of Présumé's children quickly followed suit, and one of them died less than a month later, two days after Présumé himself succumbed. A boy hired to tend the Lasniers' cows took sick in mid-September; he died less than a week later, but not before infecting his mother, who became the eleventh patient. Finally, on October 1, a woman who lived in a cottage on the Lasniers' land fell ill; she had helped out in the Lasnier house during the various family members' illnesses. Twelve cases and four deaths, all traceable to one house.[30]

What made this house such a hot zone for dysentery infection was the family's careless handling of patients' excretions, according to Dr. Marquézy, the local epidemic doctor:

> Despite the recommendations of [the treating physician] the most elementary measures of cleanliness were not taken in this house. . . .
>
> The Lasnier family had taken no precautions; the patients let go of their excretions in their bed or, if they had the time to get up, they did not bother to go in a bowl, but rather just squatted and dropped their filth [*faisaient tomber leurs ordures*] on the stone floor in every corner of their rooms; when they went in a bowl, despite the doctor's recommendations, they threw the haphazardly disinfected excretions into the garden on top of their vegetables.

When the house was cleaned, Marquézy continued, the cleaning water was simply pushed out through the front door into the same garden. The garden sloped downward to the street, where its runoff drained.[31]

Although epidemic doctors, subprefects, and prefects generally affected a tone of matter-of-fact administrative efficiency in their correspondence, Marquézy and the subprefect to whom he sent his report seemed taken aback by this flagrant example of hygienic depravity. To infect others through neglect or carelessness was one thing, but to sink so low into the beastly depths of filth and thereby cause the deaths of three innocent people crossed another line altogether. When it came time to recommend remedial action for the authorities to pursue, Marquézy was flummoxed: what could be done in such a situation? "Unfortunately," he wrote, "the measure that seems best also seems difficult to accomplish, but I think I must suggest it to you: it would be to house the Lasniers elsewhere and *to burn the house that they have so thoroughly poisoned.*" He also called for the departmental disinfection tank for the linens and furniture of the other stricken families.[32] Medical science was all but powerless in the face of such foulness, the report seemed to suggest. Disinfection, a prebacteriological technique, could help around the edges of the problem, but an even older technique was the only thing capable of confronting backwardness of such magnitude.

It is difficult to overstate the pervasiveness of excrement and its management in discussions of infectious disease and public health in the late nineteenth century. The 1895 annual report of the fourteenth arrondissement health commission in Paris hints at the fatigue that could eventually set in among hygienists: "Each of [our] monthly sessions is devoted to the examination of pending matters, and among these [especially] the eternal and interminable question of toilets—poorly maintained, unclean, soiled, [consisting simply of] gaping holes, or fitted with malfunctioning apparatuses. . . . [It is a] long, fastidious enumeration that one finds every year and that one will continue to find for a long time in the reports of the [commission]."[33] This weariness was matched by a predisposition to assign excrement as a cause—somehow—to cases or outbreaks of disease. A creative example of this tendency can be seen in the 1888 epidemic report of the Academy of Medicine. An epidemic doctor named Bertrand submitted a report, praised and quoted at length by the academy's Auguste Ollivier, on an outbreak of dysentery at the naval base in Toulon (Var) on the Mediterranean coast. Bertrand noted that the toilets in the sailors' quarters were poorly designed and channeled excrement into storm sewers, which eventually emptied into the sea. "Stinking," "mephitic" odors permeated the toilets, the sewers, and the area near the sewers' outflow. No clear origin or direct cause of the dysentery epidemic could be isolated, but neither Bertrand nor Ollivier had any doubt as to its ultimate cause: "It is impossible that, whether as generators of fetid gases, workshops producing ptomaines, or culture media for microbes, the putrid matter of the sewers did not exert a harmful effect."[34] In other words, call it what you will, whether you believe diseases are caused by miasmas, specific chemicals, or bacteria, this powerfully foul-smelling substance *must* somehow be to blame. Without the evidence of a specific microbe (matching a specific disease) found in the substance or place in question, the link could be plausibly asserted. With that evidence, which was increasingly available in later years, the link was irrefutable.

In the twenty-first century, it is difficult to look at this material without thinking that of course the nineteenth-century hygienists were concerned about fecal contamination, because there really were (and are) deadly germs in excrement and infected excrement really was (and is) a predominant cause of disease. This interpretation is attractive, but simplistic and ahistorical. For one thing, disease-causing germs can be found nearly everywhere, in a huge variety of places and substances, not all of them related to human excretion and not all of them disgusting (then or now). Furthermore, the hygienic anxiety and denunciation surrounding excrement long predated the science of germs, and even well into the Bacteriological Revolution, it was not easy for scientists to isolate the actual microbes associated with major diseases in samples of fecal matter. To conclude that the concern about excrement was a result of the actual magnitude of disease traceable to that cause, one would have to imagine a scenario in which hygienists somehow knew the true proportion of the total burden of disease attributable to each conceivable "cause" and apportioned their professional attention accordingly. Did nineteenth-century public health authorities pay attention to poverty or malnutrition, for example, in proportion to their "true" contribution to the landscape of disease? Such objective truths are unknowable even today; nineteenth-century medical and public health knowledge should be evaluated according to the scientific, political, and cultural contexts that produced it, not according to hypothetical transhistorical absolutes. Individual texts must also be read contextually, their arguments, evidence, and tone assessed critically in order to develop a deeper understanding of the various factors that shaped both popular and professional responses to disease at the time. Viewed in this light, the obsessive focus on human excrement as a health hazard is neither right nor wrong; it is simply an accurate portrayal of acute cultural anxieties translated into scientific discourse and public policy.

Curiously, the late nineteenth-century hygienic crusade for cleanliness paid relatively little attention to the cleansing of the human body itself. When the issue was raised, most authorities agreed that Frenchmen bathed less often and less thoroughly than they should, but this shortcoming failed to rise to the degree of urgency accorded to other aspects of the cleanliness question. Armaingaud advocated bodily cleanliness in his popular instructions for avoiding various diseases, and all agreed that patients' caregivers should always wash their hands after touching sick bodies and handling bodily substances. In 1884, the Ministry of Education (*Ministère de l'Instruction publique*) issued a set of guidelines designed to make all French schools more hygienic places. The guidelines placed a premium on teaching students proper personal hygiene—setting an ambitious goal of one full bath per week per child—and encouraged teachers to set a good example for children with their own physical appearance.[35] Nevertheless, in the broader corpus of public health literature and policy debates, the cleanliness of the individual body enjoyed a far lower profile as a defensive strategy against infectious disease than did cleanliness in dwellings and streets.

Filth was so powerful as a cause of disease that in some circumstances, disgust could even trump bacteriology. In this fact lies a key to understanding the enduring strength of the sanitary-bacteriological synthesis, which normally ensured that the two elements went hand in hand. What happened when filth was present but germs appeared to be absent? One such instance occurred in 1896, when twenty-six-year-old Henri Combes died in a Montpellier (Hérault) hospital of a diarrheal disease initially diagnosed as cholera. After more than six decades of cholera scares, rumors, and actual epidemics, France had an established set of procedures that were set in motion whenever a suspicious case or death was reported. The prefect of Hérault directed Dr. Hamelin, the epidemic doctor for Montpellier, to investigate immediately. Combes, Hamelin discovered, had lived in a filthy apartment on the chemin de Sept-Camps but had also spent time since the onset of his illness at his aunt's house on the boulevard de Strasbourg, and had defecated in the yard belonging to the aunt's neighbors. If Combes had indeed died of cholera, the thorough (and expensive) disinfection required in such circumstances would have had to encompass not only Combes's apartment, but also the aunt's house and the aunt's neighbors' yard.[36]

Hamelin found, however, that Combes had been "profoundly debilitated" and malnourished for some time, and had lost much of his appetite not long before he fell ill. Meanwhile, carefully administered bacteriological tests at the hospital (presumably on stool samples taken from Combes) proved negative. (Hamelin's report does not detail exactly what tests were performed nor whether the sample tested negative only for the comma bacillus of cholera or for all known pathogens.) Combes had died, Hamelin concluded, of "simple gastrointestinal troubles, [which had been] fairly common lately." Disinfection was therefore unnecessary—at least for the aunt's house and her neighbors' yard. "As for the apartment occupied by Combes . . . we deemed it useful, given how filthy it is [vu son état de saleté], to disinfect it again." Hamelin ordered a full treatment with a variety of chemical disinfectants for all floors, walls, ceilings, furniture, toilets, and salvageable belongings; he had the piles of old clothing and rags that cluttered the apartment burned.[37] The epidemic doctor's decision could be justified on the grounds of prudence, but policy called for government-initiated disinfection only during or after a case of infectious disease. The bacteriological tests ostensibly established that this case did not belong in that category, but the apartment's filthy state provided more eloquent evidence than did the hospital's laboratory. Once again, the agenda of "not everything that stinks kills"—according to which only the laboratory, not the senses, could detect true health hazards—failed to provide a convincing framework for public health policy. Even as late as 1896, bacteriology did not have the last word; the evidence of the senses could not be denied.

The training of the senses that made the crusade against filth possible must be attributed principally to long-term cultural change, although medical science certainly added to its momentum by finding new reasons to denounce transgressions against the hygienic code of separation and containment. But there were still other historical forces that shaped the cleanliness impulse in late nineteenth-century public health. Chief among them were the social renegotiation that attempted to integrate the peasantry fully into a modern French national identity, and a national political shift away from accommodation with conservatism and toward aggressively anticlerical republicanism.

THE POLITICS OF FILTH

The question of the peasantry's health consciousness was a relative one; each observer's assessment depended on his expectations. A few optimists believed that the hygienic movement was making considerable headway in rural France. In 1878, Gaston Bourrée, epidemic doctor for the arrondissement of Châtillon-sur-Seine (Côte-d'Or), echoed Villermé's claim that civilization was steadily and inexorably improving sanitary conditions in the countryside: "Well-being is penetrating even into the smallest villages, and general health is much better than it was twenty years ago. Better nourished, comfortably clothed in winter, country people are beginning to understand the usefulness of following the laws of hygiene. It is not yet perfection (which is not of this world, they say), but accepting the results as they are, we can only rejoice to see the efforts of those who work for the happiness of their fellow men begin to bear fruit."[38] This view, however, was in the distinct minority. The Academy of Medicine observed that epidemics usually caused more devastation in the countryside than in the cities because of the "worse than rudimentary" hygienic conditions that prevailed in most villages, and that offered up "no obstacle to the assault of contagious diseases." One epidemic doctor in eastern France carefully enumerated peasants' "deplorable" living conditions—manure piles and "streams" of manure runoff in front of houses, few windows, small and dirty rooms, refuse-strewn courtyards, wells infected by manure piles and cesspits ("if cesspits even exist!")—and commented, "At least they have the fresh air of the fields to counterbalance so many noxious influences!"[39] After reading this litany alongside so many others, one can only wonder how fresh the air of the fields actually was.

Many observers also argued that hygienists could not ask too much of peasants. "It is not possible to ask country folk to practice disinfection," concluded the local epidemic doctor in response to an 1899 measles epidemic in Elesmes (Nord). The most one could expect was for them to wash their laundry and their floors.[40] Not everyone would have agreed with such a pessimistic judgment, but the underlying truth could not be denied: peasants were different from the rest of the population, and everybody involved in public health knew it. The world's most advanced medical science would prove fruitless unless something could be done to bring the peasantry into the mainstream of French society.

The goal was a social one, pursued over the long term, but it intersected with some shorter-term political agendas in the last quarter of the century. The consolidation of republican authority in the 1880s operated in concert with the attempted integration of the rural population into a genuine national identity, and public health was a crucial battleground in both efforts. Some felt that only the power and prestige of the national government could drag peasants into the modern age. The mayor of Buffon (Côte-d'Or), for example, tried in 1884 to implement "the work of the immortal Pasteur" in his town by ordering refuse, manure, and animal corpses to be disposed of in safe and approved places. He encountered nothing but resistance, as he noted in a plea to the prefect: "The difficulty of convincing country people is such that it would be good for at least an extract of the health board's instructions to be posted *officially*—that is, *bearing your signature*." Marked publicly as the prefect's official instructions, the mayor added, "this advice . . . would surely be followed."[41] Whether the mayor truly believed this or was simply trying to evade the responsibility for enforcing an unpopular measure, the fact remains that efforts to make the countryside cleaner and healthier were closely associated with the institutions and authority of the republic.

Nearly every aspect of public health could be imbued with political significance in the tense and uncertain environment of the early Third Republic. As standards of cleanliness were changing, so were expectations concerning the government's responsibility for protecting its citizens' health and the scope of state action. Just as the town of Bessan (Hérault) was preparing to celebrate the new national holiday of July 14 in 1881, an unusually severe measles epidemic began sickening and killing local residents. Solicitous of the fragile emotional state of grieving and fearful families in the "very re-publican" town, the mayor and city council canceled their carefully planned celebration of republican ascendancy, and limited the official observance to the illumination of public buildings at night. The curtailed festivities emboldened the mayor's political opponents (according to whom "all of the dead belong to notoriously republican families") to claim the epidemic as "vengeance from the good Lord" in response to a recent ban on religious processions.[42]

Mindful of the danger of such subversive propaganda, the subprefect in Béziers made sure to keep himself regularly updated by the mayor of Bessan and two other political allies, including the local epidemic doctor. The mayor ordered a variety of antimeasles measures, including street cleaning, disinfection, the lighting of fires in the streets, and recommend-ing scrupulous cleanliness to the population. He even "inflicted some exemplary punishments" on those who failed to heed instructions. The epidemic doctor, referring alternately to "miasmatic emanations" and to "the infectious organisms that are regarded today as the element of a large number of diseases," praised the mayor's diligence in his reports to the subprefect.[43] Whatever the ultimate effect of the mayor's policies, by the time the measles epidemic had run its course less than a month after it had started, the subprefect could certainly congratulate himself on the quality of his political informants.

Epidemics were not just an occasion for political reconnaissance; they were also an affront to a central republican value: the duty of protection. Also in Hérault, the inspector of indigent asylums in the city of Montpel-lier protested to the mayor about hygienic conditions in the facilities, which he said were unworthy of a modern civilized nation.[44] Another unusual measles epidemic in Hérault, this time in the upland village of Le Caylar in 1883, raised the same issues in the mind of Dr. Lapeyre, the epidemic doctor in Lodève. This outbreak presented what Lapeyre called a "typhoid" character, with "irregular" symptoms and especially severe complications. Lapeyre blamed the "foul air" and typically filthy conditions of the towns' streets and homes for the gravity of the epidemic. In his report to the sub-prefect, he urged the local authorities not to shy away from bold and intru-sive measures:

> In matters of health, we must constrain people to do what is helpful for them, and to avoid what can harm them. In this respect, the residents of a locality can be treated like minors. . . .

> Poor and rich alike have the right to expect from city officials clean air, good water, clean streets, and a good enforcement of health regulations [*une bonne police de salubrité*]. This is the first duty of the mayor and city council.[45]

Lapeyre articulates here a perspective on government and social welfare that is surprisingly modern for a relatively remote French subprefecture in 1883: the state has a duty to provide sanitary living conditions for its citizens, and in the performance of this duty it should treat them essentially as children, who often need to be forced to do what is good for them. Citizens, in turn, have a right to expect the various organs of the state to be vigilant in the protection of public health, in the provision of clean water, air, etc. This is precisely the prevailing expectation that expressed itself in the outrage of Parisians during the Great Stink three years earlier. After receiving Lapeyre's report, the subprefect immediately wrote to the mayor of Le Caylar, expressing dismay at not having received any news from him about the epidemic and any remedial measures. The letter insisted on the necessity of removing manure piles from all public spaces and cleaning and disinfecting streets, "the uncleanliness of which is one of the principal causes of the epidemic." The subprefect reinforced his demand for action with a dire warning: "I ask you to make sure that these hygienic measures take place daily at times that you will designate. You will be held responsible if the health of [your town's] residents continues to suffer from the unhealthy state of the streets and public squares, over which you alone have policing authority."[46] This aggressive directive took a step beyond the usual missives from prefects or subprefects to mayors urging hygienic remediation. The subprefect of Lodève threatened real consequences if action was not taken; the threat may well have been a bluff, but it still testifies to shifting expectations and advancing thresholds for government accountability.

Jules Cambon, prefect of the Rhône department, adopted a similarly hard line in 1889, when reports reached him of seriously unhygienic conditions in the Guillotière quarter of Lyon. Cambon (who would later gain renown as a diplomat during the Spanish-American War and World War I) minced no words in the circular he sent to all neighborhood police precincts demanding "strict enforcement" of "all health measures," particularly where courtyards, stairways, and toilets were concerned: "To this effect, you will see to it that the officers under your orders make the rounds [through your precinct] as frequently as . . . possible, and you will not hesitate to write up citations against any landlord . . . who, after receiving due warning, violates the provisions of the municipal ordinances."[47] There is no evidence indicating how aggressively Cambon's crackdown was pursued by the police. Even if enforcement was not as assiduous as the prefect would have liked, however, the circular testifies to the atmosphere of heightened expectations that surrounded state sanitary policy during the 1880s and 1890s. Progress and reform, guided by science, lay at the very heart of the republic's self-image.

Equally central to the identity of the Third Republic in its formative years was anticlericalism. The line separating religion from politics was always a thin one in nineteenth-century France, and it often disappeared altogether. While Catholic traditionalists saw the secular republic as a transgression of divine law and of the eternal essence of Frenchness, anticlerical republicans saw the church as not only oppressive and obscurantist, but as the single greatest obstacle to progress in the modern world. The two reports on typhoid epidemics in the early 1880s cited at the beginning of this chapter concerned two very different regions and populations. The filthy, typhoid-ridden peasants of the arrondissement of St.-Malo were Breton; the filthy, typhoid-ridden industrial workers of Hazebrouck were Flemish. The dominant French culture had long stereotyped Bretons as tradition-bound, illiterate, alcoholic, and dirty.[48] There was no comparably common stereotype of Flemings. The dominant trait of the Flemish people in the eyes of French officials was their devout Catholicism—perhaps the only significant characteristic other than a foreign language that they shared with Bretons.[49] To epidemic doctors and their republican allies in the late nineteenth century, to be devout was to be backward, and to be backward was to be dirty.

Epidemic reports often accused religious institutions of being hotbeds of disease as well as of political subversion; in fact, it seems that republican officials tended to see these two threats as two sides of the same coin. Less than a year after Cambon's circular demanding stricter enforcement of the sanitary code in Lyon, Dr. Louis Bard (the epidemic doctor responsible for that city and its surrounding area) urged the prefect to enact a similar crackdown against a related health hazard: religious schools. Faced with a steadily increasing incidence of diphtheria, Bard complained that provisions calling for a school to be closed whenever a student came down with a serious contagious disease were too often ignored. Furthermore, he alleged, Catholic schools routinely hid cases that occurred among their pupils out of a spirit of "sectarian competition" and as part of a stubborn resistance to government intervention in church affairs. "No disciplinary repression has been undertaken against this systematic failure," Bard lamented. "A few severe examples would be needed to overcome it, and would certainly be welcomed by public opinion."[50]

The degree of mistrust and antipathy between church and state on the local level can be gauged by incidents such as the controversy over the diphtheria epidemic in Montigny (Seine-Inférieure). Beginning in December 1894, the disease attacked 30 of the village's 520 inhabitants. Emile Roux's new diphtheria antitoxin seemed to be effective on most patients, but either six or ten of them died (depending on which account is to be believed). Dr. Pennetier, the epidemic doctor, managed to identify the village slaughterhouse—surrounded by pools of stagnant water and manure piles—as ground zero of the outbreak. As he attempted to encourage disinfection and other preventive measures during the epidemic, he also identified a potentially deadly spreader of the disease: school books. Schools not only needed to be closed during an epidemic, they needed to be thoroughly disinfected as well; and a comprehensive disinfection of a school entailed the destruction of possibly infected books. In Montigny, the public boys' and girls' schools complied with these procedures, but on May 14, 1895 (nearly five months after the epidemic first broke out), the nun in charge of the Catholic school refused to surrender students' textbooks unless Mayor J. Périer would sign a reimbursement guarantee. The mayor replied that he would replace the books after a verified inventory was submitted. After consulting a lawyer in Rouen, the nun refused, and gave all school books back to the students' parents. Périer then had to contact each family individually (twenty-seven in all) to demand the books' return. Finally, on May 20, he collected the last books, and burned them all.[51]

Even then, however, the diphtheria epidemic had apparently still not run its course. Despite repeated visits to Montigny from the department's mobile disinfection tank, five new cases in four previously healthy families were reported in the last week of June 1895. When the prefect was informed of this latest resurgence, he demanded to know whether the four households involved had received school books from the uncooperative nun. The mayor responded immediately with the answer that the prefect had anticipated: indeed, the four families were among those to whom the nun had returned the possibly contaminated books. No new cases had appeared in public school families, whose books had been promptly destroyed.[52]

Extinguishing the epidemic itself was only one of the administration's priorities. It was important to establish for the record who had helped and who had hindered the battle against disease. Even before learning of the last five cases, the prefect wrote to the mother superior of the religious community to denounce the conduct of the nun who had refused to surrender her school's books. "She incurred a grave responsibility toward those families in whom she might have sowed the germ of the illness." The prefect concluded that "she deserves a most severe reprimand." On the other hand, the public school teachers received praise for their cooperation and hygienic good sense. Both the prefect and the epidemic doctor saved their greatest enthusiasm for Mayor Périer, who had gone above and beyond the call of duty in his handling of the diphtheria epidemic. "He showed the greatest zeal" and "constantly proved his devotion" to the republic, wrote Pennetier to the prefect. These terms were echoed in the prefect's citation awarding the mayor a silver medal for his dedicated service in time of crisis. The medal was presented, appropriately enough, at a special session of the Montigny town council on July 14, the republican national holiday.[53]

Contaminated books cannot have been the most serious public health threat facing France in the nineteenth century. Nevertheless, the tug of war over the school books in Montigny symbolically enacted a much larger and more important battle: the *Kulturkampf* that aggressively reasserted secular authority in every aspect of French society, and pointed an accusing finger at the Catholic church as all but synonymous with backwardness, uncleanliness, and disease.

The official reaction to the 1892 typhoid epidemic in the village of Mesnières (Seine-Inférieure) in Normandy also illustrates with unusual clarity the intertwining trajectories of the crusade against filth, anticlericalism, electoral politics, and public health. After several cases of typhoid fever broke out at the boarding school run by the Fathers of the Holy Spirit in Mesnières, the priests sent all students home to their families. Because the epidemic doctor of the arrondissement was thought to be associated with the reactionary clerical milieu, subprefect André Régnault himself reported directly to the prefect on this episode. Régnault began his own investigation after residents of Neufchâtel complained that the school was spreading typhoid fever into their city by sending possibly infected students home. He found that there had been a similar outbreak at the same school a year earlier, which a local physician (also known to be "a zealous champion" of "clerical ideas") had attributed to construction-related excavations. Régnault had reason to believe otherwise: "Numerous more impartial observers who are familiar with the Mesnières establishment have told me that everything there is but disorder and filth, and that the students live in very poor hygienic conditions. . . . I feel that hygienic measures observed in lay educational establishments should also be observed in schools that, under the cover of religion, too often [foster] only disorder and carelessness."[54]

Régnault's duty did not end at investigating the epidemic's causes and recommending remedial measures. Two weeks after his initial report, he sent the prefect an update. Thirty teachers—half of the school's staff—had left Mesnières since the beginning of the outbreak. This created an interesting political serendipity, Régnault noted, inasmuch as one of the prefect's local republican allies was running for election, and if the teachers returned before the election, "every one [of them] would vote for your friend's opponent." Given that it would be "very much in the interest" of the republicans that the teachers not return soon, Régnault recommended that the prefect designate "a doctor friend, member of the health board," to visit the school. (The implication was that the friend could keep the school closed until after the election.) "In any case," Régnault added, "it would have a very good effect for the fathers of Mesnières and especially the director to see that the administration is watching the establishment." He went on to discuss the election chances of other republican "friends" and their "reactionary" opponents.[55]

It would be a mistake to view this episode as an example of the unfortunate corruption of public health by political agendas. Rather, it ought to serve as a reminder that it is impossible to separate "objective" health concerns from "subjective" political ones. That priests were implacable foes of progress was as much an empirical fact (to an observer like Régnault) as was the notion that filth caused typhoid fever. How could one separate these two truths, and why would one want to? If one was interested in improving public health, then undermining the chances of antirepublican candidates in the upcoming election could only be a good thing. Medicine, religion, culture, politics—everything was of a piece. The Mesnières typhoid epidemic also shows indirectly how the public health surveillance system in France was meant to function, under the centralized bureaucratic system that dated back to the Napoleonic era and even (in incipient form) to the Old Regime.[56] National governments appointed prefects, each of whom was responsible for ensuring order and tranquility in his department. Prefects appointed subprefects to take care of administration on the very local level. In consultation with subprefects, prefects also appointed epidemic doctors to investigate and respond to local public health problems in each arrondissement. Epidemic doctors acted as supplemental political eyes and ears for the subprefects to whom they reported; the subprefects played the same role for the prefects to whom *they* reported; and the prefects fulfilled the same function for the national authorities in Paris. Surveillance and police power flowed outward from Paris to, for example, Rouen (capital of Seine-

Inférieure), then to Neufchâtel (the subprefecture), and then to Mesnières (and countless other remote villages). Information, in turn, flowed in the opposite direction.[57]

The Civilizing Imperative, at Home and Overseas

The intersection of these various historical tendencies and agendas—increasing intolerance of filth, positivist republicanism, secularization, and the drive to turn "peasants into Frenchmen"—put provincial hygienists and other reformers in a crucial position in the 1880s and 1890s. Responsibility for education, exhortation, cajolery, and other remedial action on the ground in remote towns and villages fell to subprefects, mayors, local notables, and especially epidemic doctors. Tireless soldiers in the battle to clean the dirty, moralize the dissolute, and heal the sick, epidemic doctors perceived their task as difficult and at times nearly hopeless, but never as something they chose to do. It was their responsibility, their patriotic duty, as educated Frenchmen.

The struggle to prevent epidemics by encouraging cleanliness has deep historical roots, and transcends changes in medical knowledge about disease transmission. A large part of this history is the history of disgust. The most ambitious and comprehensive vision of the historically shifting boundary between the acceptable and the unacceptable has been that of the German sociologist Norbert Elias (1897–1990). It is possible to see in the marriage of filth and germs the observable traces of the centuries-long series of cultural shifts that Elias called the "civilizing process." It was an uneven and gradual process, whose precise course is exceedingly difficult to discern. Beginning with the world of courtiers and the nobility, but eventually reaching haltingly throughout society, elaborate social codes constrained instinctual and what Elias called "animalic" behavior into increasingly restricted channels of acceptability. External social constraints gradually became internalized, and proscribed behaviors came to be accompanied by feelings of shame directed inward and of repugnance directed toward others.[58]

It has been written of Elias that "it is a trait of great works to be able to be proven wrong in particulars and still manage to offer a truth about the larger picture that would not have been achievable if all the particulars were right."[59] Critiques of the details of Elias's thesis have not convincingly challenged the notion of the civilizing process itself, which represents a potential blueprint for cultural historians: that between the fifteenth and nineteenth centuries in Europe, certain kinds of behavior associated with bodily functions and/or "instincts" came to be strictly regulated; that their regulation was accompanied and reinforced by strong emotional affect, social resonance, and stigma; and that external prohibitions in these realms eventually became internalized, while violations occasioned shame in the transgressor and disgust in others. The task facing cultural historians is to map carefully and critically the development of this process, to identify the who, what, where, when, how, and why of these changes, and to identify which practices and substances were proscribed under which circumstances.

Elias's own writings allude to but do not explore in depth the multiple historical meanings of disgust directed toward bodily substances. In the course of the civilizing process, he argued, the progressive muting of bodily expression and hiding of bodily functions was accompanied by a shift of outward physical conflict inward, to the individual psyche: "Social life ceases to be a danger zone in which feasting, dancing, and noisy pleasure frequently and suddenly give way to rage, blows and murder, and becomes a different kind of danger zone if the individual cannot sufficiently restrain himself, if he touches sensitive spots, his own shame-frontier or the embarrassment-threshold of others. . . . The danger-zone now passes through the self of every individual." New frontiers of sensibility also opened up new possibilities for gratification—and abjection: "Just as nature now becomes, far more than earlier, a source of pleasure mediated by the eye, people too become a source of visual pleasure or, conversely, of visually aroused displeasure, of different degrees of repugnance. The direct fear inspired in men by men has diminished, and the inner fear mediated through the eye and through the super-ego is rising proportionately."[60] One can just as well substitute other senses—smell in particular—for vision in this assessment. The "inner fear" signaled by disgust has become a powerful historical engine.

Following Elias's lead, several historical sociologists have attempted to apply the template of the civilizing process to the history of medicine and public health. Most of this work has focused on establishing that various practices and injunctions that today are associated with the rational avoidance of disease can in fact be traced to cultural and behavioral changes that took place long before there was any medical or hygienic justification for them. These rational justifications were then grafted onto the changed behaviors only in retrospect. In an overview of European responses to leprosy, plague, syphilis, and cholera, Johan Goudsblom has found "little evidence" that traumatic experiences with epidemic disease prompted significant changes in bodily conduct or even in the social meanings assigned to bodily conduct. In the mid-nineteenth century, for example, "the cholera scare only speeded up a [sanitary-reform movement] that already had a momentum of its own, propelled by disgust of stench and filth on the one hand, and by the rise of a class of engineers and administrators . . . on the other."[61]

Patrice Pinell has identified the late nineteenth century as a crucial stage in the civilizing process in France, as the secular educational system championed by Jules Ferry and his republican allies assumed responsibility for improving the behavior of the poor at the same time that germ theory revolutionized public health; as a result, according to Pinell, schools made hygienic education a central part of their curriculum, and "the neutralization of microbes . . . meant implementing a series of practical measures to civilize the lower classes."[62] The antituberculosis crusades of the Belle Epoque, recent research has also suggested, were animated to a considerable degree by the imperative of eliminating flagrantly disgusting public practices such as spitting, which was cast as the primary culprit in the spread of the tubercle bacillus throughout society.[63] Prohibitions against spitting in polite society, Elias showed, predated the medical anathema pronounced against the practice in the nineteenth century.[64] To the extent that there were causal influences at work in this case, then, it is more likely that cultural proscriptions shaped medical knowledge than the reverse.

The civilizing process might have started in Western Europe, but it eventually became a global phenomenon. It is difficult to witness the earnest, disgusted paternalism of the epidemic doctors and others who were fighting filth among the French peasantry and working classes without thinking of similar battles that were being waged in France's overseas colonies. Similarly loyal, dogged warriors in the service of republican ideals sought to clean up and lift up similarly backward and ignorant peoples for the benefit of the nation as a whole. In fact, it was the government of Jules Ferry, who first became prime minister during the Great Stink of 1880 and led the effort toward universal secular education in France, which inaugurated the wave of colonial expansion that brought most of West Africa and much of Southeast Asia into the French Empire during the succeeding decades.

In Senegal as in Brittany, civilized Frenchmen dedicated themselves to the seemingly endless task of impressing upon human beings who lived like animals the importance of cleanliness, order, and education. Their campaign proclaimed and reenacted their own superior, civilized status and the moral and physical degradation of the target populations, even as it sought to rescue the savages from their backwardness. Domestic reformers and colonizers alike invoked the intertwined ideals of republicanism and science as the driving forces behind their crusade. The work of civilization, they fervently believed, was undertaken in the mutual interests (whether they realized it or not) of the indigenous people of the colonies, French workers and peasants at home, and the nation as a whole. Only civilized peoples could assume the full rights and benefits of republican citizenship and of membership in the community of healthy, hard-working human beings.[65]

Science in general, and bacteriology in particular, served an important auxiliary function in the colonial enterprise just as it did in the civilizing imperative at home. Seven Pasteur Institutes were established in the French colonies between 1891 and 1914—in part to perform research on tropical diseases in their natural settings, but also to bring the practical gifts of French civilization to primitive populations, thereby demonstrating the essential beneficence of the colonial enterprise. Belief in what they called the "civilizing mission," along with the notion that colonized peoples could and would be assimilated into a culture of Frenchness allowed the colonizers to justify violent conquest within a discourse of rights and democracy.[66]

The chief differences between the backward populations at home and in the colonies were that the filthy Frenchmen stood closer to the bourgeois ideal on the scale of civilization than did their colonial counterparts, and because of their spatial proximity, represented a more immediate threat to the sensibilities and health of their compatriots. Less exotic, they were therefore even more disgusting. Moreover, the tremendous energy expended on educating uncivilized peoples overseas made it all the more difficult to accept the continued existence of persistent pockets of savagery at home.

Civilizing the poor was never a mere policy choice that could be abandoned in favor of others in case of poor results. To give up would have been to abandon one's community and one's homeland to a future of squalor, desolation, and ultimately extinction. In the face of daunting obstacles and popular apathy, French hygienists clung to a dogged faith in science, progress, and the republic. Elias's "process" connotes a misleading degree of impersonal inevitability, rather than a deliberate undertaking. Although Catholic missionaries were involved in French colonial expansion, to call the domestic enterprise a "civilizing mission" belies its fundamentally secular nature. Alice Bullard has referred to the French "civilizing project" in the South Pacific colony of New Caledonia.[67] "Process," "mission," "project": all capture a different aspect of this historical phenomenon. Those who were on its front lines did not consider it to be something as impersonal and automatic as a process, and they certainly would not have been flattered to be called missionaries. They approached their work as an imperative.

Even before bacteriology was widely hailed as ushering in a new era of public health based on disease-specific preventive and therapeutic advances, hygienic reformers expressed a mixture of optimism about future progress and acute frustration about seemingly insurmountable obstacles in the present. They appeared to view their project in part as a historical inevitability, and in part as a challenge to their personal sense of duty. Each setback, each disgustingly filth-ridden village represented another outrageous affront to the bourgeois sense of decency, but also another mountain to climb on the long journey to civilization. Epidemic doctors and other officials could and should bring the benefits of scientific medicine (whether old, like disinfection and isolation, or new, like diphtheria antitoxin) to every corner of France, but it was even more important in their minds that they communicate the message of cleanliness and public hygiene, lest a town be rid of one epidemic only to witness its stubbornly backward way of life give rise to another.

On this score, urban and rural hygienists sounded remarkably similar themes, even though they faced somewhat different challenges in their everyday labors. In 1881, for example, the health commission of the tenth arrondissement of Paris, found itself overwhelmed with complaints regarding the filthy state of stairways and courtyards in apartment buildings. Landlords blamed tenants, and tenants blamed landlords. Concierges reported seeing children sent by their parents to dump the family's waste on the stairway landing outside their door. Whom to blame? The parents were taught to do the same when they were children, and if evicted from their building would simply take their bad habits elsewhere, and be replaced by another family who would do the same thing. Faced with this "insurmountable barrier," the commission found itself "obliged to prescribe cleanliness without being able to show the way to obtain it": "In the current state of things, we are disarmed, but if we think of the future, a great deal of progress can be achieved. It is through instruction and education given to the child that we must attack the problem. Different habits must be inculcated starting at an early age, so that later on order and cleanliness appear to be natural." Schools could help in this effort, the commission believed, by teaching children to "reject [and keep] far away from them all that offends their sight and their smell."[68] In 1881, the bacteriological doctrine of "not everything that stinks kills" was just beginning to take shape. It was an aggressive and probably necessary assertion of scientific authority, but it could never colonize the hearts and minds of the broader population in the way that the SBS eventually did. The manifesto of the tenth arrondissement health commission would have been as timely and as apt in 1900 as it was in 1881.

While the health commissioners in Paris wrestled with their frustration and clung to their faith in progress, their counterparts in Ille-et-Vilaine were doing the same. They had heard yet another report on yet another typhoid epidemic in which basic cleanliness had been neglected and patients had not been isolated. Epidemic doctor Charles Delacour of Rennes could contain his anger no longer. "When will we obtain these vital precautions?" he burst out. "I have been submitting official requests that children's reading books contain, instead of absurd fairy tales, such summary instructions [regarding disease prevention], so that beginning in childhood our populations can be educated with notions essential to the conservation of life, just as with elementary agricultural science."[69] When it mattered (as was the case with farming), Delacour seemed to be saying, the community's values came to the fore, and progress was possible. The task at hand was to hasten the day when human public health was seen to matter.

Delacour returned to the same themes repeatedly in his annual epidemic reports for Ille-et-Vilaine. "How important it is," he wrote in 1885, "that appropriate books be made available to children in the primary schools, to publicize the danger and enlighten the population" at the age when education is relatively easy. "How important it is that we repeat everywhere we go: do not throw patients' excretions out the front door, bury them after disinfecting them, or [they] will leak into your well and poison you." Delacour added a revealing coda to this injunction: "Everyone must [understand] the immense progress that science is making for our age, [and] the new duties that result for the administrators of a country."[70] The direct antecedent in this case was typhoid fever, but the pattern holds more generally: the most advanced medical science in the world reinforced the familiar hygienic plea for cleanliness, and for a careful containment of bodily substances.

After Delacour delivered his 1888 annual report to the Ille-et-Vilaine health council, another member read a subcommittee report that called attention to two especially common causes of epidemics in the department, "so that each of us can educate those around him, and protect against" future outbreaks. The first danger was the dumping of garbage and manure near houses and wells, which contaminated water supplies and spread "various contagious diseases." The second was a common habit in Brittany "about which [the council] should warn our residents of the countryside": the keeping of henhouses inside the home. Because of recent research suggesting a similarity between a common fowl disease and diphtheria in humans, the subcommittee recommended "encouraging our rural populations" to keep henhouses as far away from human houses as possible, "to the great benefit of cleanliness and hygiene."[71]

It was fairly banal as far as health council reports go, but beyond the hygiene of cleanliness and separation, it suggests a special role for hygienists and a special relationship between them and their "populations." Each member of the council was to "educate those around him," "warn our residents," "encourage our rural populations." The epidemic doctor and his allies most often saw their duty not as bringing the benefits of medical science to the isolated corners of France as much as coaxing, uplifting, and civilizing their unenlightened fellow citizens. The conscientious epidemic doctor certainly administered medication when necessary, arranged for the departmental disinfection tank to be sent, and ensured that isolated diphtheria patients received antitoxin treatments in a timely manner. But he also laid the groundwork for a healthier future society through education on a one-to-one, everyday basis, even when the students showed little interest in the lesson.

Hence the response of Dr. Chartier, epidemic doctor in Nantes (Loire-Inférieure), to the prefect's request to investigate two reported cases of typhoid fever in the adjoining town of Doulon in 1891. "As soon as I received [your] letter," Chartier assured the prefect, "I went to the place [in question]." A three-story building in Doulon housed twenty working-class families and featured the same leaks, puddles, piles, stains, and stenches that pervaded the investigative sorties of every epidemic doctor, rural or urban. Chartier made detailed inquiries inside the two affected households concerning the health status of all family members and the care of the patients and their excretions. In the first household, where both husband and wife had recently taken ill and were being cared for (along with their two young children) by the wife's mother and another elderly woman, Chartier "recommended that [the caregivers] drink only boiled water, wash their hands and face when leaving the patients' room, never eat in [that room], keep all other people away [from the patients], and disinfect the linens and the vessels containing all excretions." The second affected apartment was that of the building's concierges, who lived on the ground floor with their three children, one of whom had recently shown symptoms of typhoid fever. "I gave the [mother] the same instructions that I had just given to her neighbors," Chartier reported dutifully. "I also urged her to keep her other children away [from their sick sibling], and to keep the courtyard in the cleanest possible state by washing it every day with a heavy flow of water." For good measure, Chartier asked the prefect to require the landlord to provide a direct conduit for all household wastewater to the cesspit, to ask the mayor to ensure that disinfectant would be added to the cesspit every day, and to enforce a prompt burial and complete disinfection if any of the patients died.[72]

The same advice could be found in the official instructions distributed by the national Comité consultatif d'hygiène publique as well as in countless other books and brochures. Dozens of other epidemic doctors throughout France probably gave the same advice every week. In fact, Chartier's recommendations were bound to be largely ignored, whether through carelessness or lack of means to carry them out. Nevertheless, it was important that he at least make the effort, and deliver the message promptly and forcefully. At his follow-up visit, he would probably express frustration at how little had been done, but eventually, in Doulon or in another town, he would take a measure of satisfaction in small hints of hygienic progress—a day's worth of garbage carefully disposed of, a relatively clean courtyard, a well-maintained toilet.

Success and failure in the campaign to civilize French workers and peasants can only be seen as relative. The continuing litany of complaints lasting well into the twentieth century on the part of epidemic doctors and ordinary citizens denouncing rural (and urban) filth might reasonably lead one to conclude that the hygienic message of cleanliness and containment had fallen on deaf ears. But if such denunciations reveal a continuing lack of public and private cleanliness, they also signify a refusal to tolerate the status quo. Those who passively accept filth as part of life do not lodge complaints about it, and there are scattered signs that intolerance was spreading. In any case, nobody was under any illusions that the battle would be quickly won.

The Academy of Medicine's Auguste Ollivier told the story of a terrible eighteenth-century epidemic in the village near Vannes (Morbihan) in Brittany in order to illustrate what hygienists were up against in that region. The investigating doctor visited in the spring of 1785 and found the gravedigger in the church cemetery, burying the most recent victims of the unnamed disease in already-occupied gravesites last used only four months earlier. The incredulous doctor railed against this flagrant abuse of hygiene, and after pleading his case to the residents, the priest, and the bishop, he had to appeal to royal authorities in Paris before the churchyard was officially closed to further burials. The epidemic "ceased immediately," but the residents never forgave what they considered an "insult . . . to their religion." Several years later, the doctor learned that the villagers had seized on the disruption caused by the revolution in order to reopen their traditional graveyard for burials, no matter how crowded it might be.[73]

In Ollivier's view, the churchyard affair symbolized Breton peasants' timeless "intellectual apathy" and "resigned fanaticism": "They vegetate in hovels without thinking to rid them of their refuse, to keep them clean, [or] to give them a bit of air and light, because they have always lived there or because the parents and the ancestors lived there as well. [Their] mental acuity is insufficient to conceive of improvement, [and] the sum of intellectual activity is too weak for any serious efforts to be made toward that goal."[74] Though Ollivier's explanation is fundamentally cultural, it almost sounds racial in its fatalism. It is possible to see a larger lesson in the episode, however—one that applies just as well to 1885 as to 1785. The Breton villagers did not resist hygiene and progress out of inertia or passivity, but rather out of a set of affirmative cultural decisions, clinging to a bodily esthetic of protective clustering and enclosure. The same could be said of parents who refused to impose strict isolation on a sick child. A coherent logic motivated their ostensibly backward and ignorant behavior; it was not a hygienic nor a scientific logic, but it was rooted in a consistent set of values that reformers ignored at their peril. The epidemic doctor saw only the logic of science and progress, and therein lay the key to his remarkable perseverance. Resistance to the civilizing imperative took many forms, and some could be rooted in affirmative adherence to alternative values rather than in apathy or intellectual insufficiency.

As the nineteenth century drew to a close, years of frustration and resistance from the public had not dampened the confidence of French hygienic reformers. In Paris, neighborhood health commissioners congratulated themselves in 1897 on the "irreproachable" quality of the municipal disinfection program, and predicted that with "perspicacity and energy," the public health movement would finally "force recalcitrant residents to understand the self-interest that results from a rigorous observation of hygienic measures." In the same year, the Academy of Medicine called attention to improvements in rural health due to "diet, housing, lifestyle, [and] wages." "Even though poverty and filth too often reign supreme," the annual report read, "they are tending to get better." Enhanced means of communication, easier transportation, and greater "material well-being" were reaching even into "the most isolated villages." Furthermore, doctors themselves were more competent, in the academy's view. Their education had become more scientific, and thanks to the recent "influence of Pasteurian doctrines," their search for the causes of epidemics was more likely to result in "serious prophylaxis."[75] Progress consisted jointly of scientific advancement and the conquest of poverty and filth.

From the crowded streets of Paris to the forgotten byways of Brittany, hygienic conditions left much to be desired, but they were moving in the right direction, according to the officials charged with their improvement. Epidemic doctors and their allies were fighting a long and uphill struggle not just to popularize disinfection or diphtheria antitoxin, but also to tear down age-old mores and rebuild new ones on hygienic foundations. The signs of failure that surrounded them every day only fueled their determination to soldier on.

6

Odors and "Infection," 1880 and Beyond

The tireless efforts of provincial epidemic doctors in the 1880s and 1890s to convert the rural populace to the civilized standards of bacteriological hygiene produced mixed results. Like Parisians, provincial families embraced specific technologies promising immediate protection—such as disinfection and diphtheria antitoxin—while for the most part rejecting isolation of their loved ones and adopting new standards of cleanliness only hesitantly. In the capital, where foul odors were blamed for spreading deadly germs in 1880, similarly equivocal changes took place during the years that followed.

THE GREAT STINK IN A MINOR KEY, 1895

If the government's goal in 1880 was to purify the urban milieu, prevent further vitiation, and eventually revitalize the nation through the physical and moral regeneration of its citizenry, its success even in the most limited of these aims is difficult to judge. The Great Stink of 1880 faded into memory in October, and the government commission issued its report the following spring. It warned of the presence of disease-causing germs in foul-smelling emanations and recommended against the *tout-à-l'égout* system, which would evacuate all Parisian waste through the city's sewers. In spite of sustained and forceful opposition, *tout-à-l'égout* remained the official policy stance of the local government, and finally became the law of the land in 1894 when parliament voted to mandate the new system for all buildings in Paris. (Fig. 12.) The replacement of the cesspit and *vidange* system by direct sewer hookups was a long, slow process, however, and debate continued into the early years of the twentieth century.[1] Although Parisians continued to complain periodically about summertime odors in

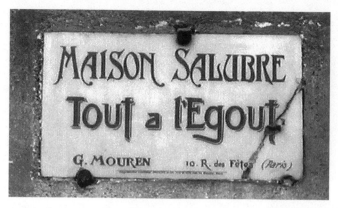

Fig. 12. "Healthy house—Tout à l'égout." Some apartment buildings in Paris advertise their hygienic modernity to this day, although the system was extremely controversial in the 1880s and 1890s. Photo by author.

the years after 1880, it was not until 1895—ironically, a year after the final legislative triumph of *tout-à-l'égout*—that a full-fledged stench in the capital grabbed headlines again.

"Fetid emanations," "nauseating" and "disgusting" odors, "Paris again turning putrid"—the noisy complaints that began in early June 1895 sounded like a reprise of August and September 1880.[2] Reaching peak volume this time in June but persisting into August, disgusted and indignant reactions to the odors of Paris again emphasized their intolerability and the urgent imperative of remedial action. Once again, the search for the culprits focused on the sewers and on suburban treatment plants, and once again local government officials were harshly criticized for inaction and complacency. Only the certainty of impending epidemics and the search for germs in the foul miasmas were missing from the response to the odors of 1895.

"A dull pestilence, penetrating and tenacious, weighs heavily on our great city, where one can no longer go out without holding one's nose," lamented *Le Figaro* on June 26: "It is impossible to stand on one's balcony, impossible to sit on the terrace of one of the busy, joyful cafés that are the pride of our boulevards, without thinking that one must be downwind from some uncouth, invisible giant. What's worse is that, the nicer the weather, the warmer the weather, and therefore the more pressing the need for fresh air—the more despotically this sneaky stench makes itself felt."[3] *Le Temps* also emphasized the stark contrast between the civilized Parisian pleasure of outdoor leisure time in late springtime and the repugnant unpleasantness that interrupted it in June 1895: "Few Parisians have been spared the unpleasant surprise, when strolling the boulevards or taking a breath of fresh air on the balcony, nose to the breeze, in the quiet of the evening, of suddenly breathing in a dull odor whose origin is impossible to tell: 'What a bad smell!' they think, disgusted and sickened."[4] Complaints in other newspapers similarly accentuated the degree to which the foul odors disturbed and spoiled various rituals of civilized life, such as the bourgeois family dinner.[5]

As in 1880, most experts in 1895 blamed the stench on either the sewers or the suburban waste treatment plants, or both. The press tended to side with what it called the "general" or "majority" opinion among Parisians, which ascribed the odors to emanations from "the thousand kilometers of sewers that carry under our feet, in a continuous flow, the digested residue of two-and-a-half million stomachs." Once again, the departmental prefecture (with administrative responsibility over the sewer network) insistently denied that the odors were coming from the sewers, and pointed with pride to the increased flow of water within the network, which it claimed rendered any significant and sustained odor impossible. "The administration to which we owe the genius of the 'tout-à-l'égout,'" mocked Le Figaro, "keeps too careful a watch over the cleanliness of its underground network, and floods . . . our refuse with too copious a volume of water, for there to be anything to worry about in that regard." The same newspaper printed an imaginary dialogue between an ordinary Parisian complaining about the offensive stench and an engineer who adamantly defended the sewers against any imputation of blame:

THE ENGINEER: Well, I'll have you know that the Paris sewers are the most beautiful in the world.

THE GENTLEMAN: That doesn't prevent them from smelling bad. . . .

THE ENGINEER: And not only are they beautiful sewers, but their cleanliness is also beyond reproach.

THE GENTLEMAN: I never said that—

THE ENGINEER: Much cleaner than the stairways in your home. . . . I would much rather live in a Paris sewer than in certain buildings in Montmartre or in the Mouffetard quarter. . . .

THE GENTLEMAN, scoffing: So perhaps we should start saying, "as clean as a sewer," then! . . .

THE ENGINEER: I know Paris from top to bottom. These odors that have been spreading out in the evening over the capital, I smell them just as well as you, and perhaps even better. Well, then, take this as a fact: there is only one place in Paris where it never smells bad!

THE GENTLEMAN: Tell me where, and I'll hurry there!
THE ENGINEER: The sewers![6]

Obviously, there were still many skeptics in 1895 who could not bring themselves to associate cleanliness—much less odorlessness—with the circulating "digested residue of two-and-a-half million stomachs."

Others pointed, as in 1880, to the suburban towns, and to the distasteful raw material treated by their industries. Bondy, Aubervilliers, Pantin, Saint-Denis: the list of suspects was a familiar one, and again some observers pointed to the geography of the odors to support their belief that certain prevailing winds ushered the putrid smells into the city. The northeast wind, usually associated with good weather, brought the industrial emanations of these northern and northeastern suburbs into the eighth, ninth, seventeenth, and eighteenth arrondissements of Paris, residents complained. It had become almost a proverb in Montmartre, several wits remarked: "It smells bad, so the weather will be good"; "When the weather turns rainy, Paris is spared."[7]

A final parallel between the responses to the odors of Paris in 1880 and 1895 can be seen in the indignant demands for government intervention. Parisians felt that aggressive remedial action of some kind—any kind—needed urgently to be taken, and that anything short of such action represented intolerable dereliction of duty. As one journalist put it: "I have to wonder what purpose is served by the health commission and the inspectors who are supposed to report to it. Frankly, we pay enough taxes to demand that our lungs have access to breathable air."[8] Members of the departmental Conseil général castigated the departmental prefect and the prefect of police, accusing each of shifting the responsibility for the odors onto the other's administration. Moreover, the councilmen claimed that as soon as an official protest was lodged with the local government or the question was placed on the council's agenda, the odors died down for several days. The insinuation was that Prefect of Police Louis Lépine had ordered his inspectors to crack down temporarily on the suburban treatment plants, curtailing their activity and thereby taking the political heat off of his administration for the time being. In the words of one council member: "The residents of Paris cannot tolerate the fact that, unless one of their representatives happens to force the inspection services into action, it is impossible for them to open their windows in the summertime."[9] This last remark was greeted with laughter in the council chamber—presumably the rueful laughter of assent, as several other councilmen shared similar opinions. The conviction was deeply held on the Conseil général that the government must, and could, stop the odors. At the close of the nineteenth century, taxpaying citizens of the French republic had a right to breathe air free of disgusting smells.

The Conseil général succeeded in prompting Lépine (under whose responsibility fell the public health council) to appoint another expert commission to study the odors and to recommend appropriate policy measures. This commission went even further than had its predecessor in 1880 to pin down the facts behind the elusive odors of Paris. The Commission to Study the Odors of Paris held meetings in plenary session and in "administrative" and "technical" subcommittees over a period of fifteen months, before issuing a lengthy and extraordinarily detailed final report, accompanied by a large fold-out map of the department (indicating the locations of potentially malodorous industrial establishments). The commission attempted to take advantage of recent scientific work on a "putridity index" that measured odors in different places and at different times with quantitative precision.[10] It solicited detailed information from every arrondissement's police headquarters and from every arrondissement's local public health council on all possible sources of bad odors in the entire department—street by street, block by block, house by house. The resulting list of "sources odorantes" (which takes up thirty-nine pages just for the city itself) includes the locations of, among other things:

poorly maintained buildings;
defective paving;
poorly maintained gutters;
garbage in the streets;
stagnant pools of wastewater;
certain sewer vents and manholes;
poorly maintained urinals;
garbage dumps;
markets;
washhouses;
stables and horse-drawn carriage stations;
workshop chimneys;
dye plants;
pigsties;
butcher shops;
hospital operating rooms;

innumerable commercial and industrial establishments dealing in animal parts or products;

cheese shops;

coffee roasters;

and building walls and street corners that served as "improvised urinals," in the euphemistic language of the commission.[11]

All of the enumerated sources of odors, the commission concluded, should be regularly inspected and brought under increased surveillance. The report also called for stricter laws and regulations governing hazardous industries, as well as for more rigorous application of unsanitary housing legislation and for popular education in personal hygiene.[12]

The commission's deliberations and final report also highlight the only area in which the reaction to the odors of 1895 differed significantly from that of 1880. In 1895, virtually nobody mentioned the possibility that foul smells or fecal emanations might contain microbes or cause disease. The commission's reporter, Dr. Alexandre Le Roy des Barres of the Seine departmental public health council, cited Henri Bouley's familiar axiom "tout ce qui pue ne tue pas," and even stated flatly that odors "do not engender, as was once believed, infectious diseases such as typhoid fever, typhus, and other epidemic diseases." It was indeed possible, the report suggested, for especially sensitive people to "experience real health troubles after continually breathing in fetid exhalations." More importantly for Le Roy des Barres and his colleagues on the commission, however, the disgust alone that foul smells cause "can be enough to disturb [a person] to the greatest degree."[13]

The fact that odors could not directly and specifically cause disease, moreover, was not a reason for physicians and hygienists to ignore them, in the commission's view: "The hygienist cannot be satisfied, in the presence of such a painful assault on the sense of smell, with negative solutions; on the contrary, he must make every effort to ensure . . . the cleanliness of the ground and the purity of the air and the water, the three elements of a city's health."[14] This sense of a wider mission beyond the immediate causes and health effects of bad smells informed the commission's entire work, and suggests that in 1895, as in 1880, the wave of offensive odors was but a trigger for an anxious reevaluation of the cleanliness and safety of the broader physical milieu of Paris. In an early commission meeting in 1895, one member complained that the odors of Paris were nothing new, and that previous attempts to solve the problem had failed because they had addressed only certain aspects of the question, without undertaking "a complete study of the air, the housing, the ground, and the underground" of the city and surrounding towns.[15] The temporary atmospheric disruption represented by the stench, it was urged, must serve as an opening to the real agenda of the commission—a thorough scientific assessment of the biological and chemical environment within which Parisians lived and died. Out of this impulse toward exhaustiveness grew, among other things, the commission's lengthy inventory of odor sources in the city.

Only one member of the commission in 1895 dissented from the consensus that the odors were unpleasant but not directly harmful to human health. Chemist and hygienist Armand Gautier refused to dismiss entirely the possibility that disgusting smells could either spread germs directly or testify to the presence of some other disease-causing influence. Where his colleagues focused on suburban industries and waste treatment plants, Gautier focused on the streets and sewers of Paris proper; where the other members saw disgust and discomfort, Gautier saw germs and illness. His reasoning was as follows: in order to isolate the locations and causes of the worst odors in a city permeated by a profusion of different smells, the commission should attempt to map the relative presence of ammonia in the air throughout the city; the smell of ammonia, he said, was both the odor most bothersome to the population and a "sure sign of the presence of putrefactive microbes." If, as he expected, the measurable proportion of ammonia declined as one moved from the narrow streets and slums of Paris to the open air of the parks and the suburbs, then the causes (and remedies) of the truly dangerous odors would be shown to be inside the city, in its streets and sewers. Similarly, Gautier argued, if it could be proven that odors can in certain circumstances emanate from the ground, and that the ground contains microbes "capable of giving off unhealthy emanations," then the commission would have to assume that it was possible for pathogenic germs to be spread by odors coming from the ground.[16]

Gautier's fellow commission members, however, neither believed that microbes or diseases could be spread in this way nor needed this claim as a justification for studying the odors of Paris. They warned against rhetorical excesses and public rumormongering as potential sources of panic: "What we must tell the public," argued Dr. Octave du Mesnil of the departmental public health council, "is that while it is justifiably complaining about a nuisance, it must in no way believe in the *harmfulness* of these emanations." Steadily repeated reminders of Bouley's dictum and of the remarkable progress made in recent years in public health reform and education would keep public attention where it belonged, du Mesnil hoped, and prevent irrational overreactions to unpleasant odors.[17]

Others on the commission urged a slightly different approach. One of Lépine's top aides at the Prefecture of Police noted that in this case, public opinion was mobilized not because of any putative health danger from the odors, but simply because they were unpleasant. Moreover, not all odors provoked public complaints, but only "one odor, almost always the same one, which is coming from a known source"—by implication, the excremental odor emanating from the suburban treatment plants, which were subject to the prefect of police's regulation. Why not simply address the complaints directly, and continue to crack down on the plants? This suggestion met with approval from Dr. Alfred Lamouroux:

> What the public is preoccupied with is the odor itself and not its more or less harmful effects on . . . health. What we should do, then, is to draft a classification of odors, taking as a scale of measurement the greater or lesser repulsion they provoke, and attempt to make those that are most intolerable and most nauseating disappear, or at least attenuate them.
>
> We would then have an immediate result that would be greatly appreciated, while continuing the long-term experiments called for by the commission.[18]

According to this approach, the allied sciences of biology, chemistry, medicine, and public health would join forces to adopt the protection of civilized sensibilities as an integral part of their mission, alongside the prevention of disease and in pursuit of an improved quality of life. Although it is unclear how many of the recommendations discussed by the commission were ever put into practice, the anecdotal evidence of newspaper reports and the Conseil général proceedings suggests that the Prefecture of Police took a more aggressive stance toward regulating the waste treatment plants during the summer of 1895.

One cannot exactly say of the odors of Paris that the tragedy of 1880 repeated itself as farce fifteen years later. Indeed, perhaps because of the memory of the vehement public outcry in 1880, authorities in science, medicine, and government took the odors of 1895 quite seriously. Yet it is noteworthy that many of the press accounts in 1895 adopted an ironic, even humorous voice of complaint, compared to the tone of urgency and danger that animated the complaints in 1880. Even more significant is the fact that nearly all of the reports in 1895 stressed the unpleasantness of the phenomenon and the discomfort it caused, rather than any potential or actual health effects. Foul odors had ceased to be a vehicle for deadly germs, although they remained a public nuisance of the first rank and a problem whose solution was politically imperative. No longer life threatening, the odors of Paris remained a threat to a way of life—the civilized urban life.

Although regulatory vigilance might have kept the odors of Paris at bay for a time, or attenuated their worst episodes, the smells could never, it seems, be eliminated entirely. Even in the first decades of the twentieth century, after both cesspits and plants treating human waste had begun to fade from the Parisian scene, disgusting odors continued to disrupt life in the capital periodically. At least twice more, in 1911 and in 1926, the summertime stench was bad enough to provoke further attention from the press, official investigations, and scientific reports. Parisians complained, pointed fingers, and demanded governmental action, as they had in 1880 and in 1895. Diseases and microbes remained absent from the discussion of intolerable odors.[19] Alongside the gradual switch from the cesspit system to the *tout-à-l'égout*, the fertilizer industry in the suburbs of Paris was undergoing change in the early twentieth century. Where treatment plants had previously handled primarily human waste, animal products (especially bones) and mineral phosphates were increasingly the raw material of choice. Studies on the odors of 1911 and 1926 incriminated the treatment of animal products for fertilizer production as the leading cause of the foul stench plaguing Paris. Temperature, humidity, wind direction, and barometric pressure were also seen as playing important roles in the spread of the smells.[20]

Although the phenomenon continued to be referred to generically in official reports as "the odors of Paris," without further description—as if the category was universally familiar and needed no qualification—human excrement (whether raw or treated) no longer figured centrally in the causation or prevention of the offensive smells. Here again, it is impossible to perceive exactly what the odors of Paris smelled like, but the examples of 1911 and 1926 suggest an interesting possibility: that a qualitatively distinct olfactory event was fitted into an administrative and scientific template derived from an earlier era and a different smell, and that the odors were understood (and perhaps even sensorially experienced) accordingly, as belonging to the familiar existing category "odors of Paris." Meanwhile, despite the disappearance of the causal link between putrid smells and disease, and despite the possibly changing nature of the odors themselves, the phenomenon known as the odors of Paris continued to be perceived as disgusting and intolerable, and it remained the government's responsibility to eliminate the smells and prevent their return.[21]

The Cemetery of the Innocents and the Long History of Parisian Odors

Looking backward from the late nineteenth century, the persistence of the odors of Paris is even more remarkable. Foul smells and residents' complaints about them were nothing new at the time of the Great Stink of 1880. In fact, complaints about the capital's stench could already claim a storied heritage of annoyance dating back seven centuries. King Philippe Auguste inaugurated a long series of royal attempts to regulate waste disposal in 1184, when he ordered the major thoroughfares of Paris paved with cobblestones to facilitate cleaning. Injunctions against the dumping of chamber pots and other waste into the streets were routinely ignored, as a 1270 report by the city's superintendent of streets (*voyer de Paris*) and a new royal edict in 1348 noted with exasperation. Every edict, every decree, every ordinance fell on deaf ears, it seemed. Parisians urinated and defecated in doorways and dumped their waste into the streets with impunity. The increasingly dense traffic of pedestrians, animals, and vehicles in the growing city served only to stir up the putrescent stew further, and to multiply the dangers posed to passersby in the rubble- and offal-clogged streets. The new esthetic of the Renaissance remade the architectural face of Paris and intensified demands for cleaner streets, but it did little to change the city's scent. In a 1539 edict, King François I voiced his "displeasure at the considerable deterioration visited upon our good city of Paris" and evoked the "great horror and greater displeasure" felt by "all valiant persons of substance" when contemplating the state of the city's streets. The edict mandated the installation of cesspits in every residence in the kingdom and reiterated the prohibition against dumping "refuse, offals, or putrefactions" into the street. Once again, the official pronouncement went unheeded and unenforced. Even the eventual proliferation of cesspits in the capital did little to solve the problem of unpleasant odors, inasmuch as the receptacles' contents had to be regularly emptied and carted through the city for dumping.[22]

By the middle of the eighteenth century, the city's population had outgrown its old walls, and bodily waste was not the only foul-smelling result. Among the noxious byproducts of urban agglomerations that needed careful disposal were human bodies themselves. Twenty or more parish churches and three hospitals buried their dead in a single graveyard: the Cemetery of the Innocents, adjacent to the central market of Les Halles. Between two and three thousand Parisian corpses were deposited in the cem-

The Great Stink of Paris

etery every year. A huge new pit destined for around 1,500 bodies opened up every six months or so; it remained open, the corpses sprinkled with lime, until it was full, when a new pit would be dug. In warm weather, the stench was insufferable, according to visitors and residents alike. When the cemetery was established in the late twelfth century, it was outside the city's walls. By the eighteenth century, the much more populous cemetery found itself at the very center of a much more populous city. Neighbors complained with increasing regularity about the odors coming from the piles of decaying bodies. Local authorities fielded organized protests in 1724, 1725, 1735, 1746, and 1755, but the stop-gap measures they proposed had little long-term effect. Open pits containing hundreds of decomposing bodies continued to plague the heart of Paris. When a new pit was dug, it inevitably disturbed older pits, some of which contained incompletely decomposed corpses. Eventually, the soil itself, "full of grease and decay," "lost its substance" entirely.[23]

Late in 1779, a new pit was dug in the Cemetery of the Innocents on the side abutting the rue de la Lingerie. Not long thereafter, residents of this street began reporting unusual phenomena in their cellars. The odors were worse than ever. Candles and lanterns were spontaneously extinguished; wine stored along the walls adjoining the cemetery turned bad, while bottles stored along the facing walls retained their flavor. More menacingly, an increasing number of workers and residents who dared to descend into the fetid cellars were struck down as if they had drunk a deadly poison. Headaches, trembling, vomiting, delirium, and fainting—even strong and healthy men were not immune. Finally, on May 30, 1780, a wall separating the cemetery's current pit from a house on rue de la Lingerie collapsed, spilling corpses into the building's cellar. This proved to be the last straw. Faced with a new chorus of complaints, the police asked Antoine-Alexis Cadet de Vaux of the Royal Academy of Sciences to investigate. Cadet de Vaux carefully documented all of the reported instances of illness and indisposition attributed to the "cadaverous gas," and experimented with protective measures such as a large "flame ventilator," mounted on a tripod, to move air through the cellars. Although his experiments proved effective, their efficacy was only temporary, and he concluded that the only safe solution was the complete closure of the cemetery and the removal of its contents to a safer location on the outskirts of Paris. The Cemetery of the Innocents was officially closed to new burials on December 1, 1780, and five and a half years later, the transportation of human remains to the former limestone quarry later known as the Catacombs of Paris began.[24]

The cemetery crisis of 1780 bears some striking similarities to the Great Stink of 1880. Foul odors exceeded a threshold of tolerability, resulting in both illness and outrage, and provoked an official response through which science validated the perceived danger. Both episodes testify to the perils of rapid urbanization, to a modern intolerance of proximity to bodily substances, and to an equally modern tendency to seek relief from nuisances by recourse to governmental authorities. The nature of the odor had changed in 1880, but the alarm and affront experienced by Parisians bore a distinct family resemblance to that of a century earlier. It is worth noting that given the population density and waste disposal practices of the time, the Cemetery of the Innocents' neighbors must have lived surrounded by the smell of excrement on an almost constant basis, but they do not appear to have complained publicly about it. Parisians' tolerance for this most familiar of odors declined noticeably over the century that followed.[25] The Great Stink of 1880 was noteworthy not only for the mobilization of scientific authority and the political outcry it occasioned, but also for the geographically generalized nature of the complaints. Other odor crises were intensely local in their origins, in their scope, and in the protests they generated. It took either exceptionally dramatic details (e.g., cadavers spilling into cellars, neighbors losing consciousness) or a stench that was both intense and widespread (1880) to galvanize public opinion enough to gain the authorities' attention.

It is probably wise not to exaggerate the differences between 1780 and 1880. The long history of complaints about all kinds of smells in Paris—especially those generated by cadavers and excrement, but also urine, animals and their excretions, foodstuffs, tanneries, and other industries—together with the city's rapid population growth in the nineteenth century, suggest (somewhat prosaically) that tolerance of such smells declined gradually over several centuries, while the gross amount of odoriferous material in Paris increased gradually, then more rapidly, over the same period of time. The pervasive stench of 1880 might not have been possible in the smaller city of 1780, and if it had occurred, the resulting protests might have been less loud and less intense. What we are left with in the end is what did in fact happen. Parisians complained about foul odors periodically for several centuries, and their complaints increased in intensity between the late eighteenth and the late nineteenth centuries, as population density increased dramatically and as cultural norms consigned bodily substances to ever deeper realms of anathema.

"*Infection*": Stench and Disease Transmission Together

It is significant that even in 1895 and subsequent years, after foul-smelling emanations had ceased to be blamed for the spread of contagious diseases, episodes of disgusting odors continued to be referred to with the term "*infection*," just as in 1880. In this durable and multivalent term can be found some clues to the changing meaning of foul smells in French medicine and culture. Medical historian Owsei Temkin has shown that the concept of infection, with its multiple connotations and strong moral overtones, has informed Western attitudes toward health since antiquity.[26] When French newspapers featured the headline "The Parisian Infection" in August and September 1880, they alluded simultaneously to a disgusting stench and to the spread of disease. In doing so, they drew upon centuries of linguistic tradition, and (whether consciously or not) drew the incipient germ theory of disease into the orbit of that tradition. Since the fourteenth century, in effect, the documented usage of the verb *infecter*, the noun *infection*, and the adjective *infect* has continuously encompassed both foul smells and the propagation of disease, as table 2 illustrates.

It is clear from this history that infection has been a bimodal concept in France—denoting both offensive smell and transmission of disease—for centuries. Central to this dual valence is the notion of vitiation or corruption, a poisoning that signals itself by its odor and causes illness. Although contagion had been associated with "infection" since the fifteenth century, the nature of that association changed in the late nineteenth century. The kind of infection that was contained within and transmitted by miasmas tended to be localized, either in place or in time, or both; it was also generally identifiable, if not by smell then by other telltale markers, such as stagnant water, geological features, or meteorological phenomena. In the years around 1880, the dangerous (and foul-smelling) vitiation that could be poisonous also became contagious in a new way.

"Infection" now came to be embodied in living microorganisms, which eventually provided the basis for a new science and new strategies for therapeutic and preventive intervention in the process of illness. Moreover, the danger of infection was now constant, not always clearly localized in place nor in time, and not only invisible but imperceptible entirely: "Not everything that stinks kills, and not everything that kills stinks." To put it differently, the proponents of germ theory borrowed from and capitalized upon time-honored ways of understanding vitiation and illness—including the link between disgusting smells and deadly disease—in order to explain

Table 2. A Lexical History of "Infection"

Word	Date of Usage	Meanings
infect, infecte (adj.)	ca. 1361	"placed in" [e.g., a dye bath], "impregnated," "poisoned"; [of tastes] "depraved"
	1363	"full of miasmas," "stinking," "poisoned," "tainted"
	ca. 1500	"engendering moral disgust"
	16th c.	"contagious"
	1552	"having an ignoble . . . [tainted] odor"
	1636	[of meat] "full of worms"
	mid-19th c.	"appalling, dreadful," "repulsive"
infect, infecte (adj.)	1987	"vile, loathsome," "revolting," "filthy, foul," "disgusting," "rotten, appalling"
odeur infecte	1987	"stench; vile, foul, or loathsome smell"
infecter (v.t.)	1416	"to impregnate [the air or water] with unhealthy emanations"
	1431	"to corrupt" [e.g., by vice]
	1520	"to communicate infection to [someone, something]"
	1530	"to poison [the air, a place] with a foul odor"
	1987	"to infect," "to contaminate," "to poison"
infection (n.f.)	end of 13th c.	[in plural] "impure thought"
	1314	the penetration into the organism of pathogenic germs and the resulting disorders
	1416	"great stench"
	1484	a contagious disease
	1552	the propagation of a disease
	1616	"putrefaction," "unhealthy emanations"
	1987	"infection," "stench"

Sources: Alain Rey, ed., *Dictionnaire historique de la langue française* (Paris: Dictionnaires Le Robert, 1993), 1022; for those entries marked "1987," *Collins-Robert French-English, English French Dictionary* (London: Collins, 1987).

the dangers of microbes that could be odorless and hidden, and to justify new means of intervention. The warnings of Pasteur and Brouardel in
1880 can be seen as the first step in the recasting of this old relationship
into the new language of bacteriology.

These meanings of "infection" are particular to the French language.
Likewise, the political, scientific, and social circumstances that shaped the
response to the Great Stink of 1880 were uniquely French. Yet the cultural
phenomenon at the core of that episode—the perception that certain odors,
especially the odor of human excrement, were disgusting and intolerable—
was by no means exclusive to France. Throughout the industrializing and
urbanizing world in the nineteenth century, increasingly large and crowded
concentrations of human beings generated more and more unmanageable quantities of garbage, urine, excrement, and other stinking effluvia.
Meanwhile, the threshold of tolerance for the smell of such refuse was declining in these same societies, precipitating crises that involved cultural
self-image as much as the technical, economic, and political considerations
involved in urban waste disposal. In addition to Corbin's pioneering work
on eighteenth- and nineteenth-century France, scholars have shown that
intolerance of offensive odors provided a significant impetus to advances
in sanitary engineering and municipal health policies, particularly during
the last half of the nineteenth century.[27]

In the summer of 1858, London was beset by a stench that revolted
residents and even disrupted the operations of Parliament. Disgusted and
fearful Londoners predicted an imminent epidemic, and local authorities
anxiously weighed various measures in response to the crisis. In these
respects, London in July 1858 resembled Paris in September 1880. But
there was no debate whatsoever in London about the causes of the stench:
everyone agreed that it came from the Thames. Since the late 1840s, in
effect, London's own version of *tout-à-l'égout* prohibited cesspits and required each building to hook up to the city's sewers; these sewers emptied
into the river at various points including some in central London, producing odors that varied in intensity and location based on temperature and
water level. An exceptionally dry season brought the Thames to a level so
low by the early summer of 1858 that the odors were worse than ever. In
contrast to the French reaction in 1880, few in London questioned the wisdom of human waste disposal through the sewers, even after this offensive
display of the consequences of this policy. Remarkably, even physicians who
acknowledged that the river odors might spread disease defended the system, claiming that it would never kill as many Londoners or cause as much

illness as had the old system of manual waste removal. On the other hand, inaction in the face of the oppressive stench was not an acceptable alternative. Even the Houses of Parliament, meeting in their normally picturesque riverside location in Westminster, were forced to adjourn by the foul odors. The widespread perception that "something must be done" eventually produced the embankments of the Thames and over one hundred miles of fully enclosed, underground brick sewer mains, which collected the sewage of London and emptied it into the river fourteen miles downstream. The massive project was completed in 1875.[28]

Similarly, a historical study of public health in Charlottetown, Prince Edward Island, has shown how disgust at putrid odors can galvanize reform movements even against considerable odds. In spite of a relatively weak structure of local government and the absence of an entrenched, vocal constituency in favor of public works, repeated assaults from disgusting smells between 1855 and 1900 contributed to the mobilization of an organized campaign that finally achieved a recognizably modern system of sanitation and public health administration.[29] In the United States, the fear of deadly "sewer gas" spreading disease into even the most respectable homes through sinks and toilets haunted urban residents in the late nineteenth century.[30]

Each of these examples, like that of Paris in 1880 (and subsequent years), is profoundly idiosyncratic, shaped by local circumstances, agendas, and imperatives. What the responses to foul odors all share is *disgust*—not a universal repulsion produced automatically by the chemical and biological processes involved in olfaction, but rather a phenomenon that is both cultural and historical. This disgust, of varying contours and intensity in different cultures and at different times, became increasingly evident in many European and North American cities during the course of the nineteenth century in reaction to the perceived problem of offensive urban smells. Although historians did not begin to take the sense of smell seriously until the 1980s (following the publication of Corbin's *Le Miasme et la jonquille*, translated into English as *The Foul and the Fragrant*), the examples mentioned here suggest that under certain conditions, olfactory disgust could move mountains, not only arousing acute dread and loathing, but also inciting collective mobilization and political change. Political and social changes can in turn alter the landscape of citizens' tolerance, expectations, and demands concerning the physical qualities of their environment. Perhaps the most salient lesson of the Great Stink of 1880 is that the simultaneously biological and cultural experience of disgust played a vital role in shaping the interplay of public health, the changing urban landscape, and politics in the nineteenth century.

The History of Disgust

A newspaper commentary that appeared in the middle of the Great Stink of 1880 provided perhaps the most vivid depiction of the mixture of disgust and indignation that gripped many Parisians during the affair. The fact that the author purported to be Emile Zola and the newspaper *Le Figaro* only underscores the political and cultural subtext of the outcry against the odors. Novelist, essayist, and occasional social and political crusader, Zola contributed commentary to various republican newspapers in between volumes of his epic Rougon-Macquart series. *Le Figaro,* long a bastion of French conservatism, had in 1880 begun to reconcile itself to the republic as a form of government, without abandoning its opposition to the republican regime then in power. As part of its gradual political shift, and in a move calculated to surprise and infuriate its rivals on the left, the newspaper recruited Zola as a commentator.[31] Shortly before it did so, however, *Le Figaro* published a parody under the novelist's byline: "We all know—or rather, we all sense—that Paris is at the moment infected by the most abominable odors. . . . People from the provinces cannot imagine how much the air of the capital is vitiated. To give them an idea, we have called upon the pen of M. Emile Zola, the only one capable of truly describing the stench of the capital." Zola's article, the editor added, would be the first chapter of his forthcoming novel, *Le Grand Collecteur* ("The Great Sewer Main").[32] In fact, the piece was almost certainly not written by Zola,[33] but the newspaper's use of his name and style perfectly encapsulates the range of emotions experienced by respectable Parisian society during the Great Stink.

Le Figaro's strange commentary reads more like a case study in Zola's literary naturalism than like the political journalism the paper normally published:[34]

> It was the summer of 1880. In the month of August. It stank to high heaven. The sewers had been uncorked, and all the filth came out in a flood. All manner of waste was on display.

The terse, laconic reporting of the commentary's opening contrasts alarmingly with the lurid excess of detail that he subsequently pours forth, reenacting in words the endless flow of stinking waste from the sewers:

In every street, the pipes gushed out where decaying rat carcasses drank everything in, tails dangling and whiskers bristling with greenish lumps. Bellies in the air, they floated amid apple peels, asparagus stalks, and cabbage cores. . . . It was like a vast infection of tooth decay, like the flatulence of a rotting stomach, like the emanations of a man who has drunk too much, like the dried sweat of wallowing animals, like the sour poison of a bedpan.[35]

This is the shocking, profuse detail of the naturalistic novel, unflinchingly observing the underbelly of urban life. The artifice of "Zola's" fiction permitted *Le Figaro* to bring the sensory experience of the Great Stink into stark relief, with vivid visual details complementing a series of horrifying olfactory similes.

Such details also allowed the commentator to focus on something that was especially offensive: the visibility of that which should remain hidden, or more broadly the perceptibility of that which should be kept imperceptible. This is the central transgression in the odors of Paris, and it offers a telling insight into the breach wrought by the Great Stink in the fundamental codes of civilized life:

All the refuse of the city went for a stroll above ground. This avalanche of excretions, tumbling down the length of the purulent streets, swollen by effluent at each broken pipe . . . rushed down the boulevards and let off its nocturnal fragrances.[36]

To disgust deliberately was in fact a common strategy for Zola; scatological details, in particular, are to be found throughout his literary work. In *La Terre*, for example, he muses on the profound connections linking peasants to their excrement. The "flagrantly anal world" of the village represents the timeless world of *la bête humaine*, the standard of earthy living whose existence a mere hour outside Paris both deflates the nation's pretense of advanced civilization and allows the capital to define itself (by opposition) as the apotheosis of refinement.[37]

As significant as the intolerability of the odors was the inaction of the authorities. Here, of course, *Le Figaro* joined the chorus of journalistic censure aimed at Alphand, Andrieux, and other Parisian administrators: "The municipal authorities were living it up on vacation and the street-cleaners couldn't have cared less. . . . Foreign visitors figured it must have been the day set aside for the cleaning of all public and private toilets. They couldn't think of any other reason that would justify the negligence of the prefecture." "Zola's" biting sarcasm gives an edge to the commentary that enhances its political critique. When the author concludes that "it's not the prefect's fault" if the sewers do not work properly and that "we shouldn't be so disgusted" by the smell of natural substances, readers are meant to learn precisely the opposite lesson.[38]

Curiously, the commentary devotes no attention to the health effects of the Great Stink, apart from one matter-of-fact aside: "There were diseases. People either succumbed or became inured to them."[39] The question of whether or not foul-smelling emanations carried germs was almost beside the point. Far more important was the fact that in the midst of an unimaginably disgusting ordeal—not just an annoyance, but an affront to civilization itself—those in power did nothing. The sight and smell of substances that belonged out of the reach of those senses signified a temporary return to a prior, inferior stage of cultural development, when such things were tolerated. Similarly, "Zola" contrasts the disgusted, indignant, civilized citizens with the local official who makes excuses and questions the seriousness of the problem. The caricature depicts the apologist not merely as negligent or insufficiently diligent, but worse still, as backward, impervious to the demands of civilization. That Emile Zola was not the author of the commentary in Le Figaro does not diminish the significance of the critique itself. Even eighteen years before "J'Accuse" (published in 1898), Zola's mordant voice had become a familiar feature of the French cultural landscape, and could be counted on to skewer the comfortable and to denounce hypocrisy at every opportunity. The newspaper capitalized on the novelist's renown by adopting his familiar critical voice to satirize a complacent government unwilling to take action in time of crisis.

There is still another aspect of Le Figaro's odd polemic that deserves comment. Might someone actually have derived pleasure from the odors of Paris? In "Zola's" fantasy, those who were strong enough to survive the diseases brought on by the smells "ended up finding a certain charm in savoring these strange stenches of liquified fertilizer and of fecal matter in motion." In what became a veritable olfactory "orgy," the author reported, there were "gourmets who sniffed out these odors as they went by and recognized them, distinguishing the rotten egg from the dead rat and the dog's corpse from the putrefying turnip." Here too the novelist wallowed in the excess of his disgusting account.

It ended up producing a kind of intense pleasure in the sense of smell. . . .
It was as if the infection made people drunk. They felt their noses turn into

snouts and, not without delight, they plunged into the thick atmosphere, they immersed themselves in the pestilential ether of the great city, which saturated their brains with pornographic scents.[40]

The references to pornography and to human noses reverting to animal snouts make clear that however fascinating he finds this phenomenon, it is fundamentally perverse, an atavism. However, the attention he devotes to this "pleasure" at least suggests that there was something less than unanimity among Parisians where the Great Stink was concerned.

Indeed, other observers expressed skepticism concerning the scope and intensity of the odors in 1880. Several newspaper and magazine columnists, while acknowledging the existence of unpleasant smells in Paris, claimed that their severity had been exaggerated. Some dissenters saw the uproar less as a natural response to foul odors than as a pose adopted by those eager to affirm their civility and social status.

The satirical press, for example, seems to have built a double edge into its humor. While mocking bureaucrats and so-called experts for their inaction and interminable studies, cartoonists also managed to poke fun at the refined sensibilities and pretensions of the bourgeoisie. Clothing, hats, pince-nez, facial expressions: all are coded in these images to identify Parisians so intent on showing themselves to be civilized and respectable that they might protest too fervently, or exaggerate their disgust. (Fig. 13.) In these instances, poking fun at the pretentious does not necessarily preclude finding the odors offensive; social commentary coexists here alongside genuine indignation.

A few other journalists and commentators, while acknowledging the existence of unpleasant smells in Paris, claimed that their severity had been exaggerated. Three weeks after Zola's commentary, Le Figaro published another article that dissented from the universal repulsion and indignation: "Without contesting [the odors'] unpleasant existence, it seems to me that there has certainly been a healthy dose of exaggeration in the complaints aroused by these infamous odors. It has become, like so many things in Paris, a veritable fashion, and he who fails to hold his nose when passing near a sewer manhole, which happens to be perfectly odorless, shows in the eyes of many people an absolute lack of decorum."[41] In the same vein, literary critic Louis Ulbach confessed in mid-September that he was having a hard time getting as exercised about the so-called infection of Paris as were his fellow city dwellers: "I do not wish to contradict the universal sense of smell . . . but I humbly admit that I am not as afflicted as most people by these alleged emanations from the sewers, the cesspits, and the

The Great Stink of Paris

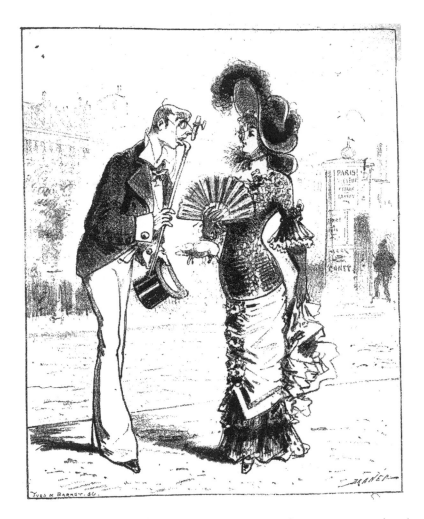

Fig. 13. "On the necessity of inventing a new system of pince-nez to combat the odors of Paris." *Le Charivari,* September 20, 1880.

waste dumps. I do not deny a very slight odor; but I imagine that it has always hung in the air of Paris and that we only notice it these days because delicacy is in fashion and because expressing our love of Paris has become outmoded."[42] This author confessed that as a youth, visiting Paris from the countryside, he positively relished the capital's earthy and bitter aromas, the smell of urban detritus and grit. "That was, I confess, somewhat depraved," he wrote, "but the sudden sensitivity that makes everybody hold their nose . . . [when] Paris [is] momentarily tormented by the heat seems to me a different kind of excess."[43]

What this jaded confession suggests is that Parisians' declining threshold of olfactory tolerance had as much to do with the Great Stink of 1880 as did the objective presence of odors in the urban air. Ulbach's ability to withstand this sensory onslaught without complaint certainly placed him in a minority in Paris, at least among those who recorded their views. However, even if his opinion was not widely shared at the time, the "sudden sensitivity" he detected in 1880 that made "everybody hold their nose" serves as a reminder of the essentially *social* nature of disgust. No individual reaction of disgust is ever purely individual; some responses may be directly influenced by the perceptions and opinions of one's peers, while others are indirectly shaped by the hidden, shifting desires and aversions of an entire cultural environment.

It is not surprising that the loudest voices raised during the Great Stink of 1880 came from the ranks of the highly class- and status-conscious Parisian bourgeoisie. In this milieu, disruptions of domestic tranquility (whether the threat was of a political or a bodily nature) did not generally go unremarked. In fact, the vigorous monitoring by newly ascendant *couches sociales* of various kinds of boundaries separating order from disorder is a recurring theme in the social history of many industrializing nations in the nineteenth century. Peter Stallybrass and Allon White, among others, have focused attention on a multifaceted and far-reaching strategy of hygienic, moral, and ideological sanitation as a critical bourgeois bulwark against the danger from below.[44]

True sanitation meant not only building sewers and carting away garbage; it also meant keeping the "lower strata" (both bodily and social) hidden. Out of sight, however—or out of smell, for that matter—proved to be far from out of mind. In fact, the aggressive and obsessive concealment of disgusting body parts, substances, and classes of people was accompanied by (and even, paradoxically, depended upon) constant and equally obsessive rhetorical invocations of the same disturbing matters. Government officials, reformers, social critics, and hygienists reinforced the increasing social distance separating the well-to-do from the poor by traversing that distance on a regular basis, observing the conditions of working-class life and reminding readers or constituents of the threat posed by the filthy and undisciplined.[45]

Moreover, far from putting an end once and for all to the perennial, anxious debates about urban waste disposal, the construction of modern sewer systems in nineteenth-century cities seemed if anything to multiply the potential sites of bourgeois coprophobia. Removed from superficial proximity aboveground, waste now circulated constantly underfoot, at once hidden and ubiquitous. Victor Hugo captured with characteristic embellishment the special place of the sewer in the nineteenth-century pantheon of fascinating horrors:

> [In the sewers] the spittle of Caiaphas encounters the vomit of Falstaff, the gold piece from the gaming house rattles against the nail from which the suicide hung, a livid foetus is wrapped in the spangles, which last Shrove Tuesday danced at the Opera, a wig which passed judgment on men wallows near the decay which was the skirt of Margoton. It is more than fraternity, it is close intimacy.[46]

In Hugo's day, even before plans were made to evacuate bodily waste through the Parisian sewers, the underground network represented a forced intimacy with the totality of the city—including its most unsavory elements. The proposed addition of urine and feces (beginning in the 1870s), intended as a safer alternative to the unhygienic cesspit system, instead called forth the threat of constant sensory contact with the entire city's excretions. The Great Stink of 1880 made that threat appallingly real, heralding the "return of the repressed"—a breakdown of the whole elaborate system of concealment and disposal on which bourgeois confidence and urban civilization rested.[47]

Although a number of satirists and critics skewered the hypercivilized refinement of the Parisian bourgeoisie, it would be rash to conclude that the Great Stink of 1880 offended only well-to-do noses. The available evidence does not allow the reconstruction of an exact social profile of Parisian disgust in 1880. However, some fragmentary clues suggest that outrage at the foul odors was not limited to social climbers and the wealthy. Angry complaints filled the columns of newspapers representing nearly the entire political spectrum in the capital, not merely those catering to the bourgeoisie. Furthermore, one of the early manifestations of popular discontent in Paris was a petition sent to the Conseil municipal signed by residents of the ninth and eighteenth arrondissements.[48] Neither was a quintessentially bourgeois district in 1880; the ninth was socially mixed, while a predominantly working-class population lived in the eighteenth.[49]

The conflicting evidence, then, suggests (at least circumstantially) two conclusions: on the one hand, it is likely that both working-class and bourgeois Parisians felt disgusted and aggrieved in the face of the odors of 1880; on the other hand, the perceived threat may have been especially acute for that segment of the population whose self-image depended on a particular kind of idealized and sanitized "urbanity." Similarly, the dissenting and satirical perspectives on the Great Stink of 1880 do not tell us that the ostentatious disgust of the status-conscious was purely phony; rather, they emphasize the extent to which disgust is always both a straightforward (even natural) reaction to sensory stimuli *and* a constituent element in elaborate strategies of self-presentation and self-fashioning.

The skeptical minority perspective on the odors of 1880 also underscores the importance of disgust as both an emotional and a historical phenomenon. Corbin, in his pathbreaking history of smell, was the first historian to address the question of how disgusting odors became disgusting, and how alluring fragrances became alluring. He argues that the years between 1750 and 1880 witnessed a "perceptual revolution," in which collective sensitivity to odors of all kinds intensified, and in which elaborate strategies of deodorization were devised for public and private spaces alike. Moreover, the changes were not merely esthetic in character, nor were they limited to a refinement of manners in polite society. The very nature of human society was at stake, as individuals and social groups struggled to form new identities and negotiate their places within a changing physical and political landscape. Corbin shows that nineteenth-century French men and women perceived threats and expressed desires through the sense of smell, which was at the foundation rather than on the periphery of their understanding of the social world around them. The nineteenth-century intensification of both disgust and allure mediated by smell, Corbin argued, "revolutionized social perceptions and symbolic references." Understanding the revolutionary nature of this perceptual change makes it possible to "measure the visceral depths to which the nineteenth-century social conflicts reached."[50]

Peter Reinhart Gleichmann has analyzed in detail architectural and engineering manuals from the nineteenth and early twentieth centuries in order to document the anxious and definitive exclusion of defecation and excrement from perceptibility (including both sight and smell) in public and private space. The increasing intolerance of certain odors in the nineteenth century required the development not only of new spatial and sanitary technologies inside the home, but also of new ways of regulating public space in the city. Governmental authorities assumed a certain "coercive role" in enforcing the new standards of sensibility when they imposed new systems of urban waste disposal. Nothing symbolized the new regime of urbanization, according to Gleichmann, more than *tout-à-l'égout*, which "signifie[d] a more refined management of human excretions." External constraints, however, were not enough. Because the act of defecation was becoming more and more hidden from view, and therefore from external control, Gleichmann argues, "the obligation of self-control" became correspondingly imperative, and Elias's formula of "the social constraint towards self-constraint" played itself out in this arena, as "the control of one's own bodily excretions" became a veritable "compulsion."[51]

Nevertheless, even if there is abundant evidence for increasing constraints on certain kinds of behavior over several centuries, that evidence does not fully explain the disgust felt by Parisians during the Great Stink of 1880. After all, blowing one's nose too loudly, eating with one's fingers, or even defecating in the wrong place may provoke disdain (and shame), but an emotional reaction of a far different order of magnitude comes into play when an entire metropolis reeks of human excrement. Violations of politeness occasion responses that may be quite strong and quite negative, but these responses are conscious judgments, or at least mediated through consciousness at some level. Even shame must be produced through a conscious awareness of one's transgression. But disgust of the sort voiced in 1880 appears to be automatic, instinctual. How can disgust at foul odors be both visceral and contingent—that is, how can responses shaped by changing cultural norms and rules through history manifest themselves in such a gut-level, seemingly unconscious way? This is the historical paradox of disgust, and smell-related disgust in particular.

Another fundamental sociological concept, Pierre Bourdieu's notion of "habitus," represents an elaborately theorized attempt to address the complex process by which the cultural products of historical contingency turn into fixed, solid bodily reality. Habitus, which has been defined as "a set of dispositions which incline agents to act and react in certain ways,"[52] is both inculcated and "generative"—that is, it is learned rather than innate, but becomes so deeply rooted in the individual or collective psyche that it can generate behaviors and reactions without being the object of conscious deliberation. The "dispositions" that constitute the habitus can be thought of as tendencies or orientations toward characteristic practices, perceptions, and beliefs rather than as strictly determined inevitabilities, since historical conditions shape the habitus in the first place and affect its manifestations in particular social contexts.[53]

The site within which the habitus expresses itself most visibly and most durably, in Bourdieu's view, is the human body itself. Beginning with the crucial formative experiences of early childhood, "the individual acquires a set of dispositions which literally mould the body and become second nature," in the words of one Bourdieu commentator; the body becomes "a repository of ingrained dispositions."[54] Bourdieu uses the term "bodily hexis" to denote a permanent style of physical carriage, deportment, and deployment of the body in society: "Bodily hexis is political mythology realized, *em-bodied,* turned into a permanent disposition, a durable manner of standing, speaking and thereby of *feeling* and *thinking.* . . . The principles em-bodied in this way are placed beyond the grasp of consciousness, and hence cannot be touched by voluntary, deliberate transformation."[55] The innocent, endlessly repeated injunctions exhorting children to adopt correct posture or polite table manners end up imprinting an entire system of values on the body, which thereafter carries and materializes those values. In Bourdieu's phrase, "Arms and legs are full of numb imperatives."[56]

In particular historical situations, certain habits and affects can accrete to the point at which they take on the quality of embodied reality—or physical responses unmediated by conscious deliberation. (Bourdieu refers to the habitus as "embodied history, internalized as . . . second nature and [thus] forgotten as history.")[57] Disgust—or, to be more specific, the visceral repulsion at the sight or smell of human excrement—can be seen as a "disposition" that, although a subjective product of cultural history, has the power to generate the objective reality of certain physical responses and to govern individual and collective behavior.

The Marriage and Divorce of Odors and Germs

The consensus of medical opinion held that the Great Stink of 1880 spread disease, while in 1895 a similar consensus reached the opposite conclusion. This does not mean, however, that all belief in pathogenic odors disappeared entirely during this period. On the contrary, claims of illness and even epidemics triggered by foul smells persisted through the late 1890s and well into the twentieth century. In June 1895, for example—in the midst of the second Great Stink in Paris—a Le Havre resident wrote the local health commission to complain about the stench caused when a neighboring cistern was pumped out into the street at night. His wife could not sleep all night, and felt sick the next day when she tried to enter her cellar. The letter added ominously that typhoid fever had swept through the street several years earlier, and the previous tenant of the author's apartment had died of it. Arthur Michel of Déville-lès-Rouen (Seine-Inférieure) filed a complaint with the state prosecutor in February 1899 against a neighbor who regularly fed his dogs a considerable amount of horse meat, which gave off sickeningly strong "emanations." The "repulsive odor that disgusts and stinks" made the neighbors sick to their stomachs, "suffocated" them, and "forced [them] to flee." After witnessing the health effects of the stinking horse meat on his children, Michel sent them off to a boarding school. In 1904, to take another representative complaint, "a group of residents" of La Madeleine (Nord) wrote the prefect to protest neighbors' accumulation of large piles of manure and fecal matter in violation of local law. Apart from the fact that the July heat made the stench "intolerable," the residents warned that "this could bring back the epidemic that held sway last year."[58]

The gut-level sense that foul odors could cause disease did not disappear after the Bacteriological Revolution and the consolidation of the SBS. The contexts in which that conviction could plausibly be expressed did change, however. After the mid-1890s, like the examples just cited, most such complaints came from private individuals or coalitions of neighbors, and did not carry the scientific sanction of the medical establishment. Their primary thrust targeted the odors' intolerability; claims about disease causation were secondary.

Why were foul smells a serious health hazard in 1880, and merely a nagging source of discomfort in 1895 and subsequent years? It is impossible to gauge the objective scope and intensity of the odors themselves; however, even though the sheer amount of public complaint in 1880 was unparalleled in the later instances, the odors of Paris had clearly not ceased to be disgusting and intolerable in 1895 and thereafter. If sensitivities had changed, they had likely only continued to become more intolerant of putrid smells. The rise of germ theory alone cannot account for the disappearance of microbes from the odors of Paris. The scientific study of the 1880 calamity had shown not only that the disciples of Pasteur were willing to consider the possibility that germs could be spread through foul-smelling emanations, but also that many believed the possibility to have been proven beyond serious doubt. Nor did a specific technical innovation or scientific advance occur between 1880 and 1895 that might have caused the medical community to discount the link between odors and microbes. Germs were certainly still believed to be airborne: researchers continued to measure the quantity of bacteria in air samples taken from different locations, and to experimentally infect laboratory animals by exposing them to air filled with microbes; meanwhile, hygienists continued to emphasize the dangers of contagion through germ-saturated air.[59]

Moreover, it is especially significant that germs were not dissociated altogether from disgusting places, practices, and substances after 1880;

far from it. In fact, the French public health literature in the two decades preceding 1900 is positively suffused with warnings about the spread of pathogenic microbes through indiscriminate excretions, domestic filth and overcrowding, poor bodily hygiene, and spitting. The same indignant and horrified tone pervades the reports of doctors and others investigating various disease outbreaks and finding them rooted in such disgusting habits.[60] And yet by the time the odors of Paris struck again in 1895, most physicians and hygienists found them nauseating, but germ free. As the science of microbes developed in the 1880s and 1890s—multiplying the diseases over which it claimed authority, refining its strategies for identifying and neutralizing pathogens, and expanding the arenas of its potential intervention in society—warning of the omnipresence of dangerous germs remained important, but specific, practical measures to fight them assumed even greater importance.

As Robert Koch and his colleagues in Germany identified the microbes responsible for tuberculosis, cholera, diphtheria, and other deadly diseases, finding and testing for specific bacteria in bodily fluids and tissues (as well as, for example, in urban water supplies) became a leading preoccupation in medicine and public health. As Pasteur followed his triumph at Pouilly-le-Fort with a successful rabies vaccination in 1885—the apotheosis of his career, and seemingly a sure sign that the science of germs would eventually conquer disease—scientists focused on ways of attenuating specific pathogens and developing "magic bullets" that would target discrete microorganisms without harming the rest of the patient's body. All tests and all preventive and therapeutic interventions came to be oriented toward the *specific* germs that, it had now been shown, caused specific diseases. Foul odors were not specific; they were diffuse, difficult to describe—much less to test scientifically—and not especially amenable to interventions aimed at individual microbes.

Excrement, of course, continued to be associated with particular diseases such as typhoid fever, and continued to preoccupy hygienists into the twentieth century. The disgusting still caused disease—as it still does today[61]—but in more distinctly identifiable ways than before. By 1895, the ideological work of medicalizing disgust had shifted from the vitiation-odors-germs nexus (itself the successor to the vitiation represented by odors and miasmas) to a new set of dangers: the contamination of water by germs contained in fecal matter and the spread of germs through spitting and through the failure to maintain clean houses and bodies. The fear of vitiation remained, and disgust still imposed a strong moral template on

The Great Stink of Paris

public health reforms, but specifically identifiable threats had supplanted the diffuse menace of odors in the hierarchy of health hazards.

From a distance, the response of bacteriological medicine's leading lights to the Great Stink of 1880 is difficult to explain. It simply does not appear to make any sense for Louis Pasteur to have invoked germ theory to explain how foul-smelling emanations can spread disease—a quintessentially miasmatist, pre-Pasteurian proposition. Likewise, for the population of a major modern metropolis in the late nineteenth century to be up in arms about unpleasant smells, and demanding urgent action from their government to stave off an imminent epidemic, seems improbable, irrational. In conventional categories of analysis, the episode can only be understood as either error, atavism, or anomaly.

But the Great Stink of 1880 has much more to tell us than such judgments would allow. It was not merely epiphenomenal, as an extreme meteorological phenomenon causing intense fear might be; nor was it simply a residue of miasmatism surviving into the age of bacteriology, or a case of great medical and scientific minds making a mistake that further research would later rectify. Even to highlight the episode as a turning point between the old regime of threatening bodies and the new regime of industrial threats to the human environment does not fully explain it.[62] The Great Stink of 1880—and the very real fears it triggered among experts and lay people alike—laid bare for all to see (and smell) a scientific world, a political world, and a cultural world in great flux. At the same time, it subtly accelerated, altered, and redirected the changes taking place in these domains, and redefined the terms of debate for future discussions of health and the urban environment.

In 1880, old habits and new possibilities combined to influence responses to disgusting smells. The age-old association of odors with corruption and disease represented by the word "infection" confronted a new science that proposed a new definition of contagion and a new way of understanding health and disease. Rather than refuting or rejecting the old set of meanings, the new science appropriated it and incorporated it into a newly scientific notion of infection. Old concerns about urban filth and sanitation combined with the recent precedent of massive public works and a new political configuration to prompt demands for remedial action and new perceptions of governmental responsibilities. Long-declining thresholds of tolerance for odors associated with bodily substances, along with a new political biology of regeneration through improvement of the social milieu, forged a new sensibility and a new imperative to cleanse the physical environment.

Germ theory redefined and reoriented, but did not eliminate, older preoccupations regarding the harmful effects of filth and contamination. Among the hazards that the new public health added to the existing repertoire was a newly scientific version of contagion, now potentially omnipresent in microbes. It lent a sense of urgency as well as optimism to the battle against killer diseases, whose causes could now be found seemingly everywhere but could also be fought with specially targeted biological weapons. The true impact of the "Pasteurian revolution" in medicine and public health, however, cannot be measured in numbers of causal bacteria discovered or of vaccines developed. Germ theory promised nothing less than a reordering of society as a whole according to hygienic principles.

Germs became metaphors for various kinds of hidden, proliferating threats in the modern world: foreigners, subversive political doctrines, unsound habits.[63] But germs were also real living microorganisms, pathogens that tended to reside in certain kinds of dangerous places and that were transmitted from person to person. The recognition of these basic facts demanded that a new, scientific attention be paid to the spaces in which germs thrived and to the contacts among people in society. It was not enough to treat the individual sick body; the social body as a whole needed healing. Claude Bernard's physiology had suggested the importance of milieu and the analogy between the healthy functioning of the organism and the healthy functioning of society.[64] The discovery of microbes as causes of disease fit this paradigm quite smoothly.

What was especially seductive about the new scientific medicine in the wake of Bernard and Pasteur, as Olivier Faure has suggested, was not its technical mastery over disease but rather its "social project." In effect, medicine had begun to claim "a sort of eminent domain over society in the name of the analogy between the human body and the social body": "Pasteur's discoveries achieved such renown only because they intersected with a series of external preoccupations that converged to find in medicine a model for describing and managing society as a whole."[65] In fact, it is impossible to separate germ theory's promise of therapeutic progress from its social ambitions; the discoveries of Pasteur and others, taken as a whole, were exciting and revolutionary precisely because they implicitly addressed both objectives. The new discipline of public health to which germ theory gave birth aspired ultimately not just to progress in the fight against specific diseases, but also to the scientific management of social space and of interpersonal contact.

In retrospect, one can see in the year 1880 key signs of change in the cultural and political realms as well as in science. Bits of old and new ways of perceiving the world combined in curious ways to shape responses to sensory phenomena. It is perhaps as a historical signpost in this regard that the Great Stink of 1880 is most illuminating. In a moment of extraordinary tension and dread, otherwise hidden manifestations of long-term historical changes suddenly crystallized and became visible. A peculiar amalgam of miasmatism and germ theory, of old aversions and new fears, the reactions to the odors of Paris in that year testify to the deep, interlocking roots that connect apparently distinct scientific, political, and cultural developments. To pronounce true or false the belief that foul smells contained germs and spread disease is to ignore the web of conditions that made that belief "true"—or at least created a consensus in its favor—at the time.

During the late summer of 1880, in the great metropolis that Walter Benjamin later called the "capital of the nineteenth century";[66] in the burgeoning city that had seen half a century of nearly uninterrupted—even cataclysmic—population growth and physical expansion; in the political tinderbox that simmered with bourgeois ambition and working-class resentment; in a culture attempting to distance itself ever further from the base demands of the body and to approach ever closer a civilized ideal of sanitized comfort while remaining haunted by the ever-present threat of murderous epidemics—in this confident yet anxious atmosphere a wave of persistent and disgusting odors triggered fearful predictions of disaster and clamorous demands for reform.

This story of foul smells and the microbes that they did or did not contain lacks a clear resolution: no devastating epidemic justified the doomsayers, no definitive scientific proof absolved the odors from a role in the spread of disease, and no single event marked their transition from health hazard to inconvenience. But perhaps this lack of clarity is appropriate for a story marked by a murky blend of enduring continuities and startling changes, a story of dimly perceptible fears and ambitions underlying ostensibly straightforward debates. Ultimately, rather than a clear denouement, the Great Stinks of 1880 and beyond provide a revealing and sometimes surprising glimpse into the overarching anxieties and dreams—personal and political, consciously articulated and darkly visceral—that transformed physical and cultural landscapes in the late nineteenth century.

Epilogue

The Legacy of the Twentieth Century

In 2001, more than a century after its founder's death, the Pasteur Institute convened an international summit to review the state of hygiene and health at the dawn of the twenty-first century. The assembled authorities noted with concern that "in the 'hygienized' world, infectious diseases have reawakened." Ironically, the chief culprit responsible for undermining decades of progress was identified as . . . progress itself. Too much technology and not enough hygiene, in the experts' view, had endangered the historical triumph over infectious disease. According to the Pasteur Institute symposium, an array of late twentieth-century developments that had made life easier for many people—from globalization to home health care and changing eating habits—had also multiplied the opportunities for people to come into contact with germs. Meanwhile, old-fashioned preventive measures such as basic cleanliness had fallen into neglect. Even the stunning successes of medical technology itself had heightened human vulnerability to infection. Blood transfusion, organ transplantation, syringes, endoscopy, dialysis—all saved lives or improved health while simultaneously creating portals of entry for microbes. Thanks to antibiotics, many infectious diseases had become treatable; those same life-saving drugs, however, had also given birth to drug-resistant strains of some diseases.[1]

The Pasteur Institute's answer to this threat, the crucial barrier against the resurgent threat of infection, could be found in a simple strategy that predated all of those scientific and technological advances: hygiene. Only what the symposium called "personal," "domestic," and "environmental" cleanliness—ranging from handwashing to sewers—could protect the population from the insidious contaminant that lurked behind so many infectious diseases: what the conference report referred to as *"the fecal peril."*[2] The future of public health, in other words, depended in part on a rediscovery of the past, and the spectacular medical victories of Pasteur and his successors since the late nineteenth century over mysterious microscopic predators could be undermined by one of the oldest and most intimate enemies of all: filth. In effect, the history of public health had come full circle: the sanitarians' obsession with cleanliness and the containment of excretions, simultaneously eclipsed by the hunt for specific microbes and appropriated as their own by the germ hunters, had reclaimed center stage in the battle against disease.

The bold claims, negotiations, and false starts that characterized the formation of the sanitary-bacteriological synthesis were not limited to France. A similar transition marked public health throughout the industrialized world during and after the Bacteriological Revolution. Its local manifestations varied according to the political, social, and cultural configurations of the countries involved, as well as their local disease ecologies. All experienced a general intensification of injunctions regarding public and private cleanliness alongside a shift toward more confident and more targeted public health campaigns rooted directly or indirectly in bacteriological laboratories.[3] What distinguished the French experience from that of other countries was the powerful valence of the SBS amid the drive to entrench republican political values among the population and the effort to integrate the peasantry into a truly national culture. In these contexts, the new scientific medicine validated preexisting agendas, but it also conferred added urgency on them, as the nation's very survival seemed to depend on using expert knowledge to increase the birth rate and decrease the death rate.

Today, well over a century after the discoveries that forever transformed medical science, the public sphere teems with warnings about the omnipresence of potentially deadly germs. News media, books, museum exhibits, and advertisements for consumer products convey lurid evocations of bodily functions, bacterial physiology, and disease symptoms. Cumulatively, they convey the titillating but terrifying message that deadly pathogens lurk all around us, awaiting only a momentary lapse in personal hygiene to wreak their devastation.[4] Television news reporters accompany scientists in white lab coats as they swab pay phones, ATM keypads, and interior surfaces in subway cars, then test them for the presence of bacteria. Invariably, multiple species of "disease-causing germs" are found, and the diseases they cause are described as if an epidemic has just been uncovered— although actual cases of the diseases in question are rarely mentioned.[5]

And the sanitary-bacteriological synthesis continues to thrive. In 2000, when the United States Centers for Disease Control issued a warning about the prevalence of infections related to home health care, the *New York Times* quoted a clinical nursing specialist about the dangers of performing medical procedures outside of the controlled hospital environment: "You have so many other issues—*sanitation, pets, rodents, insects.*"[6] Born of professional frustration, this brief comment speaks volumes. Specific etiologies are less important in this instance than the generally contaminating influence of "matter out of place," as Mary Douglas memorably defined "dirt."[7] Disgusting things and biological elements out of their proper context always threatened to spread disease. The more things change, the more they stay the same. The SBS is communicated through many different channels, but its thrust remains constant: only a vigilant policing of cleanliness, excretions, and bodily separation can protect against disease, because germs proliferate as soon as those standards are violated.

The sanitary-bacteriological synthesis is not a thing. It is neither an institution, a school of thought, nor a doctrine. Rather, it is a deeply ingrained framework that structures perceptions, knowledge, and behavior concerning bodies and disease. Before the 1880s, the SBS was impossible. It took shape gradually as a loosely connected set of ideas and practices articulated in a variety of contexts, but especially in the contacts between hygienists and the people who were the objects of their reformist enthusiasm. Eventually, it became a mental habit or patterned response, rarely questioned, whose existence did not even need to be acknowledged. Today it is common sense; we learn it and internalize it without even being consciously aware of it. It would be a mistake to view the formation of the SBS as a compromise between sanitarians and bacteriologists. It was rather the product of an ongoing tension between the old hygiene and the apostles of the hardline "not everything that stinks kills" school of germ theory. The product proved to be itself quite productive, inasmuch as an intellectual framework offering definitive scientific solutions for the thorny problems of managing bodies in modern societies can be applied to an endless array of spaces, behaviors, and diseases. It is this flexible serviceability that has allowed the SBS to endure for more than a century.

When people buy air sanitizers for their bathrooms because they kill the germs that are the cause of persistent foul odors; when they think twice about home health care because of worries about "sanitation, pets, rodents, [and] insects"; and when they watch with horrified fascination as white-coated scientists swab down pay phones and subway cars on the television news; when people do these things, they do not consciously think of Chadwick, Villermé, Pasteur, and Koch. They do not ask whether paper cup users are actually healthier than those who drink from glasses (or from their hands), nor whether patients who change their own catheters at home experience more negative health outcomes than do those in hospitals, nor whether subway riders (controlling for other variables) tend to be sicker than, say, automobile drivers. Rather, they feel a vague sense of disgust reflexively, intuitively, almost instinctively; and they simply know, on a visceral level, that germs are dirty and dirt is germy and the whole unpleasant mess can make them and their loved ones sick. This unexamined certainty—the triumphant end result of the sanitary-bacteriological synthesis—is the lasting legacy of the sanitarians of the early nineteenth century, the bacteriologists of the late nineteenth century, and the many preachers of the gospel of germs who have done missionary work at home and abroad ever since, making what was once novel and surprising feel like second nature.

Etiology matters—and not just because it can lead to vaccines and cures. There is undeniable intellectual appeal in the notion that effective disease prevention and treatment require knowledge of specific causes.[8] History tells a different story, however. Cinchona bark against malaria, Jenner's vaccine against smallpox, and antismoking campaigns against lung cancer are only the best-known of many effective strategies devised in the absence of specific causal knowledge.[9] Etiologies are always (at least implicitly) blueprints not only for prevention and treatment, but also for social and political action. Even when they influence public health policy and health-related behaviors, they often do so in an indirect, heavily mediated fashion that is far from transparent. Etiological discourse articulates mores in a language that renders them natural, scientifically sanctioned, and therefore unassailable.

Anthrax in the mail, West Nile encephalitis from mosquito bites, pandemic influenza from migrating birds—disease threats in the twenty-first century lurk everywhere. The range of health dangers seems at least as wide as it was in the premicrobial days, when swamp emanations and above-average rainfall and rotting animal corpses—not to mention fecal odors and dozens of other factors—all caused disease. Looking beyond exotic outbreaks to the more mundane realm of everyday infectious diseases, however, most people living in the developed world today inhabit the same etiological landscape whose core features took shape in the last quarter of the nineteenth century. Inattention to cleanliness facilitates the transmission of germs, thereby spreading disease, just as it did in 1900. The reality and magnitude of disease threats are measured in microbiological laboratories, just as they were in 1900. Contagion and germs continue to be closely identified with disgusting substances, places, and practices. Faced with the need to prevent and treat illness, we continue to look to the laboratory for disease-specific solutions. Nonspecific, nonpharmaceutical measures to improve health continue to be advocated here and there, but fail to attract the attention and resources that would allow them to be undertaken in a sustained manner.

Reductionism has had a lasting appeal in medicine. Perhaps the dismissively negative connotations of the term itself are unfair. After all, there is nothing wrong with reducing problems to their fundamental constitutive elements. One observer's oversimplification of complex issues is another's distillation of those same issues down to their essence. In medicine, reducing the obscure etiology and pathogenesis of a deadly disease to a single identifiable agent raises the tantalizing prospect of reliable prevention and treatment through the targeting of that agent. "The fight against this terrible plague of mankind," wrote Robert Koch after his landmark 1882 proof of the bacterial etiology of tuberculosis, "will deal no longer with an undetermined something, but with a tangible parasite, whose living conditions are for the most part known and can be investigated further."[10] Neither the epistemological nor the practical allure of reductionism should be underestimated.

Apart from a priori value judgments, however, it is important to recognize reductionist tendencies when they appear, and to explore the historical and contemporary reasons for their appeal. During the Bacteriological Revolution, reducing the vexing problem of infectious disease to the daunting but conceivable task of destroying or neutralizing microbes sparked understandable optimism. Even disregarding the practical challenge of such an endeavor, rendering such a muddled and multifarious question epistemologically clean and accessible represented a tremendous advance for hygienists and for society as a whole.

Today, the possibility of reducing a noninfectious disease such as breast cancer to a single location on the human genome holds out the promise of similar epistemological (and perhaps practical) benefits. Likewise, in a different vein, reducing a health condition such as obesity or diabetes to behavioral choices—unhealthy diet, lack of exercise—makes a complex problem seem manageable, or at least less threatening to those not currently affected. But reductionism has its pitfalls too. The hard-line bacteriological "not everything that stinks kills" style of reasoning failed to become the new guiding light of French public health at least in part because it could not articulate and incorporate the allied cultural imperatives of cleanliness and civilization. The more culturally nuanced sanitary-bacteriological synthesis proved more successful and more durable.

Genetic, behavioral, and other reductionisms today may face similar obstacles. On the one hand, purely genetic etiologies leave no room for the association of collective or individual lifestyle choices with disease. On the other hand, purely behavioral etiologies lack the promise of magic bullet–style targeted laboratory solutions. The experience of the SBS in its formative years does not necessarily provide a road map for successful navigation of these difficulties, but it does suggest that *simple* scientific reductionism speaks to entire societies less fluently and less effectively than does reductionism rooted in and inflected by cultural imperatives.

The early history of the SBS sheds light not only on the continuing vitality of the SBS and its powerful role in our lives today, but also on other (often unrecognized) cultural-scientific syntheses that shape our responses to perceived health threats. Obesity, for example, has recently been "discovered" as a serious public health problem. As was the case with infectious diseases more than a century ago, medicalizing the problem is not enough. As they are translated into a language accessible to the general public, explanations and responses derived from medical science must also undergo selective emphasis, alteration, and even rethinking in order to accommodate the changing needs of the wider culture. An approach to obesity that ignored the long-standing stigma attached to fat bodies would be unimaginable—and doomed to failure. A similar argument can be made about the connection between smoking and lung disease. Decades of scientific evidence and aggressive public health programs made relatively little impact on smoking rates; only when changing behavioral norms and clever advertising campaigns made smoking socially unacceptable, and even disgusting, did rates decline significantly.[11]

Understanding in detail the historical roots and practical workings of etiology brings with it other advantages as well. Alongside an increasing attention to genetic factors, the landscape of disease causation today is marked by the interplay of two lingering tendencies: a continuing focus on proximate causes (especially specific microbes) as exotic, alien invaders; and the moralizing reflex of rationalizing disease and inequality by assigning blame, especially to their victims.[12] The combination of these two tendencies routinely deflects attention—and diverts limited resources—away from health problems that appear to be "caused" (or triggered, or aggravated) by factors that are neither disease-specific nor particularly exotic, such as poverty, social dislocation, and environmental degradation. This deflection and diversion is not inevitable, however. A critical reflection on the dynamics of culturally sanctioned health knowledge is essential if public health priorities are to be reoriented, both in the wealthy nations and in the developing world.

In this regard, late nineteenth-century France can be looked upon as a "distant mirror"[13] reflecting the tensions, fears, hopes, and ambitions of our own society. Prior to the Bacteriological Revolution, public health was ambitious and thoroughly nonspecific. Villermé and his fellow hygienists pursued the audacious goal of determining patterns of disease throughout society. They combed available demographic records in order to map morbidity and mortality differentials in detail by time and place. Having identified what would today be called "at-risk communities," they studied them up close, neglecting no detail, even living among them and following their members to their workplaces. By today's standards, their etiologies were hopelessly vague, and their proposed remedies either unrealistic or ineffective. Their moralism was brutal and unyielding.

The last quarter of the nineteenth century brought dazzling progress. Most of it was theoretical rather than practical in the short term, or potential rather than actual. However, diphtheria antitoxin undoubtedly saved many lives, and the epistemological breakthroughs achieved through the germ theory (or theories) of disease laid the groundwork for a century of prophylactic and therapeutic discoveries, whose benefits are incalculable. But historians must also ask what we have lost while gaining so much. Medicine's triumphs in the twentieth century lose no luster when we contemplate the cost they entailed. The scope of Villermé's public health in the sanitarian era was in effect sacrificed on the altar of germs. Only his moralism survived. Open-ended, nonspecific epidemiology aimed at determining who is getting sick where and when has become marginalized, while the search for specific bacteria, viruses, or even genes that can be targeted by magic bullets proceeds apace. This tightly focused science of public health owes its triumph in part to developments outside of medicine. The SBS was built on the twin foundations of bacteriological discovery and cultural change. Recognizing the contingency of this historical marriage does not diminish its significance. It is, however, a precondition to being able to evaluate health threats based on other, deliberately formulated criteria.

In the middle of Philippe-le-Bon Square in the northern city of Lille, just a block from the university where Louis Pasteur served as dean in the 1850s, there stands a larger-than-life-size monument to the great scientist. On April 9, 1899, the scientific elite of France and several other nations joined other French dignitaries at the dedication of the statue. The ceremony coincided with the inauguration of a new Pasteur Institute in Lille, and provided yet another occasion for a grateful nation to pay tribute to the late master, already lionized as the hero of the new scientific medicine. What distinguished this celebration from the others was the esthetic eloquence of the tribute. The monument expressed in a series of three-dimensional images the impact of science on French society at the close of the nineteenth century. Two companion statues flanking the central piece represented, on the left, a young brewer holding the tools of his trade and looking gratefully toward Pasteur and, on the right, a woman giving an injection to a child cradled in her lap. Three smaller bas-relief scenes graced Pasteur's pedestal: the master studying fermentation with a microscope, the vaccination of a sheep against anthrax, and the administration of the first rabies vaccine to young Joseph Meister. All eyes were drawn, however, to the centerpiece, in which Pasteur gazes downward intently at a laboratory flask while a young mother reaches upward imploringly, holding a baby out toward him.[14] (Fig. 14.)

Inaugurated eighteen years after the triumph at Pouilly-le-Fort, fourteen years after the rescue of Joseph Meister from rabies, and four years after Pasteur's death, the monument captures a moment in time and freezes it for eternity. It is not an actual moment in Pasteur's life, but rather the symbolic representation of a historical moment: the apotheosis of one scientist's personal glory and the definitive triumph of his science in the world of medicine and public health. One can see clearly in the central statue Pasteur's single-minded focus on his flask, his task, his scientific vision. It is slightly harder for a passerby at ground level to see the expression on the young mother's face. She seems desperate, certainly, but there must be some hope in her eyes, even some optimism, as she confides (or sacrifices) the care of her beloved child to science. The spectators at the monument's inauguration knew that the mother had chosen wisely, and knew that the nation as a whole was in the process of making the same wise choice. What they might not have understood quite as clearly was that the historic triumph of bacteriological knowledge was predicated upon a carefully negotiated accommodation between scientific authority and cultural imperatives. Not everything that stank killed, perhaps, but hygienists continued to direct their attention primarily to that which was filthy and disgusting. Odors per se no longer caused disease, but the microbes that did could more often than not be found if one followed one's nose.

If the Lille monument represented only the salvation of rabies victims, it would be a historical curiosity. Rabies killed only a few hundred people per

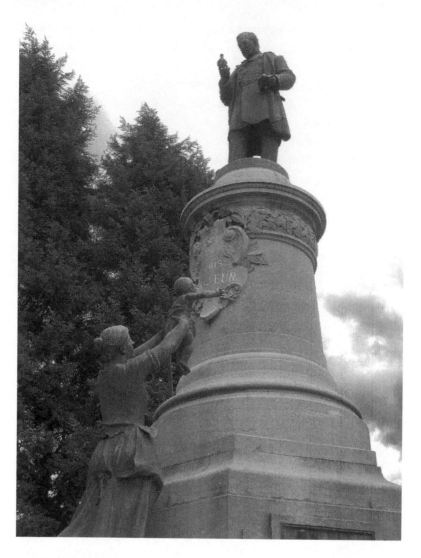

Fig. 14. The Pasteur Monument in Lille, inaugurated in 1899. Photo by author.

year in nineteenth-century France, a mere fraction of the number claimed by typhoid, diphtheria, and the other infectious diseases battled by hygienists throughout the country at the time.[15] Pasteur's triumph transcended anthrax and rabies, and even the diphtheria antitoxin, which his deputy Emile Roux had helped to produce. The monument commemorated an even greater triumph: that of a new science and a new way of understanding health and disease.

The Great Stink of Paris

The young mother in the statue represents the French nation as a whole struggling with the clash between familiar certainties and the promise of unprecedented breakthroughs. She stands in for the families visited by Villermé and his colleagues, who clung to their hygiene of protective clustering and enclosure rather than adopt the new ideal of bodily separation and aeration. She also embodies the families who grudgingly adopted the custom of disinfection but stubbornly refused to give up all contact with their family members during a potentially infectious illness. All were faced with limited choices, none of which seemed risk free. All made their decisions based on an obscure calculus in which demonstrated scientific efficacy played only a minor role. All took part, however unwittingly, in a great cultural shift, as Frenchmen gradually began to adopt the styles of bodily comportment associated with hygienic modernity. Bodies came to be more rigorously separated from one another in domestic space; excretions were more carefully policed and contained inside and outside the home; and those who faced illness increasingly turned to medical science for interventions ranging from bacteriological testing and home disinfection to antitoxin treatment for diphtheria.

In the early twenty-first century, patients and those who hope to avoid becoming patients face a very different health landscape. In much of the world today, AIDS, malaria, and deficiency diseases decimate populations, although contaminated water supplies continue to spread infections widely. In wealthy countries, chronic afflictions such as heart disease and lung cancer long ago supplanted infectious diseases as the leading causes of death, although exotic epidemics (both actual and hypothetical) still claim an outsized share of public attention.[16] Diet and exercise loom much larger than they did a century ago, as do genetic predispositions, which may or may not be medically remediable. What has not changed, however, is the fruitlessness of health-related knowledge that is not rooted in the values, beliefs, and practices of the communities that are its object. Medical truth must resonate with cultural truth; both have been reshaped by the winds of historical change. Parents in the industrialized world today may have a more highly developed sense of scientific and technological possibility than did the young mother in the Lille statue, but their choices continue to be guided by a confused blend of confidence, hope, fear, and desperation. Unspoken desires and visceral aversions shape medical science and public understanding of health today just as surely as they did a century ago. Physicians, policymakers, and others seeking to improve public health may be tempted to dismiss such considerations as extraneous to the science of health. They will be better equipped to confront the many dimensions of health-related knowledge and behavior, however, if they resist that temptation.

Historian Christopher Hamlin has called attention to the profound "contingency" that characterized the development of public health in nineteenth-century Britain. Individual and social choices, rather than externally imposed conditions, caused some hygienists' concern about the link between poverty and disease to be erased from the new profession's agenda. "To go back to the beginning, to recover possibility in the past," Hamlin argues, "is one very important way to open our eyes to the possibilities we confront in the present."[17] Recognizing that bacteriologically oriented public health triumphed for a variety of reasons other than simple truth or practical efficacy does not diminish the significance of that triumph. On the contrary, it reveals the thoroughgoing nature of a historical transformation that transcended science and medicine. It also shows that the shape of public health today is neither a natural nor an inevitable result of historical change. Recovering the lost multiplicity of etiologies and the contingency of their disappearance may open our eyes to new possibilities in understanding disease causation and prevention in the present.

Notes

ABBREVIATIONS

ACL: Archives communales de Lille
ADC: Archives départementales de la Charente
ADCdO: Archives départementales de la Côte-d'Or
ADEL: Archives départementales de l'Eure-et-Loir
ADH: Archives départementales de l'Hérault
ADIV: Archives départementales de l'Ille-et-Vilaine
ADLA: Archives départementales de la Loire-Atlantique
ADM: Archives départementales de la Mayenne
ADN: Archives départementales du Nord
ADR: Archives départementales du Rhône
ADS: Archives départementales de la Somme
ADSM: Archives départementales de la Seine-Maritime (formerly Seine-Inférieure)
ADV: Archives départementales de la Vienne
AHPML: Annales d'hygiène publique et de médecine légale
AMB: Archives municipales de Bordeaux
AMH (F.C.): Archives municipales du Havre, Fonds contemporain
AML: Archives municipales de Lille
AMLy: Archives municipales de Lyon
AMM: Archives municipales de Montpellier
AN: Archives nationales
AP: Archives de Paris
APP: Archives de la Préfecture de Police, Paris
BAM: Bulletin de l'Académie nationale de médecine
BHM: Bulletin of the History of Medicine
CAP, RA: Commission de l'assainissement de Paris instituée . . . en vue d'étudier les causes de l'infection signalée dans le département de la Seine ainsi que les moyens d'y remédier, Rapports et avis de la Commission, 94–96, in APP, DB¹: 434.
CGS: Conseil général de la Seine: Procès-verbaux
CHPS: Conseil d'hygiène publique et de salubrité du Département de la Seine
CMPP: Conseil municipal de Paris: Procès-verbaux
CMPR: Conseil municipal de Paris: Rapports et documents

CRAS: *Comptes rendus de l'Académie des sciences*
JHMAS: *Journal of the History of Medicine and Allied Sciences*
RGE: Commission des épidémies, Académie nationale de médecine, *Rapport général à M. le Ministre de l'Intérieur sur les épidémies qui ont régné en France pendant l'année* . . .
RHMC: *Revue d'histoire moderne et contemporaine*
RHPS: *Revue d'hygiène et de police sanitaire*

INTRODUCTION

1. "Sur la longue durée de la vie des germes charbonneux et sur leur conservation dans les terres cultivées," *CRAS* 92 (1881): 209–11 (session of January 31, 1881); CAP, *RA*, 94–96.

2. "Pasteur at Notre Dame: Obsequies of the Man of Science Attended by National Homage," *New York Times*, October 6, 1895; Patrice Debré, *Louis Pasteur*, trans. Elborg Forster (Baltimore: Johns Hopkins University Press, 1998), 495–96.

3. Ann F. La Berge, "Edwin Chadwick and the French Connection," *BHM* 62 (1988): 23–41. Christopher Lawrence and Richard Dixey, "Practising on Principle: Joseph Lister and the Germ Theory of Disease," in Christopher Lawrence, ed., *Medical Theory, Surgical Practice: Studies in the History of Surgery* (London: Routledge, 1992), 153–215.

4. Michael Worboys, *Spreading Germs: Disease Theories and Medical Practice in Britain, 1865–1900* (Cambridge: Cambridge University Press, 2000); Anne Hardy, "On the Cusp: Epidemiology and Bacteriology at the Local Government Board, 1890–1905," *Medical History* 42 (1998): 328–46; Nancy J. Tomes and John Harley Warner, eds., *Rethinking the Reception of the Germ Theory of Disease: Comparative Perspectives,* a special issue of the *Journal of the History of Medicine and Allied Sciences* (vol. 51, no. 1, January 1997); Nancy Tomes, *The Gospel of Germs: Men, Women, and the Microbe in American Life* (Cambridge: Harvard University Press, 1998); Paul Weindling, *Health, Race and German Politics between National Unification and Nazism, 1870–1945* (Cambridge: Cambridge University Press, 1989), 158–88; and Elizabeth A. Hachten, "Science in the Service of Society: Bacteriology, Medicine, and Hygiene in Russia, 1855–1907" (Ph.D. diss., University of Wisconsin–Madison, 1991).

5. On French regional variation in general, see Eugen Weber, *Peasants into Frenchmen: The Modernization of Rural France, 1870–1914* (Stanford: Stanford University Press, 1976) and Fernand Braudel, *The Identity of France*, trans. Siân Reynolds (London: Collins, 1988). An exemplary approach to accounting for regional differences while studying a national phenomenon on the local level can be seen in Michael Burns, *Rural Society and French Politics: Boulangism and the Dreyfus Affair, 1886–1900* (Princeton: Princeton University Press, 1984).

6. Among the many historical studies of what has been called the "social construction" of medicine, some of the most noteworthy and influential titles include Peter Wright and Andrew Treacher, eds., *The Problem of Medical Knowledge: Examining the Social Construction of Medicine* (Edinburgh: Edinburgh University Press, 1982); Charles E. Rosenberg and Janet Golden, eds., *Framing Disease: Studies in Cultural History* (New Brunswick: Rutgers University Press, 1992); Charles E. Rosen-

berg, *Explaining Epidemics and Other Studies in the History of Medicine* (Cambridge: Cambridge University Press, 1992); and Allan M. Brandt, *No Magic Bullet: A Social History of Venereal Disease in the United States since 1880* (Oxford: Oxford University Press, 1985).

7. For example, Michel Foucault, *Discipline and Punish: The Birth of the Prison*, trans. Alan Sheridan (New York: Pantheon, 1977), and Foucault, "Questions of Method," in Paul Rabinow and Nikolas Rose, eds., *The Essential Foucault* (New York: The New Press, 2003), 246–58:

> Programs, technologies, apparatuses—none of these is an "ideal type." I try to study the play and development of a set of diverse realities articulated onto each other; a program, the connection that explains it, the law that gives it its coercive power, and so on, are all just as much realities—albeit in a different mode—as the institutions that embody them or the behaviors that more or less faithfully conform to them.
>
> You say to me: Nothing happens as laid down in these "programs," they are no more than dreams, utopias, a sort of imaginary production that you aren't entitled to substitute for reality. . . .
>
> To this I would reply: . . . the fact that ["real life"] isn't the same thing as the theoreticians' schemes doesn't entail that these schemes are therefore utopian, imaginary, and so on. One could only think this if one had a very impoverished notion of the real. For one thing, the elaboration of these schemas corresponds to a whole series of diverse practices and strategies. . . . For another thing, these programs induce a whole series of effects in the real (which isn't of course the same as saying that they take the place of the real): they crystallize into institutions, they inform individual behavior, they act as grids for the perception and evaluation of things. . . .
>
> These programmings of behavior, these regimes of jurisdiction and veridiction aren't abortive schemas for the creation of a reality. They are fragments of a reality that induce such particular effects in the real as the distinction between true and false implicit in the ways men "direct," "govern," and "conduct" themselves and others. To grasp these effects as historical events . . . this is more or less my theme. You see that this has nothing to do with the project . . . of grasping a "whole society" in its "living reality." (253–54)

The "program" or "schema" at issue in this book is the cumulative efforts of hygienic reformers to implement the lessons of germ theory in everyday life and to civilize the filthy and backward elements of French society.

8. Pierre Bourdieu, *The Logic of Practice*, trans. Richard Nice (Stanford: Stanford University Press, 1990), esp. 52–65; Bourdieu, *Outline of a Theory of Practice*, trans. Richard Nice (Cambridge: Cambridge University Press, 1977), esp. 93–94; and Bourdieu and Loïc J. D. Wacquant, *An Invitation to Reflexive Sociology* (Chicago: University of Chicago Press, 1992), esp. 149, 172–73.

9. Norbert Elias, *The Civilizing Process*, trans. Edmund Jephcott (1939; repr., London: Blackwell, 1994).

10. Mary Douglas, *Purity and Danger: An Analysis of Concepts of Pollution and Taboo* (1966; repr., London: Routledge, 2002).

11. On the history of *mentalités*, see Roger Chartier, *Cultural History: Between Practices and Representations*, trans. Lydia G. Cochrane (Ithaca: Cornell University Press, 1988), 21–37. For definitions of the "history of meaning," see William J. Bouwsma, "Intellectual History in the 1980s: From the History of Ideas to the History of Meaning," *Journal of Interdisciplinary History* 12 (1981): 279–91, and Thomas R. Cole, *The Journey of Life: A Cultural History of Aging in America* (Cambridge: Cambridge University Press, 1992).

12. For example, Carlo Ginzburg, *The Cheese and the Worms: The Cosmos of a Sixteenth-Century Miller*, trans. John and Anne Tedeschi (Baltimore: Johns Hopkins University Press, 1980); Clifford Geertz, *The Interpretation of Cultures: Selected Essays* (New York: Basic Books, 1973); Natalie Zemon Davis, *Society and Culture in Early Modern France: Eight Essays* (Stanford: Stanford University Press, 1975).

13. Alain Corbin, *The Foul and the Fragrant: Odor and the French Social Imagination* (Cambridge: Harvard University Press, 1986); *The Lure of the Sea: The Discovery of the Seaside in the Western World, 1750–1840*, trans. Jocelyn Phelps (Berkeley: University of California Press, 1994); and *Village Bells: Sound and Meaning in the Nineteenth-Century French Countryside*, trans. Martin Thom (New York: Columbia University Press, 1998).

14. Stéphane Gerson, "Introduction: The Virtue of Idiosyncrasy," Special Issue: Alain Corbin and the Writing of History, *French Politics, Culture & Society* 22, no. 2 (Summer 2004): 5–6. The internal quotation comes from Jacques Revel, *Jeux d'échelles: La micro-analyse à l'expérience* (Paris: Gallimard and Le Seuil, 1996), 28.

15. On urban infrastructure, see William B. Cohen, *Urban Government and the Rise of the French City: Five Municipalities in the Nineteenth Century* (New York: Saint Martin's Press, 1998), esp. 147–240. It is risky to generalize about disease-specific death rates in the absence of any reliable nationwide data covering the period in question. However, large French cities do seem to have experienced declining rates of many infectious diseases during the last quarter of the century. See, e.g., ibid., 172; and for Paris, Jean-Noël Biraben, "Pasteur, Pasteurization, and Medicine," in R. Schofield, D. Reher, and A. Bideau, eds., *The Decline of Mortality in Europe* (Oxford: Clarendon Press, 1991), 220–32 (esp. the table at 232).

16. John Waller, *The Discovery of the Germ: Twenty Years That Transformed the Way We Think about Disease* (New York: Columbia University Press, 2002), 2.

17. See, for example, Paul de Kruif, *Microbe Hunters* (1926; repr., San Diego: Harcourt Brace, 1996), in particular his chapters on Pasteur and Koch, 54–177.

18. See, for example, Worboys, *Spreading Germs*, and the articles in Tomes and Warner, eds., *Rethinking the Reception of the Germ Theory of Disease*.

19. Rosenberg, *Explaining Epidemics*.

20. See, for example, the exchange between Judith W. Leavitt and J. Andrew Mendelsohn: Leavitt, "'Typhoid Mary' Strikes Back: Bacteriological Theory and Practice in Early Twentieth-Century Public Health," *Isis* 83 (1992): 608–29; Mendelsohn, "'Typhoid Mary' Strikes Again: The Social and the Scientific in the Making of Modern Public Health," *Isis* 86 (1995): 268–77; and Leavitt's letter to the editor, *Isis* 86 (1995): 617–18.

21. Allan Mitchell, *The Divided Path: The German Influence in French Social Reform after 1870* (Chapel Hill: University of North Carolina Press, 1991).

22. Lion Murard and Patrick Zylberman, *L'Hygiène dans la république: La Santé publique en France, ou l'utopie contrariée, 1870–1918* (Paris: Fayard, 1996).

23. See chapters 2 and 4 for detailed discussions of these specific questions.

24. The establishment of the "healthy carrier" phenomenon in the later stages of the Bacteriological Revolution is only one example of this style of reasoning. One can see this kind of thinking at work in the periodic coverage of germ scares on nightly television news shows—for example, the series of special reports on CBS Evening News's "Eye on America" segment during the week of May 12, 1997.

25. David S. Barnes, *The Making of a Social Disease: Tuberculosis in Nineteenth-Century France* (Berkeley: University of California Press, 1995); Pierre Darmon, *La Longue Traque de la variole: Les Pionniers de la médecine préventive* (Paris: Perrin, 1986); Patrice Bourdelais and Jean-Yves Raulot, *Une Peur bleue: Histoire du choléra en France, 1832–1854* (Paris: Payot, 1987); François Delaporte, *Disease and Civilization: The Cholera in Paris, 1832,* trans. Arthur Goldhammer (Cambridge: MIT Press, 1986); Catherine J. Kudlick, *Cholera in Post-Revolutionary Paris: A Cultural History* (Berkeley: University of California Press, 1996).

26. Barnes, *Making of a Social Disease;* Pierre Guillaume, *Du Désespoir au salut: Les Tuberculeux aux XIXᵉ et XXᵉ siècles* (Paris: Aubier, 1986).

27. Darmon, *Longue Traque de la variole.*

28. Kudlick, *Cholera in Post-Revolutionary Paris;* Bourdelais and Raulot, *Peur bleue.*

CHAPTER 1. "NOT EVERYTHING THAT STINKS KILLS"

1. Emile Trélat, "Rapport sur l'évacuation des vidanges," *RHPS* 4 (1882): 119. (All translations by author unless otherwise noted.)

2. This term is intended to denote both the odors themselves and the "stink," or public outcry, that arose in response to the odors. The name Great Stink has also been applied to an episode of foul odors in London in 1858, which is discussed in chapter 6. See, for example, Stephen Halliday, *The Great Stink of London: Sir Joseph Bazalgette and the Cleansing of the Victorian Capital* (Stroud: Sutton, 1999) and, more recently, a novel by Clare Clark set in London in 1858 and entitled simply *The Great Stink* (New York: Harcourt, 2005).

3. *Paris-Journal,* September 11, 1880 (quoting the newspapers *Le Gaulois* and *Le Soleil*); *Paris-Journal,* September 28, 1880 (quoting the newspaper *Le XIXᵉ Siècle*).

4. CAP, *RA,* 15 (emphasis added).

5. *Le Siècle,* September 3, 1880.

6. *Paris-Journal,* September 4, 1880.

7. Alain Corbin, *Le Miasme et la jonquille* (Paris: Aubier, 1982), translated as *The Foul and the Fragrant* (Cambridge: Harvard University Press, 1986).

8. Gérard Jacquemet, "Urbanisme parisien: La bataille du tout-à-l'égout à la fin du XIXᵉ siècle," *RHMC* 26 (1979): 505–48; Andrew R. Aisenberg, *Contagion: Disease, Government, and the "Social Question" in Nineteenth-Century France* (Stanford:

Stanford University Press, 1999), 105–12; Lenard Berlanstein, *The Working People of Paris, 1871–1914* (Baltimore: Johns Hopkins University Press, 1984), 56; Donald Reid, *Paris Sewers and Sewermen: Realities and Representations* (Cambridge: Harvard University Press, 1991), 78–83.

9. Robert Darnton, *The Great Cat Massacre and Other Episodes in French Cultural History* (New York: Basic Books, 1984), 75–104; Edward Berenson, *The Trial of Madame Caillaux* (Berkeley: University of California Press, 1992), 6–8.

10. William Ian Miller discusses the impoverished lexicon of smells in *The Anatomy of Disgust* (Cambridge: Harvard University Press, 1997), 67–68.

11. *Gazette des tribunaux*, August 6, 1880; *Le Figaro*, August 7, 1880; *Le Temps*, August 7, 1880.

12. CAP, *RA*, 158–59; *CMPP*, session of October 9, 1880, 2: 339.

13. *CMPP*, session of July 27, 1880, 2: 148.

14. *Le Siècle*, August 21, 1880.

15. The following discussion of the complaints about odors in 1880 is based on a compilation of coverage from July through October 1880 in five Parisian daily newspapers: *Le Siècle, Paris-Journal, Le Figaro, Le Petit Journal*, and *Le Temps*. These newspapers often reprinted material from other newspapers as well.

16. *Le Siècle*, August 22, 1880.

17. *Le Siècle*, September 4, 1880; *Paris-Journal*, September 4, 1880.

18. *Paris-Journal*, September 28, 1880 (quoting the newspaper *Le XIXᵉ Siècle*).

19. On the relationship between body, environment, and disease in a different cultural context during the early nineteenth century, see Conevery Bolton Valencius, *The Health of the Country: How American Settlers Understood Themselves and Their Land* (New York: Basic Books, 2002).

20. *Paris-Journal*, September 9, 1880 (quoting *Le XIXᵉ Siècle*).

21. *Paris-Journal*, September 11, 1880 (quoting the newspaper *Le XIXᵉ Siècle*).

22. *Paris-Journal*, September 27, 1880 (quoting the newspaper *Le Gaulois*).

23. *Paris-Journal*, September 9, 1880.

24. *Paris-Journal*, September 11, 1880 (quoting the newspaper *Le Gaulois*).

25. *Paris-Journal*, September 12, 1880 (quoting a letter to the editor from the newspaper *Le National*).

26. Corbin, *Foul and the Fragrant*; Caroline Hannaway, "Environment and Miasmata," in W. F. Bynum and Roy Porter, eds., *Companion Encyclopedia of the History of Medicine* (London: Routledge, 1993), 1: 292–308; George Rosen, *History of Public Health*, expanded ed. (Baltimore: Johns Hopkins University Press, 1993), 263–66.

27. *Paris-Journal*, September 9, 1880.

28. *Le Siècle*, August 22, 1880, and September 4, 1880.

29. *Paris-Journal*, September 4, 1880 (quoting *Le Rappel*).

30. *Le Siècle*, September 4, 1880 (emphasis in original).

31. *Paris-Journal*, September 4, 1880.

32. *Le Siècle*, September 15, 1880.

33. These figures are drawn from the first three volumes (1880–1882) of the *Annuaire statistique de la ville de Paris*, which began publication in 1880. Although the annual reports contain some retrospective data, they do not provide figures for

specific causes of death prior to 1880. Deaths from dysentery (one of the diseases that some observers attributed to foul odors) were relatively negligible throughout the period in question, and show no clear correlation either with the chronology of the Great Stink or with the districts of Paris most often mentioned in complaints about the odors.

34. This geographical information is based on a review of five Parisian daily newspapers (*Le Siècle, Paris-Journal, Le Figaro, Le Petit Journal,* and *Le Temps*) from July through October 1880, including material that these newspapers reprinted from other publications. Each instance in which a location of any kind was mentioned as being affected by the odors—whether a street, a landmark, an arrondissement, or a general area of the city—was counted as a single datum for the purposes of the map in figure 1. A specific location mentioned once is indicated by a single symbol on the map. In addition to specific locations, the first arrondissement in general, for example, was mentioned once in the complaints, the fourth not at all, and the ninth six times; the thickness of these arrondissements' boundaries in figure 1 reflects these proportions. I am grateful to Martin von Wyss of the Harvard Map Collection for his invaluable assistance.

35. *Le Siècle,* September 15, 1880.

36. Again, the figures are taken from *Annuaire statistique de la ville de Paris,* vols. 1–3 (1880–1882). This source does not provide month-by-month figures for specific causes of death in each arrondissement.

37. David H. Pinkney, *Napoleon III and the Rebuilding of Paris* (Princeton: Princeton University Press, 1958), 151–73; T. J. Clark, *The Painting of Modern Life: Paris in the Art of Manet and His Followers* (New York: Alfred A. Knopf, 1984), 44–46; David Harvey, *Consciousness and the Urban Experience: Studies in the History and Theory of Capitalist Urbanization* (Baltimore: Johns Hopkins University Press, 1985), 89–92, 103–6, 164–68.

38. Louis Chevalier, *Laboring Classes and Dangerous Classes in Paris during the First Half of the Nineteenth Century,* trans. Frank Jellinek (Princeton: Princeton University Press, 1973).

39. For quantitative data and maps concerning the social geography of Paris in this period, see Berlanstein, *Working People of Paris,* 11–15; Toussaint Loua, *Atlas statistique de la population de Paris* (Paris: J. Dejey, 1873), 67–76, maps 33–37.

40. For examples of complaints about cesspits during the Great Stink of 1880, see *Le Siècle,* September 12 and October 4, 1880, and *Paris-Journal,* September 13, 1880.

41. For example, see *Le Siècle,* September 6, 9, 19, and 22, 1880; *Paris-Journal,* September 20, 1880.

42. For example, see *Le Siècle,* September 6, 1880; *Le Figaro,* September 9 and 26, 1880.

43. *Le Siècle,* September 28, 1880; see also *Le Siècle,* September 4, 5, and 7, 1880.

44. For example: Procès-verbaux de la Commission d'hygiène et de salubrité du 6e arrondissement, session of October 28, 1880, in AP, Vbis 6 I^5: 1; "Discussion sur l'épidémie de fièvre typhoïde," session of June 19, 1883, *BAM,* 2d ser., 12 (1883): 791.

45. Complaints about odors in suburban towns are shown in figure 2 according to the same procedures (and on the same underlying map) used in figure 1. The waste treatment plants shown in figure 2 are those mentioned in newspaper coverage of the Great Stink of 1880, as well as in the official government reports.

46. *Le Temps*, August 7, 1880.

47. *Paris-Journal*, September 11, 1880 (quoting *Le Soleil*); *Paris-Journal*, September 11, 1880 (quoting *Le Gaulois*); *Paris-Journal*, September 12, 1880; *Le Siècle*, September 11, 1880.

48. *Paris-Journal*, September 28, 1880 (quoting *La Lanterne*).

49. *Paris-Journal*, September 12, 1880 (quoting *L'Evènement*).

50. Georges Grison, "Les Pestiférés de Paris," *Le Figaro*, September 28, 1880.

51. *Le Siècle*, August 21, September 26, and September 28, 1880.

52. Robert A. Nye, *Masculinity and Male Codes of Honor in Modern France* (New York: Oxford University Press, 1993), 191–200; Berenson, *Trial of Madame Caillaux*, 169–207.

53. *Paris-Journal*, September 28, 1880.

54. *Paris-Journal*, September 17, 1880 (quoting *Le Soir*).

55. *Paris-Journal*, September 9, 1880.

56. These were the principal complaints addressed by the health committee of the tenth arrondissement in 1880. "Rapport sur les travaux de la Commission d'hygiène et de salubrité du 10ᵉ arrondissement pendant l'année 1880," AP, Vbis 10 I⁵: 5. The records of most of the district health committees (including those of the ninth and eighteenth arrondissements, where the odors of 1880 were particularly intense) have not survived.

57. Procès-verbaux de la Commission d'hygiène et de salubrité du 6ᵉ arrondissement, session of October 28, 1880, in AP, Vbis 6 I⁵: 1.

58. *CMPP*, session of July 27, 1880, 2: 148.

59. *CMPP*, session of October 7, 1880, 2: 302–306.

60. Ibid.

61. *CMPP*, session of October 9, 1880, 2: 324–33.

62. *CMPP*, sessions of October 9 and 12, 1880, 2: 338–41, 367.

63. *CGS*, session of October 26, 1880, 42–82, quotations at pp. 42, 43.

64. Ibid.; the specific allegations regarding political influence in the contrasting cases of Nanterre and Hautes-Bornes are at pp. 45–47, 61, and 66; *CMPP*, session of October 12, 1880, 2: 354–55.

65. *CGS*, session of October 26, 1880, 66–70, 77–78.

66. CHPS, "Commission spéciale pour l'étude des causes de l'infection de Paris," report to prefect of police, September 29, 1880, in *Journal officiel de la République française*, October 7, 1880, 10333.

67. Ibid., 10333–37.

68. CAP, *RA*, 5–6. On Brouardel, see Lion Murard and Patrick Zylberman, *L'Hygiène dans la république: La Santé publique en France, ou l'utopie contrariée, 1870–1918* (Paris: Fayard, 1996), 198–203; Olivier Faure, *Histoire sociale de la médecine, XVIIIᵉ-XXᵉ siècles* (Paris: Anthropos, 1994), 180; Jacques Léonard, *La Médecine entre les pouvoirs et les savoirs* (Paris: Aubier, 1981), 252–54, 292–95; and George Weisz,

The Medical Mandarins: The French Academy of Medicine in the Nineteenth and Early Twentieth Centuries (New York: Oxford University Press, 1995), 79–80.

69. CAP, RA, 13–14.

70. Ibid., 23.

71. Ibid., 15.

72. Out of the voluminous literature on Pasteur, the most significant contributions include Gerald L. Geison, The Private Science of Louis Pasteur (Princeton: Princeton University Press, 1995); Bruno Latour, The Pasteurization of France, trans. Alan Sheridan and John Law (Cambridge: Harvard University Press, 1988); Pierre Darmon, Pasteur (Paris: Fayard, 1995); René J. Dubos's classic Louis Pasteur: Free Lance of Science (Boston: Little, Brown, 1950); and the somewhat offbeat, provocative volume by Daniel Raichvarg, Louis Pasteur: L'Empire des microbes (Paris: Gallimard, 1995).

73. The original report of the episode was published as "Compte rendu sommaire des expériences faites à Pouilly-le-Fort, près Melun, sur la vaccination charbonneuse," CRAS 92 (1881): 1378–87. On the Pouilly-le-Fort demonstration, see Latour, "Give Me a Laboratory and I will Raise the World," in Karin D. Knorr-Cetina and Michael Mulkay, eds., Science Observed: Perspectives on the Social Study of Science (London: Sage, 1983), 141–70; Geison, Private Science of Louis Pasteur, 145–76; and Raichvarg, Louis Pasteur, 78–81.

74. "Compte rendu sommaire des expériences faites à Pouilly-le-Fort."

75. "Sur la longue durée de la vie des germes charbonneux et sur leur conservation dans les terres cultivées," CRAS 92 (1881): 209–11 (session of January 31, 1881). Pasteur's study was quoted in the final report of the commission studying the Paris odors of 1880: CAP, RA, 94–96. Interestingly enough, the Rosières experiment does not appear in even the most thorough and detailed biographies of Pasteur. The village's name is spelled Rozières in Pasteur's study, but today's standard spelling Rosières is used here.

76. CAP, RA, 95 (emphasis added).

77. Ibid., 95–96 (emphasis added).

78. Ibid., 96.

79. Although improbable, it is theoretically conceivable that anthrax spores could be inhaled under the circumstances Pasteur described at Rosières. After all, what was called "wool-sorters' disease," a rare pulmonary form of anthrax in humans, was known to occur in textile workers who manipulated animal hairs or hides and inhaled virulent spores from infected animals. However, wool-sorters' disease involved direct, close contact with animal remains and manifested itself differently than did other forms of anthrax. See Lise Wilkinson, "Anthrax," in Kenneth F. Kiple, ed., Cambridge World History of Human Disease (Cambridge: Cambridge University Press, 1993), 582–84.

80. This discussion of spontaneous generation and the Pasteur-Pouchet debate is drawn from the following sources: Gerald L. Geison, "Louis Pasteur," in Charles C. Gillispie, ed., Dictionary of Scientific Biography (New York: Charles Scribner's Sons, 1981), 10: 366–72; John Farley and Gerald L. Geison, "Science, Politics and Spontaneous Generation in Nineteenth-Century France," Bulletin of the History of Medi-

cine 48 (1974): 161–98; Nils Roll-Hansen, "Experimental Method and Spontaneous Generation: The Controversy between Pasteur and Pouchet, 1859–64," *JHMAS* 34 (1979): 273–92.

81. See Pierre Miquel, *Les organismes vivants de l'atmosphère* (Paris: Gauthier-Villars, 1883).

82. Geison, *Private Science of Louis Pasteur,* 177–256.

83. CAP, *RA,* 31–32.

84. Ibid.

85. Ibid., 78–84; quotation at 84 (emphasis in original).

86. *Le Siècle,* September 3, 7, and 27, 1880.

87. The full quotation reads: "There are two doctrines which I think these conclusions, and my own investigations, would establish: one is in respect to the sanatory condition of towns, that all smell is, if it be intense, immediate acute disease, and eventually we may say that, by depressing the system and rendering it susceptible to the action of other causes, all smell is disease; and I think the other conclusion will be established as to agricultural districts, that all smell of decomposing matter may be said to indicate the loss of money. Certainly that extent of dilution that prevents the escape of any offensive emanations, indicates the best state in which the manure is preserved, and the state in which it is best applied." "Minutes of Evidence taken before Select Committee on Metropolitan Sewage Manure," June 26, 1846, in House of Commons, *Parliamentary Papers,* 1846, 10: 651.

88. See, for example, Rosen, *History of Public Health,* 260–66, 270–319; Paul de Kruif, *Microbe Hunters* (1926; repr., San Diego: Harcourt Brace, 1996). For more recent and more subtle analyses, see the contributions to the special issue of the *Journal of the History of Medicine and Allied Sciences* (vol. 51, no. 1, January 1997) devoted to "rethinking the reception of the germ theory of disease," edited by Nancy J. Tomes and John Harley Warner; Tomes, *Gospel of Germs;* and Michael Worboys, *Spreading Germs: Disease Theories and Medical Practice in Britain, 1865–1900* (Cambridge: Cambridge University Press, 2000).

89. Roy Porter, *The Greatest Benefit to Mankind: A Medical History of Humanity* (New York: W. W. Norton, 1998), 442.

90. Ibid., 259–60, 262, 411; Rosen, *History of Public Health,* 263–66; John Duffy, *The Sanitarians: A History of American Public Health* (Urbana: University of Illinois Press, 1990), 67–68, 129.

91. CHPS, "Commission spéciale pour l'étude des causes de l'infection de Paris," 10334.

92. *Le Siècle,* October 6, 1880.

93. Unsigned notes from Rosières dated November 24, 1880, in Pasteur's laboratory notebook, 10ᵉ cahier, November 10, 1880–April 10, 1882, Bibliothèque nationale de France, manuscrits occidentaux, Nouvelles acquisitions françaises 18016.

94. Although some of this growth can be attributed to the city's annexation of adjacent suburban towns in 1860, the vast majority of the population increase came from provincial migration to the capital; see Pinkney, *Napoleon III and the Rebuilding of Paris,* 151–52.

95. In addition to Pinkney's classic *Napoleon III and the Rebuilding of Paris* and

Jeanne Gaillard's *Paris, la ville, 1852–1870: L'Urbanisme parisien à l'heure d'Haussmann* (Paris: Honoré Champion, 1977), there are important discussions of Haussmann's program and its critics in Anthony Sutcliffe, *The Autumn of Central Paris* (Montreal: McGill–Queen's University Press, 1971); Clark, *Painting of Modern Life*; Harvey, *Consciousness and the Urban Experience*; and David P. Jordan, *Transforming Paris: The Life and Labors of Baron Haussmann* (New York: Free Press, 1995).

96. Anthony Vidler, "The Scenes of the Street: Transformations in Ideal and Reality, 1750–1871," in Stanford Anderson, ed., *On Streets* (Cambridge: MIT Press, 1978), 91; see also Harvey, *Consciousness and the Urban Experience*, 178.

97. Vidler, "Scenes of the Street," 91; Jordan, *Transforming Paris*, 48; Pinkney, *Napoleon III and the Rebuilding of Paris*, 30–31.

98. Jordan, *Transforming Paris*, 267–84; Pinkney, *Napoleon III and the Rebuilding of Paris*, 94–150; Faure, *Histoire sociale de la médecine*, 181.

99. Clark, *Painting of Modern Life*, 23–78; Jordan, *Transforming Paris*, 185–210.

100. G. M. Young, *Victorian England: Portrait of an Age* (London: Oxford University Press, 1936), 11, as cited in Pinkney, *Napoleon III and the Rebuilding of Paris*, 127.

101. On the increased sensitivity to odors and the intensifying "olfactory vigilance" that marked the nineteenth century, see Corbin, *Foul and the Fragrant*.

102. Clark, *Painting of Modern Life*, 66.

103. Harvey, *Consciousness and the Urban Experience*, 204.

104. *Paris-Journal*, September 9, 1880.

105. *Le Siècle*, September 28, 1880.

106. *Le Siècle*, September 12, 1880, citing *Le Gaulois*, September 11, 1880.

107. Reid, *Paris Sewers and Sewermen*, 36; CAP, *RA*, 86. Reid's book documents especially well the conflicting reactions provoked in contemporaries by the sewers.

108. Reid, *Paris Sewers and Sewermen*, 12–15, 25–30.

109. The following discussion of the *tout-à-l'égout* controversy is based in large part on Jacquemet, "Urbanisme parisien," 505–48, as well as Reid, *Paris Sewers and Sewermen*, 58–65, 79–83, 118–20, and Roger-Henri Guerrand, "La bataille du tout-à-l'égout," *L'Histoire*, February 1983, 66–74.

110. Jacquemet, "Urbanisme parisien," 517–19, 527–45.

111. Jules Brunfaut, *Les Odeurs de Paris: Assainissement* (Paris: J. Baudry, 1880), 29; Léon Le Fort, "Discussion sur l'épidémie de fièvre typhoïde," Academy of Medicine, session of June 12, 1883, *BAM*, 2d ser., 12 (1883): 763.

112. *Paris-Journal*, September 12, 1880 (quoting *Le Soir*).

113. *Le Siècle*, August 22, 1880 (quoting *Le Gaulois*). Both sentences in this quotation end with ellipses in the original. The last sentence reads: "Il suffit de passer à côté d'un *regard* d'égout pour se convaincre de l'évidence de cette vérité, qui saute *au nez* . . . " (emphases in original).

114. CAP, *RA*, 19.

115. Ibid., 85. Brouardel attributed this "energetic" turn of phrase to the Bavarian physician Franz von Gietl (although Brouardel gives his name as "Gielt"), to whose research on typhoid fever Brouardel referred to support his opposition to the *tout-à-l'égout*. My thanks to Ed Morman for helping me track down von Gietl.

116. CHPS, *Rapport sur les questions posées au Conseil d'hygiène par la commission du Sénat relativement à l'assainissement de la Seine* (Paris: Chaix, 1888), 14, 20; Corbin, *Foul and the Fragrant*, 224–25; Reid, *Paris Sewers and Sewermen*, 81; Jacquemet, "Urbanisme parisien," 514–15.

117. Jacquemet, "Urbanisme parisien," statistics at 543.

118. *Gazette des tribunaux*, September 27–28, 1880; *Le Petit Journal*, September 28, 1880.

119. *Gazette des tribunaux*, September 27–28, 1880; *Le Figaro*, September 27 and October 11, 1880.

120. *Le Siècle*, September 29, 1880; *Le Petit Journal*, September 28, 1880; *Le Figaro*, September 29 and 30 and October 2 and 11, 1880. I have been able to find no evidence of the criminal investigation of the *vidangeurs* proceeding beyond the evidence-gathering stage, nor of any final judicial determination in the matter.

121. *Gazette des tribunaux*, September 27–28, 1880; *L'Illustration*, October 2, 1880; see also *Le Figaro*, September 27, 1880, and *Le Petit Journal*, October 1, 1880.

122. Reid, *Paris Sewers and Sewermen*, 39–52; quotations at 39, 41, 47.

123. I use the term "positivist" not to refer to the specific school of philosophical thought associated with Auguste Comte's *"philosophie positive,"* but rather in its more general sense, designating a characteristic late nineteenth-century faith in progress through science.

124. See Catherine J. Kudlick, *Cholera in Post-Revolutionary Paris: A Cultural History* (Berkeley: University of California Press, 1996), and Richard J. Evans, "Epidemics and Revolutions: Cholera in Nineteenth-Century Europe," *Past and Present* 120 (1988): 123–46.

125. Judith F. Stone, *Sons of the Revolution: Radical Democrats in France, 1862–1914* (Baton Rouge: Louisiana State University Press, 1996), 88–96.

126. Jean-Marie Mayeur, *Les Débuts de la Troisième République, 1871–1898* (Paris: Seuil, 1973), 105; R. D. Anderson, *France, 1870–1914: Politics and Society* (London: Routledge & Kegan Paul, 1977), 12.

127. On Ferry's intellectual and philosophical debt to positivism, see Claude Nicolet, "Jules Ferry et la tradition positiviste," in François Furet, ed., *Jules Ferry, fondateur de la république* (Paris: Editions de l'Ecole des hautes études en sciences sociales, 1985), 23–48.

128. *Le Siècle*, September 4, 1880.

129. *Le Siècle*, September 11, 1880.

130. Francisque Sarcey, *Les Odeurs de Paris: Assainissement de la Seine* (Paris: Gauthier-Villars, 1882), 6–7.

131. Philip Nord, *The Republican Moment: Struggles for Democracy in Nineteenth-Century France* (Cambridge: Harvard University Press, 1995), 133; see also Judith F. Stone, *Sons of the Revolution: Radical Democrats in France, 1862–1914* (Baton Rouge: Louisiana State University Press, 1996), 88ff.

132. See Sanford Elwitt, *The Making of the Third Republic: Class and Politics in France, 1868–1884* (Baton Rouge: Louisiana State University Press, 1975), 208–15; Elwitt, *The Third Republic Defended: Bourgeois Reform in France, 1880–1914* (Baton Rouge: Louisiana State University Press, 1986), quotation at 292; David S. Barnes,

The Making of a Social Disease: Tuberculosis in Nineteenth-Century France (Berkeley: University of California Press, 1995), esp. 174–214.

CHAPTER 2. THE SANITARIANS' LEGACY, OR
HOW HEALTH BECAME PUBLIC

1. Erwin H. Ackerknecht, *Medicine at the Paris Hospital, 1794–1848* (Baltimore: Johns Hopkins University Press, 1967); Michel Foucault, *The Birth of the Clinic: An Archeology of Medical Perception,* trans. A. M. Sheridan Smith (New York: Pantheon, 1973); Jacalyn Duffin, *To See with a Better Eye: A Life of R. T. H. Laënnec* (Princeton: Princeton University Press, 1998).

2. Ann F. La Berge, "Edwin Chadwick and the French Connection," *BHM* 62 (1988): 23–41.

3. Among others: Erwin H. Ackerknecht, "Hygiene in France, 1815–1848," *BHM* 22 (1948): 562–93; Ann F. La Berge, *Mission and Method: The Early Nineteenth-Century Public Health Movement* (Cambridge: Cambridge University Press, 1992); Bernard-Pierre Lécuyer, "L'Hygiène en France avant Pasteur," in Claire Salomon-Bayet, ed., *Pasteur et la révolution pastorienne* (Paris: Payot, 1986), 67–139; Lécuyer, "Démographie, statistique et hygiène publique sous la monarchie censitaire," *Annales de démographie historique,* 1977, 215–45; William Coleman, *Death Is a Social Disease: Public Health and Political Economy in Early Industrial France* (Madison: University of Wisconsin Press, 1982); Patrice Bourdelais, ed., *Les Hygiénistes: Enjeux, modèles, et pratiques, XVIIIe–XXe siècles* (Paris: Belin, 2001).

4. Ackerknecht, "Hygiene in France"; La Berge, *Mission and Method.*

5. La Berge, *Mission and Method.*

6. Alain Corbin, "Présentation," in Alexandre Parent-Duchâtelet, *La Prostitution à Paris au XIXe siècle* (Paris: Seuil, 1981), 9–47; Lécuyer, "L'Hygiène en France avant Pasteur."

7. Coleman, *Death Is a Social Disease.*

8. La Berge, *Mission and Method,* 318; Coleman, *Death Is a Social Disease;* Lécuyer, "L'Hygiène en France avant Pasteur" and "Démographie, statistique et hygiène publique."

9. A. J. B. Parent-Duchâtelet, "Des obstacles que les préjugés médicaux apportent dans quelques circonstances, à l'assainissement des villes et à l'établissement de certaines manufactures," *Hygiène publique,* 2 vols. (Paris: J. B. Baillière, 1836), 1: 12–58; on Montfaucon, see also Donald Reid, *Paris Sewers and Sewermen: Realities and Representations* (Cambridge: Harvard University Press, 1991), 71–83.

10. Parent-Duchâtelet, "Des obstacles que les préjugés médicaux," 42–43.

11. Ibid., 29–44; quoted passage at 44 (emphasis in original). It is difficult to determine precisely whom Parent-Duchâtelet was addressing in this text. Many professors taught surgery and pathological anatomy at the time of his studies in Paris (he received his degree in 1814). Among the most prominent were Alexis Boyer, Philippe Pinel (who gained fame as one of the fathers of modern psychiatry), and Philippe Pelletan. Ackerknecht, *Medicine at the Paris Hospital;* Françoise Huguet, *Les Professeurs de la faculté de médecine de Paris: Dictionnaire biographique, 1794–1939* (Paris: Editions du CNRS, 1991).

12. Parent-Duchâtelet, "Des obstacles que les préjugés médicaux," 44–45.

13. Ibid., 45 (emphasis added).

14. On the Paris clinical school see: Ackerknecht, *Medicine at the Paris Hospital;* Foucault, *Birth of the Clinic;* Russell Maulitz, *Morbid Appearances: The Anatomy of Pathology in the Early Nineteenth Century* (Cambridge: Cambridge University Press, 1987); John Harley Warner, *Against the Spirit of System: The French Impulse in Nineteenth-Century American Medicine* (Princeton: Princeton University Press, 1998).

15. A. J. B. Parent-Duchâtelet, "Essai sur les cloaques ou égouts de la ville de Paris, envisagés sous le rapport de l'hygiène publique et de la topographie médicale de cette ville" (1824), in *Hygiène publique*, 1: 156–307; quoted passages at 157–60 (emphasis in original).

16. Ibid., 160.

17. Parent-Duchâtelet, "Des obstacles que les préjugés médicaux," 46.

18. Louis-René Villermé, *Tableau de l'état physique et moral des ouvriers employés dans les manufactures de coton, de laine et de soie*, 2 vols. (Paris: Jules Renouard, 1840), 1: v–vi.

19. Alphonse Guérard, "Notice sur M. Villermé," *AHPML*, 2d ser., 21 (1864): 162–77.

20. E. Vallin, review of Adrien Proust, *Traité d'hygiène publique et privée* (G. Masson, 1877), *AHPML*, 2d ser., 48 (1877): 389.

21. Villermé, *Tableau*, 2: 350–52.

22. Claude Lachaise, *Topographie médicale de Paris* (1822), quoted in Louis Chevalier, *Laboring Classes and Dangerous Classes in Paris during the First Half of the Nineteenth Century*, trans. Frank Jellinek (Princeton: Princeton University Press, 1973), 151.

23. Ann F. La Berge, "The Paris Health Council, 1802–1848," *BHM* 49 (1975): 339–52.

24. "Rapport du Conseil de salubrité," *AHPML* 2 (1829): 331–32.

25. Villermé, *Tableau*, 1: 5–6. Villermé singled out Lille as the city in which this working-class self-segregation was most marked.

26. Louis-René Villermé, "Sur les cités ouvrières," *AHPML* 43 (1850): 241–61, quotation at 245–46.

27. Louis Chevalier's sprawling *Laboring Classes and Dangerous Classes in Paris* paints a lurid and thorough landscape of this fear. While Chevalier purports to demonstrate that the Parisian working poor were in fact menacingly criminal and disease-ridden, what he actually shows beyond a doubt is that they were almost universally *seen* (in the eyes of bourgeois observers) as being so.

28. Honoré de Balzac, *César Birotteau*, quoted in Chevalier, *Laboring Classes*, 152–53. (I have edited Jellinek's translation slightly.)

29. Vicomte de Launay (1838), quoted in Chevalier, *Laboring Classes*, 152.

30. Henri Lecouturier, *Paris incompatible avec la République* (1848), quoted in Chevalier, *Laboring Classes*, 155–56.

31. On medical attitudes toward contagionism before the Bacteriological Revolution, see Erwin H. Ackerknecht, "Anticontagionism between 1821 and 1867," *BHM* 22 (1948): 562–93; Roger Cooter, "Anticontagionism and History's Medical

Record," in Wright and Treacher, eds., *Problem of Medical Knowledge*, 87–108; Margaret Pelling, *Cholera, Fever, and English Medicine, 1825–1865* (Oxford: Oxford University Press, 1978); Peter Baldwin, *Contagion and the State in Europe, 1830–1930* (Cambridge: Cambridge University Press, 1999).

32. Léon Colin, "De l'influence pathogénique de l'encombrement," *AHPML*, 2d ser., 45 (1876): 233–35.

33. Ibid., 235–41; quotations at 239, 240. Colin's general argument represented a "contingent contagionist" viewpoint that was widespread and generally uncontroversial in medicine at this time. See, for example, Pelling, *Cholera, Fever, and English Medicine;* Cooter, "Anticontagionism and History's Medical Record"; Charles E. Rosenberg, "Florence Nightingale on Contagion: The Hospital as Moral Universe," in Rosenberg, ed., *Healing and History: Essays for George Rosen* (New York: Science History Publications, 1979), 116–36.

34. Colin, "De l'influence pathogénique de l'encombrement," 241–42.

35. A. J. B. Parent-Duchâtelet, "Rapport sur le curage des égouts Amelot, de la Roquette, Saint-Martin et autres," in *Hygiène publique*, 1: 308–437.

36. A J. B. Parent-Duchâtelet, "Recherches et considerations sur la riviere de Bievre, ou des Gobelins, et sur les moyens d'ameliorer son cours, relativement a la salubrite publique et a l'industrie manufacturiere de la ville de Paris" (1822), in *Hygiène publique*, 1: 98–155.

37. "Urinoirs," *AHPML* 44 (1850): 470–71.

38. A. J. B. Parent-Duchâtelet, "Rapport sur les améliorations à introduire dans les fosses d'aisances, leur mode de vidange, et les voiries de la ville de Paris," in *Hygiène publique*, 2: 351.

39. Alphonse Guérard, "Observations sur le méphitisme et la désinfection des fosses d'aisances," *AHPML* 32 (1844): 342–43.

40. H. Gaultier de Claubry, "De la suppression de la voirie de Montfaucon," *AHPML* 40 (1848): 306–308.

41. Adolphe Chevallier, "Observations sur l'hygiène publique," *AHPML* 8 (1832): 214–16.

42. M. Bricheteau, "Extrait d'un rapport de la Commission des épidémies de l'Académie Royale de Médecine pour l'année 1839 et une partie de 1840," *AHPML* 25 (1841): 272, 276, 278.

43. Dr. É. Beaugrand, "Mortalité produite par les émanations putrides s'exhalant d'un dépôt de paniers à poisson," *AHPML*, 2d ser., 16 (1861): 222–23, citing an article by A. Chevallier in *Journal de chimie médicale*, December 1860.

44. For example, an 1861 medical thesis purported to show that emanations from the decaying corpses of animals that had died of noncontagious causes were harmless, and that studies claiming the contrary had confused simple asphyxiation for actual morbid effects. É. Beaugrand, "Des miasmes provenant des matières animales en putréfaction," *AHPML*, 2d ser., 17 (1862): 457–60.

45. Ambroise Tardieu, *Dictionnaire d'hygiène publique et de salubrité*, cited in Beaugrand, "Des miasmes provenant," 458.

46. Parent-Duchâtelet, "Recherches et considerations sur la riviere de Bievre," 151–52.

47. Parent-Duchâtelet, "Des obstacles que les préjugés médicaux," 14.

48. Ibid., 14–18.

49. Bricheteau, Chevallier, and Furnari, "Note sur les vidangeurs," *AHPML* 28 (1842): 46–55; Guérard, "Observations sur le méphitisme."

50. Villermé, *Tableau*, 1: 5–6.

51. Bricheteau, "Extrait d'un rapport de la Commission des épidémies," 269–71.

52. See, for example, Norbert Elias, *Civilizing Process*, trans. Edmund Jephcott (1939 repr., London: Blackwell, 1994), 3–41.

53. William Coleman has emphasized the economic/material dimension of civilization in Villermé's work (*Death Is a Social Disease*, 284–95, 300–302). This reading is valuable but, in my view, underestimates the cultural and moral dimensions of the concept throughout Villermé's most important hygienic writings.

54. Louis-René Villermé, "Des épidémies sous les rapports de l'hygiène publique, de la statistique médicale et de l'économie politique," *AHPML* 9 (1833): 5–8.

55. Ibid., 9–10.

56. Coleman, among others, demonstrates clearly that Villermé was at heart a liberal in matters of political economy, and that he found himself constitutionally incapable of drawing the radical conclusions that might seem to others implicit in his findings about socioeconomic inequalities in health. *Death Is a Social Disease*, 241–306.

57. Villermé, "Des épidémies," 58.

58. Louis-François Benoiston de Châteauneuf and Louis-René Villermé, "Rapport d'un voyage fait dans les cinq départements de la Bretagne pendant les années 1840 et 1841, d'après les ordres de l'Académie des sciences morales et politiques," *Mémoires de l'Académie des sciences morales et politiques* 4 (1844): 641–42.

59. Ibid., 644.

60. Ibid., 644–45, quoting Emile Souvestre in *Revue des deux mondes*, 4th ser., 4 (1835): 403.

61. Benoiston de Châteauneuf and Villermé, "Rapport d'un voyage," 647–54.

62. Ibid., 657–59.

63. Ibid., 782–84.

64. Ibid., 784–85.

65. Bricheteau, "Extrait d'un rapport de la Commission des épidémies," 269–90.

66. François-Joseph Double, "Rapport sur l'insalubrité de la plaine du Forez," *Archives générales de médecine* 14 (1827): 594, quoted in Octave du Mesnil, "Influence de l'instruction sur la santé publique et la mortalité," *AHPML*, 2d ser., 38 (1872): 103–4.

67. Du Mesnil, "Influence de l'instruction," 105–106, quoting a summary of Mêlier's study in *Archives générales de médecine* 17 (1828): 459.

68. Ibid., 111–12.

69. Chevalier, *Laboring Classes*, 11–17; Catherine J. Kudlick, *Cholera in Post-Revolutionary Paris: A Cultural History* (Berkeley: University of California Press, 1996); Richard J. Evans, "Epidemics and Revolutions: Cholera in Nineteenth-Century Europe," *Past and Present* 120 (1988): 123–46.

70. See, among others, La Berge, *Mission and Method*, 42–43, 180–83; and David S. Barnes, *The Making of a Social Disease: Tuberculosis in Nineteenth-Century France* (Berkeley: University of California Press, 1995), 38–41. The term "hygienism" comes from La Berge, *Mission and Method*, esp. chapters 1 (9–48) and 9 (316–19).

71. "Alphonse L., pedestrian," *De la salubrité de la Ville de Paris* (1826), quoted in Chevalier, *Laboring Classes*, 461–42 n. 9. Nearly identical wording can of course be found in countless nineteenth-century texts on the hygienic crisis in and/or unpleasant physical state of the capital.

72. Bricheteau, "Extrait d'un rapport de la Commission des épidémies," 284.

73. Villermé, *Tableau*, 2: 350–51.

74. Coleman, *Death Is a Social Disease*; Barnes, *Making of a Social Disease*, 31–33.

75. Mary Douglas, *Purity and Danger: An Analysis of Concepts of Pollution and Taboo* (1966; repr., London: Routledge, 2002), 36.

76. Victor Considérant, *Description du phalanstère et considérations sociales sur l'architectonique* (1848), quoted in Chevalier, *Laboring Classes*, 154–55.

77. Parent-Duchâtelet, "Des obstacles que les préjugés médicaux," 14.

78. Jules Arnould, "Considérations sur l'atmosphère de la ville de Lille et sur son influence étiologique propre," *AHPML*, 3d ser., 1 (1879): 309 (emphasis added).

79. Villermé, "Sur les cités ouvrieres," 251.

80. Ibid., 252–53.

81. Report of "une commission de l'Intendance sanitaire (conseil de salubrité) du département du Nord," April 1, 1832, quoted in Villermé, *Tableau*, 1: 86–87 n. 1.

82. Ibid.

83. Ibid.

84. Villermé, *Tableau*, 1: 80–84.

85. Thomas Laqueur, "Bodies, Detail, and the Humanitarian Narrative," in Lynn Hunt, ed., *The New Cultural History* (Berkeley: University of California Press, 1989), 176–204; Karen Halttunen, "Humanitarianism and the Pornography of Pain in Anglo-American Culture," *American Historical Review* 100 (1995): 303–34; Joan W. Scott, "'L'Ouvrière! Mot impie, sordide . . .': Women Workers in the Discourse of French Political Economy, 1840–1860," in Joan Wallach Scott, *Gender and the Politics of History* (New York: Columbia University Press, 1988), 150; Barnes, *Making of a Social Disease*, 184.

86. Villermé, *Tableau*, 1: 84–85 (emphasis added).

87. Unsigned review of J.-J. Virey, *Petit manuel d'hygiène prophylactique contre les épidémies, ou de leurs meilleurs préservatifs, AHPML* 9 (1833): 235–36; Isidore Bourdon, *Notions d'hygiène pratique* (Paris: L. Hachette, 1844), 199, 205.

88. Guérard, "Notice sur M. Villermé," 163.

89. Villermé, "Sur les cités ouvrieres," 246–47.

90. Ibid., 258–59.

91. Felix Driver, "Moral Geographies: Social Science and the Urban Environment in Mid-Nineteenth Century England," *Transactions of the Institute of British Geographers* 13 (1988): 281–82.

92. Colin, "De l'influence pathogénique de l'encombrement," 246–47, 403, 407.

93. Rodolphe El-Khoury, "Introduction," in Dominique Laporte, *History of Shit*, trans. Nadia Benabid and Rodolphe El-Khoury (Cambridge: MIT Press, 2000), xi–xii.

94. See, for example, the folk wisdom voiced by the proverbs collected in Françoise Loux and Philippe Richard, *Sagesses du corps: La santé et la maladie dans les proverbes français* (Paris: G.-P. Maisonneuve et Larose, 1978), 103, 115–26.

CHAPTER 3. TAXONOMIES OF TRANSMISSION

1. Charlemagne Pilat, *Rapport général sur les épidémies qui ont régné dans le département du Nord pendant l'année 1883* (Lille: L. Danel, 1884), 12–13; Dr. (Jacques) Botrel, "Arrt. de St.-Malo / Epidémies 1882," March 10, 1883, ADIV 5 M 70.

2. This explains why I occasionally use the relativistic phrase "caused x" instead of "was believed to cause x" for certain historical etiologies. On the implications of distinguishing belief from knowledge, see Byron J. Good, *Medicine, Rationality, and Experience: An Anthropological Perspective* (Cambridge: Cambridge University Press, 1994), 1–24. I do not do so to make some fatuous point that all etiological claims are always equally valid. Rather, I am bending over backward to emphasize that *some* bygone etiologies were true by the standards of their time and place, which were as systematic and scientific in their contexts as later epistemologies were in theirs. Many etiological claims of the prebacteriological era were based on years of careful observation and correlation, and were rooted in the most advanced medical science of the time. Today's scientific orthodoxy is tomorrow's misguided superstition; however, it is impossible to know at any given moment *which* truths will eventually be undone. Obsolete etiological beliefs or facts may not meet the standards of truth established by today's epistemologies, or even by those of 1900, but they were as true as any etiological observations could be by the standards of the time and place in which they were made. By writing "caused" instead of "was believed to cause," I am trying to call attention to the coherence and empiricism of a now-obsolete body of knowledge, and thereby perhaps to rescue the actors who produced and acted upon it, in E. P. Thompson's words, from "the enormous condescension of posterity." E. P. Thompson, *The Making of the English Working Class* (1963; repr., New York: Vintage Books, 1966), 12–13.

3. "Bulletin d'information sanitaire," distributed to prefectures by the Direction de l'Assistance et de l'Hygiène publiques in the Interior Ministry, ADH, 5 M 147. The form includes the following instruction: "This bulletin must be filled out by the prefecture based on the information furnished by mayors and epidemic doctors; it must be accompanied by the reports of these doctors."

4. E. Littré, *Dictionnaire de médecine, de chirurgie, de pharmacie, de l'art vétérinaire et des sciences qui s'y rapportent*, 15th ed. (Paris: J. B. Baillière, 1884), 484.

5. Dr. [Sigismond] Jaccoud, ed., *Nouveau dictionnaire de médecine et de chirurgie pratiques*, vol. 36 (Paris: J. B. Baillière, 1884), 563–64 (emphasis in original).

6. On illness narratives and their interpretation, see Arthur Kleinman, *The Illness Narratives: Suffering, Healing, and the Human Condition* (New York: Basic Books, 1988). On narrativity, individual and collective etiologies, and morality, see David S. Barnes, *The Making of a Social Disease: Tuberculosis in Nineteenth-Century*

France (Berkeley: University of California Press, 1995), 78–80; Hayden White, "The Value of Narrativity in the Representation of Reality," *Critical Inquiry* 7 (1980): 5–27; and White, *The Content of the Form: Narrative Discourse and Historical Representation* (Baltimore: Johns Hopkins University Press, 1987).

7. Dr. Léon Baraduc, "Contribution à l'étiologie de la fièvre typhoïde," *RHPS* 3 (1881): 33.

8. Françoise Loux and Philippe Richard, *Sagesses du corps: La santé et la maladie dans les proverbes français* (Paris: G. P. Maisonneuve et Larose, 1978), 279, 283, 300.

9. Report by Dr. Régnault to prefect on behalf of Conseil départemental d'hygiène, July 3,1873, ADIV, 5 M 40.

10. Ibid.

11. Ibid.

12. Ibid. The ultimate fate of the project is lost in the silence of the archives.

13. Dr. Briquet, *RGE,* 1875 (Paris: G. Masson, 1878), 6–18.

14. Léon Colin, *RGE,* 1881 (Paris: G. Masson, 1883), 13.

15. L. Noirot to prefect, March 10, 1880, in ADCdO, M7 f I: 16.

16. Jules Bucquoy, *RGE,* 1882 (Paris: G. Masson, 1884), 7–11.

17. "Rapport sur les maladies occasionnées par des poisons morbides humains ou telluriques," canton de Givors, January 3, 1890, in ADR, 5 M 5. Later etiologies would regard transmissibility by drinking water to be common for typhoid fever, but not for diphtheria.

18. Dr. Ferrand, for example, introduced the academy's 1896 epidemics report as follows: "Il semble que le rapport annuel a l'Académie de médecine, sur les maladies épidémiques de la France, doive être une étude susceptible d'apporter a l'oeuvre scientifique médicale, de nouvelles donnees; de jeter, surtout, quelques nouvelles clartés sur les problèmes toujours si obscurs, ou du moins si compliqués, de la pathogénie. La question des constitutions médicales, par exemple, question si dépréciée aujourd'hui, j'allais presque dire enterrée, y trouverait peut-être une sorte de renaissance, et certainement les questions d'hygiène et de prophylaxie devraient rencontrer là plus d'un enseignement." Ferrand, *RGE,* 1896 (Melun: Imprimerie administrative, 1897), 5.

19. *Création d'un Bureau d'hygiène municipal: Proposition faite par les Docteurs Givert, Fauvel et Lafaurie dans la séance du 11 février 1878* (Le Havre: Alphée Brindeau, 1878), in AMH (F.C.), I⁵ 4: 1.

20. "Discussion sur l'épidémie actuelle de fièvre typhoïde à Paris," session of November 14, 1882, *BAM,* 2d ser., 11 (1882): 1319–21.

21. Henri Guéneau de Mussy, "Rapport général sur les épidémies pendant l'année 1880," *Mémoires de l'Académie de médecine* 34 (1884): clix–clx.

22. Ferrand, *RGE,* 1896, 9–10.

23. See Barnes, *Making of a Social Disease,* 41–43.

24. Jean-Antoine Villemin, "Rapport général sur les épidémies pendant l'année 1877," *Mémoires de l'Académie de médecine* 33 (1882): cxlv–cxlvii.

25. René Vallery-Radot, *La Vie de Pasteur* (Paris: Ernest Flammarion, 1935), 351–52.

26. Félix Féréol, *RGE,* 1883 (n.p., n.d.), clxvi–clxxvi.

27. Ibid.

28. Georges Dujardin-Beaumetz, *RGE*, 1885 (Paris: G. Masson, 1887), 7.

29. Most of the annual epidemic reports appeared with a publication date two years after the year covered by the report. Soliciting, compiling, and analyzing the individual reports from the epidemic doctors and other contributors took quite a bit of time, and it is impossible to know exactly when the text as published was written. I have adopted the convention of dating the bulk of the writing of the annual reports in the year following the one covered by the report.

30. Charles Fernet, *RGE*, 1898 (Melun: Imprimerie administrative, 1900), 72.

31. On the Academy of Medicine, see George Weisz, *The Medical Mandarins: The French Academy of Medicine in the Nineteenth and Early Twentieth Centuries* (Oxford: Oxford University Press, 1995).

32. On the work of Henle: Jacob Henle, *Pathologische Untersuchungen* (Berlin: Hirschwald, 1840); K. Codell Carter, "Koch's Postulates in Relation to the Work of Jacob Henle and Edwin Klebs," *Medical History* 29: 353–74; Carter, *The Rise of Causal Concepts of Disease: Case Histories* (Aldershot, England: Ashgate, 2003). Although I am indebted to Carter's account of Henle's work, Carter would likely not endorse my characterization of Henle's germ theory as "sterile."

33. Technically, this was possible well before 1880, as Pasteur himself demonstrated in his famous refutation of spontaneous generation in the early 1860s. (See chapter 1.)

34. Commission d'étude de l'assainissement du Havre, 2eme sous-commission, minutes of the meeting of March 23, 1882; AMH (F.C.), I^5 16: 4.

35. Ibid.

36. Other texts around the same time attributed similar findings concerning the measurement of germs in Paris to the work of Pierre Miquel of the Paris Observatory.

37. Commission d'étude de l'assainissement du Havre, March 23, 1882 minutes; AMH (F.C.), I^5 16: 4.

38. Ibid.

39. Xavier Delore, *Des Microbes au point de vue de la maladie et de l'hygiène* (speech before the Académie des sciences, belles-lettres et arts de Lyon, June 15, 1886) (Lyon: Association typographique, 1886), 3–4.

40. AMH (F.C.), I^5 19: 1–2.

41. AMH (F.C.), I^5 1: 5.

42. *Compte-rendu des travaux de l'Institut Pasteur de Lille en 1900* (Lille: L. Danel, 1901), 29; *Compte-rendu des travaux de l'Institut Pasteur de Lille en 1901* (Lille: L. Danel, 1902), 23; *Compte-rendu des travaux de l'Institut Pasteur de Lille en 1902* (Lille: L. Danel, 1903), 8–9; *Compte-rendu des travaux de l'Institut Pasteur de Lille en 1903* (Lille: L. Danel, 1904), 6–7.

43. Barnes, *Making of a Social Disease*, 41–47.

44. For a discussion of Kelsch and his theory of latent germs, see Andrew R. Aisenberg, *Contagion: Disease, Government, and the "Social Question" in Nineteenth-Century France* (Stanford: Stanford University Press, 1999), 99–105.

45. Achille Kelsch, *RGE*, 1892 (Melun: Imprimerie administrative, 1894), 7–8.

46. Ibid., 127–28.

47. Achille Kelsch, *RGE*, 1893 (Melun: Imprimerie administrative, 1896), 50. Note that the word "saprophyte" is more commonly used today to designate an organism that lives off of decaying organic matter.

48. Kelsch, *RGE*, 1892, 61.

49. Nancy Tomes, *The Gospel of Germs: Men, Women, and the Microbe in American Life* (Cambridge: Harvard University Press, 1998).

50. "Société de médecine publique," *RHPS* 4 (1882): 431–32.

51. Ibid., 432–33.

52. Ibid.

53. Ibid., 433–34.

54. Mayor of Buffon to prefect, July 28, 1884, ADCdO, M7 f I: 16 (emphasis in original).

55. Emile Troisier, *RGE*, 1901 (Melun: Imprimerie administrative, 1904), 27.

CHAPTER 4. PUTTING GERM THEORY INTO PRACTICE

1. E. Affre report, January 29, 1900, ADCdO, M7 f I: 20.

2. Bacteriologists advocating disinfection in the late nineteenth century often made reference to the long pedigree of this practice, while taking pains to emphasize its newly scientific justification and efficacy. See, for example, Samuel Rideal, *Disinfection and Disinfectants* (London: Charles Griffin & Co., 1895), 2–5.

3. Pierre Larousse, *Grand dictionnaire universel du XIXᵉ siècle*, 17 vols. (Geneva: Slatkine, 1982), 6:559. This volume was originally published in 1870.

4. Christopher Lawrence and Richard Dixey, "Practising on Principle: Joseph Lister and the Germ Theories of Disease," in Christopher Lawrence, ed., *Medical Theory, Surgical Practice: Studies in the History of Surgery* (London: Routledge, 1992), 153–215; Lindsay Granshaw, " 'Upon This Principle I Have Built a Practice': The Development and Reception of Antisepsis in Britain, 1867–90," in John V. Pickstone, ed., *Medical Innovations in Historical Perspective* (New York: St. Martin's Press, 1992), 17–46. It is worth pointing out that Lister himself eschewed cleanliness, believing that only the direct chemical neutralization of germs was effective in preventing infection. "There had previously always been an annual cleaning of the wards of our infirmary. . . . I used to consider whether the patient would get more harm from the want of cleansing of the wards, or from the transportation. . . . I thought them more likely to get harm from the transport, and this being year after year my conviction, it is now three years since any cleaning took place on these wards of mine. . . . If we take cleanliness in any other sense than antiseptic cleanliness, my patients have the dirtiest wounds and sores in the world. I often keep on dressings for a week at a time, during which the discharge accumulates . . . the altered blood with its various shades of colour convey often both to the eye and to the nose an idea of anything rather than cleanliness. Aesthetically they are dirty, though surgically clean." Joseph Lister, "Address on the Effects of the Antiseptic Treatment upon the General Salubrity of Surgical Hospitals," *British Medical Journal*, 1875, ii, 769–71, quoted in Nicholas J. Fox, "Scientific Theory Choice and Social Structure: The Case of Joseph Lister's Antisepsis, Humoral Theory and Asepsis," *History of Science* 26 (1988): 367–97

(quotation at 375). In contrast, the later doctrine of asepsis, which developed more or less independently from antisepsis, emphasized strict cleanliness of room, bodies, and instruments in surgery (Fox, "Scientific Theory Choice and Social Structure"). Asepsis, far more consonant with the esthetic dimensions of the SBS, eventually won the day.

5. ADIV, 5 M 40.

6. AMH (F.C.), I⁵ 4: 1.

7. Bureau municipal d'hygiène du Havre, *Instruction sur la désinfection dans les cas de maladies épidémiques ou transmissibles* (Le Havre: Imprimerie commerciale Eug. Costey, 1880), in AMH (F.C.), I⁵ 4: 1.

8. *Rapport général sur les travaux du Conseil d'hygiène publique et de salubrité du département de la Seine depuis 1878 jusqu'à 1880 inclusivement* (Paris: Imprimerie Chaix, 1884), 63–64.

9. Ibid., 65–67; CHPS, *Etablissement, à Paris, d'étuves publiques pour la désinfection des objets de literie et des linges qui ont été en contact avec des personnes atteintes de maladies infectieuses ou contagieuses* (Paris: Charles de Mourgues Frères, 1880), 3–5.

10. Léon Colin, *RGE*, 1881 (Paris: G. Masson, 1883), 33–36; Lille city council minutes, June 27, 1884, ACL, 1D2: 83, 432–37; "Le Croup a Lambersart," *La Vraie France*, undated, in ADN, M 303: 68; H. Monod, Directeur de l'assistance et de l'hygiène publiques, to prefect of Mayenne, April 21, 1893, in ADM, 5 M 57; prefect to M. le président du Tribunal civil de Lille, November 21, 1893, in ADN, M 319: 2; Dr. Sockeel (prison physician of Maison d'arrêt de Douai) to subprefect (Douai), June 29, 1893, in ADN, M 319: 2.

11. "Rapport sur les travaux de la Commission d'hygiène du 10ᵉ arrondissement pendant l'année 1885," AP, Vbis 10 I⁵: 6.

12. *CMPP*, session of December 21, 1889, 2: 763–65.

13. *Le Temps*, December 6, 1892.

14. *Lyon Républicain*, November 9, 1889, in ADR, 5 M 5.

15. ADSM, 5 M 139.

16. Ambroise Rendu, *RGE*, 1897 (Melun: Imprimerie administrative, 1899), 57–58.

17. *Le Temps*, July 18, 1899.

18. AMLy, 1124 WP 035: 1.

19. Prefect Jules Cambon of Rhône to all mayors in department, June 12, 1889, in ADR, 5 M 5.

20. AMLy, 1128 WP 001.

21. *CMPP*, session of June 17, 1891, 1: 897.

22. Dr. Gorez to prefect, June 7, 1893, in ADN, M 319: 2.

23. Mayor of Le Tréport to subprefect (Dieppe), December 20, 1893, in ADSM, 5 M 139.

24. Dr. Georges Dumont, *Une épidémie de diphtérie* (reprinted from *Bulletin medical du Nord*) (Lille: Le Bigot Freres, 1896), 28–32 (in ADN, M 303: 74).

25. Ibid., 29–30.

26. Ibid., 30.

27. *Le Temps*, September 12, 1894; *Le Petit Temps*, January 22, 1895.

28. "Rapport general sur les travaux de la Commission d'hygiène du 14ᵉ arrondissement en 1895," AP, Vbis 14 I⁵: 2.

29. *CMPP*, session of December 5, 1898, 2: 895–99.

30. *CMPP*, session of June 24, 1898, 1: 785–86; "Rapport sur l'extension du service de la désinfection," présenté par M. Landrin, conseiller municipal, *CMPR*, 1899, no. 83. On the tipping point, see Malcolm Gladwell, *The Tipping Point: How Little Things Can Make a Big Difference* (Boston: Little, Brown, 2000).

31. Discussion of MM. Laveran et Vaillard, "De la désinfection des locaux spécialement au moyen des pulvérisateurs, et de la valeur de ce procédé," *BAM*, 3d ser., 33 (1894): 143.

32. *CMPP*, session of June 24, 1898, 1: 785–86.

33. *Annuaire statistique de la ville de Paris* (Paris: Imprimerie nationale), 1888–1901.

34. Dr. Eugène Deschamps, "Rapport sur la désinfection par l'industrie privée" (report to CHPS, November 9, 1892), 7–9, in APP, DB¹: 442.

35. Ibid.

36. Ibid.

37. Evelynn Hammonds, *Childhood's Deadly Scourge: The Campaign to Control Diphtheria in New York City, 1880–1930* (Baltimore: Johns Hopkins University Press, 1999), 95–97; David S. Barnes, *The Making of a Social Disease: Tuberculosis in Nineteenth-Century France* (Berkeley: University of California Press, 1995), 74–111.

38. ADR 5 M 25. Surviving archives contain no record of the extent of official follow-up (if any) in either case.

39. Charles Fernet, *RGE*, 1898 (Melun: Imprimerie administrative, 1900), 67–68.

40. ADS, 99 M 98598: 2.

41. Ibid.

42. Achille Kelsch, *RGE*, 1893 (Melun: Imprimerie administrative, 1896), 10.

43. Botrel report to subprefect of St.-Malo on typhoid fever epidemic in Roz-sur-Couesnon, December 23, 1881, ADIV, 5 M 70.

44. Dr. Gascon, annual epidemic report for arrondissement of Redon, 1884; ADIV, 5 M 71.

45. Auguste Ollivier, *RGE*, 1887, 58 (emphasis added).

46. Ibid., 58–59.

47. Prefect of Rhône to all mayors in department, June 12, 1889, ADR 5 M 5.

48. Jules Chauvel, *RGE*, 1891 (Melun: Imprimerie administrative, 1893), 40.

49. Achille Kelsch, *RGE*, 1892 (Melun: Imprimerie administrative, 1894), 68–69. This account is based on the report submitted to the Academy by Dr. Legée, epidemic doctor for the arrondissement of Abbeville (Oise).

50. The gloomy, nihilistic historical accounts that replicate the hygienists' frustration (e.g., Lion Murard and Patrick Zylberman, *L'Hygiène dans la république: La Santé publique en France, ou l'utopie contrariée, 1870–1918* [Paris: Fayard, 1996]) must be read in this light.

51. François Siredey, "Rapport général sur les épidémies qui ont sévi en France pendant l'année 1884" (n.p.: n.d.), ccxci–ccxcii (emphasis in original).

52. Alphonse Laveran, *RGE*, 1899, 25.

53. Daniel Pick, *Faces of Degeneration: A European Disorder, c. 1848–c. 1918* (Cam-

bridge: Cambridge University Press, 1989); Robert A. Nye, *Crime, Madness, and Politics in Modern France: The Medical Concept of National Decline* (Princeton: Princeton University Press, 1984); Barnes, *Making of a Social Disease*, 138–73; Bertrand Taithe, *Defeated Flesh: Medicine, Welfare, and Warfare in the Making of Modern France* (Lanham, MD: Rowman & Littlefield, 1999).

54. AMB, 808 R 1. On the tradition of hygiene as guide to bourgeois living, see William Coleman, "Health and Hygiene in the *Encyclopédie:* A Medical Doctrine for the Bourgeoisie," *JHMAS* 29 (1974): 399–421; and Georges Vigarello, *Le Sain et le malsain: Santé et mieux-être depuis le Moyen-Age* (Paris: Seuil, 1993).

55. AMB, 808, R 1.

56. Ibid.; Arthur Armaingaud, *Instructions populaires sur les causes et l'hygiène préventive de la fièvre typhoïde* (Bordeaux: Cours municipal d'hygiène, 1883). This pamphlet is not paginated.

57. Armaingaud, *Instructions populaires* (emphasis in original).

58. Nancy Tomes, *The Gospel of Germs: Men, Women, and the Microbe in American Life* (Cambridge: Harvard University Press, 1998), 130–32.

59. Armaingaud, *Instructions populaires*.

60. Louis Brébant, *Société industrielle de Reims: Cours public d'hygiène* (Reims: Imprimerie de Gérard, 1868); J. A. Mandon, *Cours municipal d'hygiène publique* (Limoges: Imprimerie de Chatras, 1869).

61. Conseil général du département des Pyrénées-Orientales, session of April 1887, *Rapport supplémentaire de M. Georges Lafargue sur l'organisation de l'enseignement populaire de l'hygiène* (Perpignan: Imprimerie de l'Indépendant, 1887). The report contains no information on the plan's implementation.

62. Ernest Monier, *Causeries sur l'hygiène et causeries scientifiques*, 2d ed. (Compiègne: Henry Lefebvre, 1897), 184.

63. Lawrence and Dixey, "Practising on Principle."

64. Monier, *Causeries sur l'hygiène*, 182–83.

65. Eugen Weber, *Peasants into Frenchmen: The Modernization of Rural France, 1870–1914* (Stanford: Stanford University Press, 1976); Mona Ozouf, *L'Ecole, l'église, et la république* (Paris: A. Colin, 1963); Jacques Ozouf and Mona Ozouf, *La République des instituteurs* (Paris: Seuil, 1992).

66. MM. Brouard et Ch. Defodon, *Les Nouveaux programmes des écoles primaires*, 7th ed. (Paris: Hachette, 1901), 16–17.

67. M. le Dr. Javal, "Rapport d'ensemble," in Ministère de l'Instruction publique, *Hygiène des écoles primaires et des écoles maternelles: Rapports et documents présentés à M. le Ministre de l'Instruction publique par la Commission d'hygiène scolaire* (Paris: Imprimerie nationale, 1884), 1–20.

68. Circulaire ministeriel du 15 mars 1890, signed A. Fallières, AN F 17: 1478, F 17: 11781.

69. Conseil d'hygiène de l'arrondissement de Laval, session of December 11, 1894, ADM, 5 M 39.

70. Some of the many surviving accounts of such school-closing debates can be found in: AN F 17: 1478; ADN, M 303: 60; ADIV, 5 M 40, 70, 71; Charlemagne Pilat, *Rapport général sur les épidémies qui ont régné dans le département du Nord pendant*

l'année 1883 (Lille: L. Danel, 1884), 20; AMH (F.C.), I⁵ 1: 3; ADR, 5 M 5; ADSM, 5 M 139; ADEL, 5 M 50; ADM, 5 M 39; ADH, 5 M 152.

71. Allan Mitchell, *The Divided Path: The German Influence in French Social Reform after 1870* (Chapel Hill: University of North Carolina Press, 1991), 266–75, 309–15.

72. Murard and Zylberman, *L'Hygiène dans la république*, 37, 586. The introduction of *L'Hygiène dans la république* is entitled "The Orthodoxy of the *Néant*," and its conclusion is entitled "A Provisional *Néant*." The book's subtitle is "The Thwarted Utopia" (*l'utopie contrariée*).

73. In the voluminous literature on the McKeown thesis, useful points of reference include: Thomas McKeown, *The Role of Medicine: Dream, Mirage, or Nemesis?* 2d ed. (Princeton: Princeton University Press, 1979); Simon Szreter, "The Importance of Social Intervention in Britain's Mortality Decline, 1850–1914: A Reinterpretation of the Role of Public Health," *Social History of Medicine* 1 (1988): 1–37; and the contributions to the Health Policy and Ethics forum entitled "The McKeown Thesis," *American Journal of Public Health* 92 (2002): 722–32.

74. Murard and Zylberman, *L'Hygiène dans la république*, 27.

75. ADV, M 5: 40.

76. AMLy, 1124, WP 035: 1; see, for example, Dr. Jablonski to prefect (Vienne), September 23, 1892, ADV, M 5: 40. Requests for departmental disinfection tanks seem to have been quite common; where they survive in departmental archives, they are abundant: for example, ADCdO, M7 f I: 18, 19.

77. ADEL, 5 M 50.

78. ADCdO, M7 f I: 17.

79. ADEL, 5 M 50.

80. Ibid.

81. Mayor D. Martin of Vouzailles to prefect, March 18, 1892, ADV, M 5: 40. There is no record of the prefect's response.

82. Mayor of Cuhon to prefect, September 22, 1892; Mayor Valet of Massognes to prefect, September 23, 1892; and prefect to Valet, September 27, 1892; ADV M 5: 40.

83. Dr. Jablonski to prefect, September 23, 1892, ADV M 5: 40.

84. Mayor of Mazeuil to prefect, September 27, 1892, ADV, M 5: 40 (emphasis added).

85. Martin to prefect, November 15, 1892; Jablonski to prefect, November 17, 1892; Martin to prefect, June 28, 1893; ADV, M 5: 40.

86. ADCdO, M7 f I: 17.

87. Ibid.

88. Compare, for example, the numbers of reports from epidemic doctors received by the Academy of Medicine's Epidemics Committee each year with the records of epidemic doctors' activity that survive in departmental archives. No archive I have visited contains material relating to any more than a small fraction of the number of reports sent to the academy, as disclosed in the annual report of the Epidemics Committee.

89. According to some definitions, the rabies "vaccine" was not a vaccine but a

treatment, as it was administered after infection and acted to prevent the onset of symptoms rather than to prevent infection per se. However, Pasteur self-consciously used the language of "vaccination" to link his research with Jenner's pedigree, and most contemporary observers followed his lead (as have historians).

90. Although most historians apportion credit for the breakthrough jointly to Roux, Emil von Behring, and Shibasaburo Kitasato, and German and English speakers at the time were more likely to use Behring's name to designate the antitoxin treatment, the French chauvinistically attributed the diphtheria cure exclusively to Roux, and called it "Dr. Roux's serum."

91. Claire Salomon-Bayet, "Penser la révolution pastorienne," in Salomon-Bayet, ed., *Pasteur et la révolution pastorienne* (Paris: Payot, 1986), 47–49; Bert Hansen, "America's First Medical Breakthrough: How Popular Excitement about a French Rabies Cure in 1885 Raised New Expectations for Medical Progress," *American Historical Review* 103 (1998): 373–418; Patrice Debré, *Louis Pasteur,* trans. Elborg Forster (Baltimore: Johns Hopkins University Press, 1998), 415–17; Daniel Raichvarg, *Louis Pasteur: L'Empire des microbes* (Paris: Gallimard, 1995), 89.

92. Jules Worms, *RGE,* 1890 (Paris: G. Masson, 1892), 3.

93. Subprefect of Beaune to prefect (Côte-d'Or), October 29, 1894, ADCdO, M7 f I: 18; Dr. Ernest Hiblot to subprefect of Châteaudun (Eure-et-Loir), January 6, 1896, ADEL, 5 M 50; Emile Troisier, *RGE,* 1901 (Melun: Imprimerie administrative, 1904), 20–21.

94. Maunoury report dated January 1, 1896, ADEL, 5 M 50.

95. Report from Dr. Hiblot, February 20, 1902, ADEL, 5 M 50.

96. Ibid.

CHAPTER 5. TOWARD A CLEANER AND HEALTHIER REPUBLIC

1. Dr. (Jacques) Botrel, "Arrt. de St.-Malo / Epidémies 1882," March 10, 1883, ADIV 5 M 70.

2. Ibid.

3. Eugen Weber, *Peasants into Frenchmen: The Modernization of Rural France, 1870–1914* (Stanford: Stanford University Press, 1976).

4. ADN, M 303: 60.

5. Ibid.

6. Ibid.

7. Georges Vigarello, *Concepts of Cleanliness: Changing Attitudes in France since the Middle Ages,* trans. Jean Birrell (Cambridge: Cambridge University Press, 1988), 202–14, quotation at 212.

8. Conseil central d'hygiène publique (Seine-Inférieure), session of December 4, 1869, ADSM, 5 M 141.

9. Jules Chauvel, *RGE,* 1891 (Melun: Imprimerie administrative, 1893), 28.

10. Emile Troisier, *RGE,* 1901 (Melun: Imprimerie administrative, 1904), 18–19.

11. Household pets represent the most obvious exception to this separation, but the elaborate codes in bourgeois society governing their care and control reinforce the broader argument presented here. See Kathleen Kete, *The Beast in the Boudoir:*

Petkeeping in Nineteenth-Century Paris (Berkeley: University of California Press, 1994).

12. Alphonse Mauricet, *Compte-rendu des épidémies, des épizooties et des travaux des conseils d'hygiène du Morbihan en 1882* (Vannes: Imprimerie Galles, 1883), 22–23.

13. AMH (F.C.), I^5 4: 1.

14. Arthur Armaingaud, *Instructions populaires sur les causes et l'hygiène préventive de la fièvre typhoïde* (Bordeaux: Cours municipal d'hygiène, 1883). This pamphlet is not paginated.

15. "Rapport sur les maladies occasionnées par des poisons morbides humains ou telluriques," canton de Givors, 1889, ADR, 5 M 5.

16. Conseil municipal, session of March 24, 1893, ACL, 1D2: 92, p. 115.

17. Georges Dumont, "Une épidémie de diphtérie" (extrait du *Bulletin medical du Nord*), ADN, M 303: 74.

18. Commission d'hygiène du 14e arrondissement, session of July 13, 1895, AP, Vbis 14 I^5:2.

19. Henri Guéneau de Mussy, "Rapport général sur les épidémies pendant l'année 1879," *Mémoires de l'Académie de médecine* 34 (1884): clxi–clxii.

20. Ibid. This section of the report was written as a paraphrase of the original report by Dr. Bos, the epidemic doctor investigating the Marcolez epidemic, with occasional direct quotations. It is not always clear which phrasings came originally from Dr. Bos, and which from Guéneau de Mussy.

21. Léon Colin, *RGE*, 1881 (Paris: G. Masson, 1883), 7–8.

22. ADIV, 5 M 71.

23. Troisier, *RGE*, 1901, 9–10.

24. ADH, 5 M 147.

25. ADSM, 5 M 139.

26. ADCdO, M7 f I: 20.

27. Colin, *RGE*, 1881, 6.

28. Armaingaud, *Instructions populaires* (emphasis in original).

29. Ibid.

30. ADSM, 5 M 139.

31. Ibid.

32. Ibid. (emphasis added).

33. "Rapport general sur les travaux de la Commission d'hygiène du 14e arrondissement en 1895," AP, Vbis 14 I^5: 2.

34. Auguste Ollivier, *RGE*, 1888 (Paris: G. Masson, 1890), 65.

35. Armaingaud, *Instructions populaires*; Charles Fernet, *RGE*, 1898 (Melun: Imprimerie administrative, 1900), 30–31; Ministère de l'Instruction publique, *Hygiene des ecoles primaires et des ecoles maternelles: Rapports et documents presentes a M. le Ministre de l'Instruction publique par la Commission d'hygiene scolaire* (Paris: Imprimerie nationale, 1884), 1–20.

36. ADH, 5 M 135.

37. Ibid.

38. ADCdO, M7 f I: 16.

39. Fernet, *RGE*, 1898, 8. The quotation is attributed to "Dr. Ficatier of Bar-le-Duc."

40. ADN, M 317: 1.

41. ADCdO, M7 f I: 16 (emphasis in original).

42. ADH, 5 M 145.

43. Ibid.

44. AMM, 5 I, "Inspection sanitaire des écoles."

45. ADH, 5 M 145.

46. Ibid.

47. ADR, 5 M 24.

48. Leslie Page Moch, "Migration and the Nation: The View from Paris," *Social Science History* 28 (2004): 1–18; Catherine Bertho, "L'Invention de la Bretagne: Genèse d'un stéréotype," *Actes de la recherche en sciences sociales* 35 (1980): 45–62; Ronan Dantec and James Eveillard, *Les Bretons dans la presse populaire illustrée* (Rennes: Editions Ouest-France, 2001).

49. Weber, *Peasants into Frenchmen*, 82.

50. ADR, 5 M 25. Bard is also referred to in some correspondence as the epidemic doctor for the Rhône department as a whole.

51. ADSM, 5 M 139.

52. Ibid.

53. Ibid.

54. ADSM, 5 M 141.

55. Ibid.

56. Just as administrative centralization as a whole in France traced its roots as far back as Louis XIV but took on its recognizably modern form during the empire of Napoleon I, the role of epidemic doctor was created during the ancien régime but systematized within the departmental prefectoral/subprefectoral system under Napoleon. *Recueil des travaux du Comité consultatif d'hygiène publique*, vol. 1 (Paris: J. B. Baillière, 1872), 122–33.

57. All observers agreed that the woefully underfunded system functioned imperfectly. Outbreaks were not reported to epidemic doctors, who, when they were notified, often failed to investigate, and when they investigated, often failed to file reports. *Recueil des travaux du Comité consultatif d'hygiène publique*, vol. 4 (Paris: J. B. Baillière, 1875), 127–30; vol. 10 (Paris: J. B. Baillière, 1881), 119–20; vol. 12 (Paris: Imprimerie nationale, 1883), 99; vol. 14 (Paris: Imprimerie nationale, 1885), 84; vol. 30 (Melun: Imprimerie administrative, 1901), 219–29. The surviving documentation of their work nevertheless provides a glimpse of the sustained will to bring the dark and sickly corners of the republic under administrative (and, of course, political) surveillance, and to improve the nation's health by civilizing its inhabitants.

58. Norbert Elias, *The Civilizing Process*, trans. Edmund Jephcott (London: Blackwell, 1994); the original German edition was published in 1939. A cogent summary of Elias's civilizing process and its critics can be found in Robert van Krieken, *Norbert Elias* (London: Routledge, 1998), 84–134. Sociologists and anthropologists have quarreled with one aspect or another of this model, but historians have been especially reluctant to embrace Elias's paradigm of cultural change. Some have objected

to his use of the European Middle Ages as a starting point, the "zero hour" of the civilizing process, in which behavioral constraints were by implication all but non-existent; it is not difficult for medievalists to point to the existence of quite extensive codes of conduct in that era. Other historians have cast doubt on the role of noble courts and courtiers as the principal engines of cultural change; still others question Elias's contention that state formation and a state monopoly on violence were the indispensable enabling conditions of the civilizing process. Here too scholars can identify counterexamples that seem to weaken or disprove each of these elements of Elias's hypothesis. For summary critiques of Elias, see, among others, van Krieken, "Violence, Self-Discipline, and Modernity: Beyond the Civilizing Process," *Sociological Review* 37 (1989): 193–218, and *Norbert Elias*, 118–34; R. J. Robinson, "'The Civilizing Process': Some Remarks on Elias's Social History," *Sociology* 21 (1987): 1–17; Eric Dunning, "A Response to R. J. Robinson's 'The Civilizing Process': Some Remarks on Elias's Social History," *Sociology* 23 (1989): 299–307. Historians of early modern French culture have also wrestled with the implications of Elias's work for their field: see Roger Chartier, *Cultural History: Between Practices and Representations*, trans. Lydia G. Cochrane (Ithaca: Cornell University Press, 1988), 75–94, and Daniel Gordon, *Citizens without Sovereignty: Equality and Sociability in French Thought, 1670–1789* (Princeton: Princeton University Press, 1994), 86–94.

59. Ian Miller, *The Anatomy of Disgust* (Cambridge: Harvard University Press, 1997), 170. A similar case is made in John F. Kasson, *Rudeness and Civility: Manners in Nineteenth-Century Urban America* (New York: Hill and Wang, 1990), 9–12.

60. Elias, *Civilizing Process*, 497.

61. Johan Goudsblom, "Public Health and the Civilizing Process," *Milbank Quarterly* 64 (1986): 180–81.

62. Patrice Pinell, "Modern Medicine and the Civilising Process," *Sociology of Health and Illness* 18 (1996): 11.

63. David S. Barnes, *The Making of a Social Disease: Tuberculosis in Nineteenth-Century France* (Berkeley: University of California Press, 1995), esp. 83–91.

64. Elias, *Civilizing Process*, 125–31.

65. Alice L. Conklin, *A Mission to Civilize: The Republican Idea of Empire in France and West Africa, 1895–1930* (Stanford: Stanford University Press, 1997); Alice Bullard, *Exile to Paradise: Savagery and Civilization in Paris and the South Pacific, 1790–1900* (Stanford: Stanford University Press, 2000).

66. Conklin, *Mission to Civilize*, 59–61; Bullard, *Exile to Paradise*.

67. Bullard, *Exile to Paradise*.

68. "Rapport sur les travaux de la Commission d'hygiène publique et de salubrité du 10e arrondissement pour l'année 1881," AP, Vbis 10 I⁵: 5.

69. ADIV, 5 M 50.

70. ADIV, 5 M 71. In the original text, there is one additional sentence interposed between the two quoted here: "How important it is that those to whom the administration and the application of the rules of hygiene are entrusted know that their nonobservance [of hygienic rules] creates the heaviest of taxes for the population."

71. ADIV, 5 M 71.

72. ADLA, 1 M 1335.

73. Auguste Ollivier, *RGE*, 1887 (Paris: G. Masson, 1890), 18–20.

74. Ibid., 20–21.

75. "Rapport général sur les travaux de la Commission d'hygiène du 14ᵉ arrondissement en 1897," in AP, Vbis 14 I⁵: 3; Ambroise Rendu, *RGE*, 1897 (Melun: Imprimerie administrative, 1899), 8.

CHAPTER 6. ODORS AND "INFECTION," 1880 AND BEYOND

1. Gérard Jacquemet, "Urbanisme parisien: La bataille du tout-à-l'égout à la fin du XIXᵉ siècle," *RHMC* 26 (1979): 505–48.

2. See, for example, *Le Temps*, June 4, 1895; *Le Figaro*, June 7 and 26, 1895; *Le Siècle*, June 16, 1895; *Paris-Journal*, August 4, 1895.

3. *Le Figaro*, June 26, 1895.

4. *Le Temps*, June 4, 1895.

5. For example, *Paris-Journal*, August 4, 1895.

6. *Le Figaro*, June 7 and 26, 1895; *Le Temps*, June 4, 1895.

7. *Le Temps*, June 4, 1895; *Paris-Journal*, August 4, 1895; *CGS*, session of July 8, 1895, 540.

8. *Paris-Journal*, August 4, 1895.

9. *CGS*, session of July 8, 1895, 539–44.

10. Alexandre Le Roy des Barres (Commission d'études dite des Odeurs de Paris), *Rapport préliminaire sur les causes des émanations odorantes de Paris et de la banlieue* (Paris: Chaix, 1896), 6.

11. Ibid., 39–77.

12. Ibid., 115–16.

13. Ibid., 4.

14. Ibid.

15. Commission d'études dite des Odeurs de Paris, minutes of the second meeting of the Technical Subcommittee, September 20, 1895, 6–7, in APP, DB¹: 434.

16. Ibid., 4–5, and minutes of the third meeting of the Technical Subcommittee, November 27, 1895, 10–11, in APP, DB¹: 434.

17. Commission d'études dite des Odeurs de Paris, minutes of the second plenary session, May 13, 1896, 11–12, in APP, DB¹: 434 (emphasis in original).

18. Ibid., 15, 21–22.

19. The official report of the commission set up by the Prefecture of Police to study the odors of 1926 did mention that hygienic wisdom since antiquity had incorrectly associated putrid odors with the spread of diseases and with the onset of epidemics; noting that "there is always a grain of truth in popular observations," the reporter hypothesized that in some cases, certain gases present in foul-smelling air could provide a favorable environment for the survival of pathogenic microbes, while other gases could kill them. A. Trillat, *Commission des odeurs de Paris: Rapport général* (Paris: Chaix, 1928), 7–8.

20. O. Boudouard, "Recherches sur les odeurs de Paris," *Revue scientifique* 50 (1912): 614–21; *Compte rendu des séances du conseil d'hygiène publique et de salubrité du Département de la Seine*, 1911, 2: 102–103, 1926, 164; Trillat, *Commission des odeurs de Paris*.

21. Boudouard, "Recherches sur les odeurs de Paris," 614; Trillat, *Commission des odeurs de Paris*, 3–4.

22. Martin Monestier, *Histoire et bizarreries sociales des excréments des origines à nos jours* (Paris: Le Cherche Midi, 1997), 79–103; Dominique Laporte, *History of Shit*, trans. Nadia Benabid and Rodolphe el-Khoury (Cambridge: MIT Press, 2000), 3–7.

23. Antoine-Alexis Cadet de Vaux, *Mémoire historique et physique sur le cimetière des Innocents*, presented to the Académie royale des sciences in 1781 (reprinted from *Journal de Physique*, June 1783), unpaginated; David L. Garrioch, *The Making of Revolutionary Paris* (Berkeley: University of California Press, 2002), 213–16; Jean Chagniot, *Nouvelle Histoire de Paris: Paris au XVIIIᵉ siècle* (Paris: Hachette, 1988), 177–78; Louis-Sébastien Mercier, *Panorama of Paris*, ed. Jeremy Popkin (University Park: Pennsylvania State University Press, 1999), 180–81. Sources vary on the number of parishes served by the cemetery; for example, Cadet de Vaux gives the figure as twenty-four, Garrioch as eighteen.

24. Cadet de Vaux, *Mémoire historique*; Jacques Hillairet, *Dictionnaire historique des rues de Paris*, 2d ed. (Paris: Editions de Minuit, 1964), 2: 394–96; Garrioch, *Making of Revolutionary Paris*, 216.

25. Alain Corbin, *The Foul and the Fragrant: Odor and the French Social Imagination* (Cambridge: Harvard University Press, 1986), esp. 59–61.

26. Owsei Temkin, "An Historical Analysis of the Concept of Infection," in *The Double Face of Janus and Other Essays in the History of Medicine* (Baltimore: Johns Hopkins University Press, 1977), 456–73.

27. See, among others, Douglas O. Baldwin, "The Campaign against Odors: Sanitarians and the Genesis of Public Health in Charlottetown, Prince Edward Island (1855–1900)," *Scientia canadensis* 10 (1986): 72–83; and Antonio Lafuente and Tiago Saraiva, "The Urban Scale of Science and the Enlargement of Madrid (1851–1936)," *Social Studies of Science* 34 (2004): 553.

28. David S. Barnes, "Confronting Sensory Crisis in the Great Stinks of London and Paris," in William A. Cohen and Ryan Johnson, eds., *Filth: Dirt, Disgust, and Modern Life* (Minneapolis: University of Minnesota Press, 2005), 103–29; Stephen Halliday, *The Great Stink of London: Sir Joseph Bazalgette and the Cleansing of the Victorian Capital* (Stroud: Sutton, 1999); John D. Thompson, "The Great Stench or the Fool's Argument," *Yale Journal of Biology and Medicine* 64 (1991): 529–41; Roy Porter, *London: A Social History* (London: Hamish Hamilton, 1994), 262–65.

29. Baldwin, "Campaign against Odors."

30. John Duffy, *The Sanitarians: A History of American Public Health* (Urbana: University of Illinois Press, 1990), 129, 186–87; Nancy Tomes, *The Gospel of Germs: Men, Women, and the Microbe in American Life* (Cambridge: Harvard University Press, 1998), esp. 68–82.

31. Frederick Brown, *Zola: A Life* (New York: Farrar, Straus & Giroux, 1995), 444–57.

32. "Un Chapitre inédit de M. Zola," *Le Figaro*, August 24, 1880. Zola biographer Frederick Brown dates Zola's first contribution to *Le Figaro* on September 16, more than three weeks later. Brown, *Zola*, 452–53.

33. I am grateful to Gerald Prince, Alain Pagès, and Henri Mitterand for helping me separate fact from fiction on this question.

34. On Zola's naturalism and on his political journalism—out of a truly vast biographical and critical literature—see (in addition to Brown, *Zola*): Pierre-Olivier Perl, "Les Caricatures de Zola: Du naturalisme à l'affaire Dreyfus," *Historical Reflections / Réflexions historiques* 24 (1998): 137–54; Maria Watroba, "*Thérèse Raquin*: Le Naturalisme entre mensonge et vérité," *Romantisme* 95 (1997): 17–28; Jean Kaempfer, *Emile Zola: D'un naturalisme pervers* (Paris: J. Corti, 1989); Henri Mitterand, *Zola: L'Histoire et la fiction* (Paris: Presses universitaires de France, 1990); William J. Berg, *The Visual Novel: Emile Zola and the Art of His Times* (University Park: Pennsylvania State University Press, 1992); Henri Mitterand, *Zola journaliste: De l'affaire Manet à l'affaire Dreyfus* (Paris: Armand Colin, 1962). The most exhaustive bibliography of Zola's journalistic output in these years is Henri Mitterand and Halina Suwala, *Emile Zola, journaliste: Bibliographie chronologique et analytique*, vol. 1: *1859–1881* (Paris: Les Belles Lettres, 1968).

35. "Un Chapitre inédit de M. Zola."

36. Ibid.

37. Brown, *Zola*, 571–73.

38. "Un Chapitre inédit de M. Zola."

39. Ibid.

40. Ibid.

41. *Le Figaro*, September 13, 1880; see also *L'Illustration*, September 18, 1880.

42. Louis Ulbach, "Notes et impressions," *Revue politique et littéraire* 26 (1880): 286–87.

43. Ibid.

44. Peter Stallybrass and Allon White, *The Politics and Poetics of Transgression* (Ithaca: Cornell University Press, 1986).

45. Ibid.

46. Victor Hugo, *Les Misérables*, trans. N. Denny (Harmondsworth: Penguin, 1980), 2: 369, quoted in Stallybrass and White, *Politics and Poetics*, 141.

47. Stallybrass and White, *Politics and Poetics*, 141–42. An extremely thoughtful and wide-ranging analysis of disgust as a cultural and historical phenomenon can be found in William A. Cohen, "Introduction: Locating Filth," in Cohen and Johnson, eds., *Filth*, vii–xxxvii.

48. *Le Siècle*, September 28, 1880. Although newspapers quoted from the text of the petition, I have been unable to find either copies of the petition or any indication of the names, ages, occupations, addresses, etc. of the signatories, apart from the fact that they lived in the ninth and eighteenth arrondissements.

49. For quantitative data and maps concerning the social geography of Paris in this period, see Lenard Berlanstein, *The Working People of Paris, 1871–1914* (Baltimore: Johns Hopkins University Press, 1984), 11–15; Toussaint Loua, *Atlas statistique de la population de Paris* (Paris: J. Dejey, 1873), 67–76, maps 33–37.

50. Corbin, *Foul and the Fragrant*, 229–32. As important and original as Corbin's work has been, a somewhat minor quibble is appropriate in this context. He invokes the odors of 1880 as proof that Pasteur had by that time decisively severed the connection between foul smells and the spread of disease. Quoting Brouardel's

use in 1882 of the maxim "tout ce qui pue ne tue pas," Corbin claims that "once they had become convinced that infectious germs transmitted disease, scientists no longer associated unpleasant odor with the morbific threat" (223). Clearly, the evidence presented in chapter 1—including Pasteur's and Brouardel's own warnings in 1880—shows Corbin's argument to be more applicable to the odors of 1895 (and subsequent years) than to the earlier stench.

51. Peter Reinhart Gleichmann, "Des Villes propres et sans odeur: La vidange du corps humain, ses équipements et sa domestication," *Urbi* 5 (April 1982): 95–96; Elias, *Civilizing Process,* 443.

52. John B. Thompson, "Editor's Introduction," in Pierre Bourdieu, *Language and Symbolic Power,* trans. Gino Raymond and Matthew Adamson (Cambridge: Harvard University Press, 1994), 13.

53. Bourdieu discusses habitus in many books and essays that have been translated into English; one of the more straightforward discussions of the issues raised here may be found in Pierre Bourdieu, *The Logic of Practice,* trans. Richard Nice (Stanford: Stanford University Press, 1990), 52–65.

54. Thompson, "Editor's Introduction," 12–13.

55. Bourdieu, *Outline of a Theory of Practice,* trans. Richard Nice (Cambridge: Cambridge University Press, 1977), 93–94 (emphasis in original).

56. Bourdieu, *Logic of Practice,* 69.

57. Ibid., 56.

58. June 28,1895, letter to "Commission d'hygiène, Hâvre" from P. Bouys, 15 rue Marc (but written from Paris), AMH (F.C.), I^5 1: 5; complaint sent to Procureur de la Republique, February 11, 1899, by Arthur Michel of Déville-lès-Rouen, ADSM, 5 M 62. July 9, 1904, letter to prefect from "un groupe d'habitant du quartier de Berkem," in La Madeleine (Nord), in ADN, M 303: 81.

59. See, for example, Tomes, *Gospel of Germs,* and David S. Barnes, *The Making of a Social Disease: Tuberculosis in Nineteenth-Century France* (Berkeley: University of California Press, 1995), esp. 74–111.

60. On disgust and the role of spitting in the spread of tuberculosis around the turn of the century, see Barnes, *Making of a Social Disease,* 83–85, 114–17, 184–85.

61. Johan Goudsblom, "Public Health and the Civilizing Process," *Milbank Quarterly* 64 (1986). 161–88, and Patrice Pinell, "Modern Medicine and the Civilising Process," *Sociology of Health and Illness* 18 (1996): 1–16, among others, emphasize the degree to which rational health concerns are invoked a posteriori to justify previously existing aversions or preferences.

62. Corbin relies primarily on this explanation in *Foul and the Fragrant,* 222–28.

63. On the persistent association of foreigners with germs, for example, see Alan Kraut, *Silent Travelers: Germs, Genes, and the Immigrant Menace* (New York: Basic Books, 1994); Howard Markel, *When Germs Travel: Six Major Epidemics That Have Invaded America since 1900 and the Fears They Have Unleashed* (New York: Pantheon, 2004); Markel, *Quarantine! East European Jewish Immigrants and the New York City Epidemics of 1892* (Baltimore: Johns Hopkins University Press, 1997); Christoph Gradmann, "Invisible Enemies: Bacteriology and the Language of Politics in

Imperial Germany," *Science in Context* 13 (2000): 9–30; and Paul Weindling, *Health, Race and German Politics between National Unification and Nazism, 1870–1945* (Cambridge: Cambridge University Press, 1989), 170.

64. See, for example, Jacques Michel, "Emile Durkheim et la naissance de la science sociale dans le milieu bernardien," in Michel, ed., *La nécessité de Claude Bernard* (Paris: Méridiens Klincksieck, 1991), 229–54.

65. Olivier Faure, *Histoire sociale de la médecine, XVIIIᵉ-XXᵉ siècles* (Paris: Anthropos, 1994), 177.

66. Walter Benjamin, "Paris, Capital of the Nineteenth Century," in *Reflections: Essays, Aphorisms, Autobiographical Writings*, trans. Edmund Jephcott (New York: Schocken Books, 1986), 146–62. Geographer David Harvey's term is "capital of modernity": Harvey, *Paris, Capital of Modernity* (New York: Routledge, 2003).

EPILOGUE

1. "Dossier: Pleins feux sur l'hygiène: Hygiène et santé," *La Lettre de l'Institut Pasteur,* 33 (April 2001): 7–9.

2. Ibid. (emphasis added).

3. Nancy J. Tomes and John Harley Warner, eds., *Rethinking the Reception of the Germ Theory of Disease: Comparative Perspectives,* a special issue of the *Journal of the History of Medicine and Allied Sciences* (vol. 51, no. 1, January 1997); Nancy Tomes, *The Gospel of Germs: Men, Women, and the Microbe in American Life* (Cambridge: Harvard University Press, 1998); Michael Worboys, *Spreading Germs: Disease Theories and Medical Practice in Britain, 1865–1900* (Cambridge: Cambridge University Press, 2000); Paul Weindling, *Health, Race, and German Politics between National Unification and Nazism, 1870–1945* (Cambridge: Cambridge University Press, 1989), 158–88; Elizabeth A. Hachten, "Science in the Service of Society: Bacteriology, Medicine, and Hygiene in Russia, 1855–1907" (Ph.D. diss., University of Wisconsin–Madison, 1991).

4. Many of these texts and events have legitimate and potentially important educational value: for example, the major U.S. and international traveling museum exhibits "Epidemic! The World of Infectious Disease," sponsored by Bristol-Myers Squibb (1999); "Microbes: Invisible Invaders, Amazing Allies," sponsored by Pfizer (1998–2005); and "Grossology" (2003–2005). Such exhibits, bankrolled by pharmaceutical companies, educate the public in creative, entertaining, and effective ways, but generally cannot resist the simple equations disease = germ and germ = disease.

5. For example, the series of special reports on CBS Evening News's "Eye on America" segment during the week of May 12, 1997.

6. *New York Times,* March 14, 2000 (emphasis added).

7. Mary Douglas, *Purity and Danger: An Analysis of Concepts of Pollution and Taboo* (1966; repr., London: Routledge, 2002), 36.

8. Among others, philosopher K. Codell Carter has made this case in a series of detailed historical studies focusing on the advent of bacteriological etiologies. Attention to causes that were neither necessary nor disease-specific "make[s] little sense if one is really interested in controlling disease, because prevention and treatment require necessity," he claimed in a 1991 article. Carter, "The Koch-Pasteur

Dispute on Establishing the Cause of Anthrax," *BHM* 65 (1991): 528–48. He later backed away somewhat from this aggressive stance in his 2003 book: "Recharacterizing diseases in terms of necessary causes was a major advance that made possible coherent explanations of disease phenomena as well as *systematic* treatment and prophylaxis." Carter, *The Rise of Causal Concepts of Disease: Case Histories* (Aldershot, England: Ashgate, 2003), 201, emphasis added. The addition of the qualifier "systematic" adds a degree of precision to the assertion. However, the kind of empirical nonbacteriological epidemiology championed by Villermé and the other early nineteenth-century hygienists, which produced studies like those correlating smoking with lung cancer, was nothing if not coherent and systematic. Carter's studies show persuasively that specific etiologies durably *changed* the nature of medical treatment and prevention, but they do not (and cannot) show that such etiologies were a *necessary precondition* of effective disease-fighting strategies.

9. Similarly, thirty years before Koch's identification of *Vibrio cholerae*, John Snow traced the 1854 outbreak of cholera around Golden Square in London to drinking water drawn from the Broad Street Pump, and recommended that the pump be shut down. Snow, *Snow on Cholera* (New York: The Commonwealth Fund, 1936); William Coleman, *Yellow Fever in the North: The Methods of Early Epidemiology* (Madison: University of Wisconsin Press, 1987), recounts how, in the half century preceding the Bacteriological Revolution, epidemiological studies in the absence of specific etiological knowledge inspired sophisticated and effective preventive measures.

10. Robert Koch, "The Aetiology of Tuberculosis" (1882), trans. Berna Pinner and Max Pinner, reprinted in David J. Rothman, Steven Marcus, and Stephanie A. Kiceluk, eds. *Medicine and Western Civilization* (New Brunswick: Rutgers University Press, 1995), 328.

11. It is difficult to pin down the precise timing and causes of the decline in cigarette smoking in the United States, for example. More research is needed to clarify the role of stigma in encouraging or accelerating this decline. Studies touching on this relationship include: Paul Rozin and Leher Singh, "The Moralization of Cigarette Smoking in America," *Journal of Consumer Behavior* 8 (1999): 321–37; David M. Cutler, "Behavioral Health Interventions: What Works and Why?" in Norman B. Anderson, Randy A. Bulatao, and Barney Cohen, eds., *Critical Perspectives on Racial and Ethnic Differences in Health in Late Life* (Washington, D.C.: National Academies Press, 2004), 643–74; Mark A. Hall, "The Scope and Limits of Public Health Law," *Perspectives in Biology and Medicine* 46 (2003): S199-S209; and Samuel H. Preston, "Deadweight? The Influence of Obesity on Longevity," *New England Journal of Medicine* 352 (2005): 1135–37.

12. David S. Jones, *Rationalizing Epidemics: Meanings and Uses of American Indian Mortality since 1600* (Cambridge: Harvard University Press, 2004), details the means by which inequality before death has been naturalized and explained away over the centuries.

13. Barbara Tuchman, *A Distant Mirror: The Calamitous Fourteenth Century* (New York: Knopf, 1978).

14. Henri de Parville, "Inauguration du monument Pasteur à Lille," *La Nature*,

April 15, 1899, 305–306. De Parville's article describes the "child" as having been "bitten by a rabid dog." There is nothing in the statue itself to suggest this, however, and the child in the statue is clearly a baby—not an older child, who might be more likely to be bitten by a dog. A baby, however, carries greater emotive value in the context of an artwork such as this one, and the overall effect of the baby in the Pasteur statue is to represent both an utterly helpless victim and the future France (and humanity as a whole) in need of salvation.

15. Patrice Debré, *Louis Pasteur*, trans. Elborg Forster (Baltimore: Johns Hopkins University Press, 1998), 416–17.

16. For example, Ebola and other hemorrhagic fevers, West Nile encephalitis, avian influenza, and bioterrorism.

17. Christopher Hamlin, *Public Health and Social Justice in the Age of Chadwick* (Cambridge: Cambridge University Press, 1998), 339–41.

Index

154–60, 227; of prisons, 144; by private companies, 155, 158–60; residential, 147–60, 210; resistance to, 146–51; vs. sanitation, 153, 158–59; of schools, 153, 177, 216; skepticism about, 144, 146–49, 157; stations for, 144; statistics on, 155–56, 157; stigma of, 155; tanks for, 143–46, 148, 180, 185–86, 207, 225

Double, François-Joseph, 91

Douglas, Mary, 5, 262

Driver, Felix, 102–3

Dujardin-Beaumetz, Georges, 126, 156

du Mesnil, Octave, 92, 235–36

Dumont, Georges, 153, 201

dysentery, 10, 93; etiology of, 20, 44, 77, 93, 200–201, 207; and isolation, 166; in military, 77, 166, 206–8

Eberth, Karl, 43, 105, 123, 195, 203

education, 61, 63, 64, 209; for adults, 169–74; and bacteriology, 138, 170, 174–76; civilizing effects of, 91–92, 223; by doctors and hygienists, 90–91, 106, 219, 225; health curriculum, 175–76, 224; mandatory secular public, 59, 91, 174–77, 221; and SBS, 138, 140. *See also* schools

Elias, Norbert, 5, 219–20, 222

emanations, 54, 68–70, 80, 200, 235; disease-causing, 36–49, 229; and odors, 36–49, 206; from sewers, 23–27, 44

environmental determinism, 75, 88–89

epidemic doctors, 125, 177, 178, 181, 186–87, 191, 208; as civilizers, 196, 225; on contagion, 163–69; on crowding, 120–21; definition of, 106; on disinfection, 140–54, 210, 212; as educators, 90–91, 106, 219, 224, 225; and government, 185, 213; vs. health councils, 106; history of, 106–7; on isolation, 140–41, 161–62; paternalism of, 221; on religion, 215; role of, 106–7, 218, 219, 223; on rural customs, 163, 167–68; and SBS, 107, 134; training of, 228

epidemics, decline in, 84–86, 156–57

Epidemics Committee. *See under* Academy of Medicine

etiologies, 105–39; academic, 108, 114; bacteriological, 14, 77, 126, 197; behavioral, 2, 96, 109, 220–21, 265; contagionist, 77, 122–24; folk, 108–10, 213; genetic, 265, 269; geographic, 110–16, 120; germ theory in, 3, 44–45, 124–26; individual, 108; local, 108–10, 114–16, 125, 127–28, "medical constitution" in, 116–20; miasmatic, 19, 44–45, 194–95; reductionist, 264–65; weather in, 116–17. *See also* causation; sanitary-bacteriological synthesis; *and specific diseases*

excrement, 83, 198, 223, 224; in cities, 78, 80–81; concealment of, 246, 251–53; containment of, 2, 100, 102, 202, 208, 269; and disgust, 199, 205–10; in gardens and yards, 207, 210; as infectious, 38–39, 43, 54, 67, 122, 194, 199, 205–9, 234, 256; in London, 243–44; as obsession, 208–9; odor of, 23–25, 31–33, 52–57, 94–95, 199, 205–10, 240, 254–60; and SBS, 205–11; in sewers, 52–57, 231; stockpiling of, 25–27; in waterways, 81, 187, 188

excrement, animal. *See* animals: waste from

expectations, 189

farms, sewage, 53, 54, 179

Faure, Olivier, 258

feces. *See* excrement

Féréol, Félix, 125–26

Ferry, Jules, 59, 61, 174, 221

Le Figaro, 29, 30, 230–31, 245–48

Flaubert, Achille, 198

Flemish population of France, 127, 196, 202, 215

food, 86, 201, 207, 240; adulterated, 131, 175; disease from, 93, 130; lack of, 97, 133, 210; poor, 196, 200, 264; in schools, 198–99

Foucault, Michel, 5

François I, King of France, 238

Franco-Prussian War, 58, 169

Frank, Johann Peter, 65–66

French Revolution, 13, 59, 212, 217

Freycinet, Charles de, 59

funerals, 165. *See also* cemeteries

Gailleton, Antoine, 151, 152

Gambetta, Léon, 61

garbage, 31, 76, 78, 97

Gautier, Armand, 235

Geoffroy Saint-Hilaire, Isidore, 43, 54

geography, medical, 110–20; and Bacteriological Revolution, 120, 123, 125; and Great Stink, 21–23, 26, 27, 240

Germany, 170, 178

germs: in air, 41–44, 95–96, 128–31, 135, 255; in city vs. country, 129–30, 135; and crowding, 200, 256; in dust, 41, 131, 135; in excrement, 12–23, 38–39, 43, 54, 67, 122, 194, 199, 205–9, 234, 256; in gases, 31, 35, 43, 47, 56; gospel of, 10, 169–74, 263; in hospitals, 77, 103, 136, 166; and infection, 241–43; invisibility of, 48; measurability of, 128–31; as metaphors, 258; omnipresence of, 42, 47–48, 130, 208, 261–62; as saprophytes, 133; as seeds, 45, 115, 125, 133, 196, 203; in water, 41, 119, 130, 179, 186, 199, 202–3, 269 germ theory, 7, 9, 138, 199, 255; acceptance of, 38, 132; application of, 127–32; emergence of, 36–49, 124–26; isolation in, 160–63; legacy of, 2, 266; presumptive analogy in, 160, 166; and sanitation, 120–22, 190; skepticism about, 121–22, 126, 132; and social change, 258

Gleichmann, Peter Reinhart, 252

Goudsblom, Johan, 220

government: accountability of, 59–60, 63, 87, 162, 213–14; active vs. inactive, 177–88; demands on, 12, 14, 27–36, 151–60, 181; and disinfection, 142–60; in Great Stink of 1880, 27–36, 59–63, 229; as protector, 212–13; responsive, 59–60, 62, 63, 162; role of, 7–8, 13, 29, 63, 65, 87, 131, 137–38, 151, 165, 177, 196, 212–15, 232–33, 237, 240, 252, 257; unresponsive, 28–29, 177–79, 230, 246–48. *See also* mayors; prefects

Great Stink of 1880, 10, 12–64; vs. 1895, 234, 236; causes of, 16, 23–27, 31; commission on, 1, 11–12, 29, 36–48, 54, 229; complaints in, 12, 15–23, 27–28, 53, 60, 245–55; enforcement in, 32–37; geography of, 21–23, 26, 27, 240; germ theory in, 1, 45–46; government in, 27–36, 59–63, 229; mortality in, 20–21, 31, 35; newspapers in, 12, 245–49; and republicanism, 58–63; sewers in, 52–58, 229; significance of, 13, 240, 244, 259

Great Stink of 1895, 229–37; vs. 1880, 234, 236; causes of, 231, 233–34, 254–58; commission on, 233–36; complaints in, 230–32, 236–37, 254–57; disgust in, 230–31, 241–45, 254–58; excrement in, 254–56; germs in, 254–60; government in, 232–33

Grison, Georges, 29, 30

Guéneau de Mussy, Henri, 122–23, 203

habitus, 253–54

Hamlin, Christopher, 270

Harvey, David, 51

Haussmann, Georges Eugène, Baron, 24, 49–52, 61, 64

Hazebrouck, 127, 196, 202, 215

Henle, Jacob, 127

heterogenesis. *See* spontaneous generation

Hiblot, Ernest, 181–82, 192–93

hospitals, 103, 167, 210, 233, 238; air in, 73, 131; contagion in, 77, 166; germs in, 77, 103, 136, 166; isolation in, 160, 166, 192–93

The Hot Zone (Preston), 145

housing: in Brittany, 88–91; disinfection of, 147–60; legislation on, 171, 196, 234; overcrowded, 96–100; of peasants, 97, 211; reform in, 63–64, 75–76; substandard, 49, 64, 65, 75, 84, 96–100, 136, 171, 235; urban, 14, 135; working-class, 75, 84, 96–100, 102–3, 136, 196–97, 202, 225

Hugo, Victor, 57, 251

hygiene, 84, 228; lectures on, 169–72; personal, 93, 97–99, 175, 209, 256, 260; in schools, 174, 175, 209, 217, 224. *See also* cleanliness; sanitation

hygienists, early. *See* sanitarians

industrialization, 4, 33, 74, 86, 91, 100, 243

industries, 70, 79–80, 83, 132, 240; fertilizer, 237; horse-rendering, 68–70; regulation of, 32, 234; tanning, 36, 79, 240; textile, 72–73

"infection," 134, 229–37, 247, 269; definition of, 241, 257; etymology of, 241, 242; in Great Stinks, 241–43; invisibility of, 241–43

insects, 18, 19, 40, 67, 98, 201, 262, 263

isolation, 161–67; of children, 8, 163–64, 165, 167, 168; of contagious persons, 103, 122–23; epidemic doctors on, 140–41, 161–62; in hospitals, 160, 166, 193; and placarding, 160–61; resistance to, 163–69; and schools, 123, 177

J'Accuse (Zola), 247

Jenner, Edward, 123, 190, 263

Kelsch, Achille, 132–34, 163

Klebs, Edwin, 43, 131

Koch, Robert, 9, 127, 262, 264

La Berge, Ann, 66, 68

laboratories, 126–32, 263, 264–65; animals in, 43, 255; expectations from, 189, 211; and industry, 132; and Pasteur, 2, 38, 41–42, 190; role of, 3, 9, 37, 127–35, 171; and SBS, 189–93, 197

Lachaise, Claude, 74

Lamouroux, Alfred, 236

Launay (Vicomte de), 76

Lecouturier, Henri, 76

legislation: anticlerical, 59; on burial, 137; on disinfection, 151–52; on dumping, 238; on education, 174; enforcement of, 32–37, 214–15; housing, 171, 196, 234; on industry, 32, 234; on reporting disease, 180; on *tout-à-l'égout*, 229–30; on treatment plants, 35, 236; on urination, 79

Le Havre, 63–64, 120, 131, 142, 200, 254

Lépine, Louis, 232–33

Le Roy des Barres, Alexandre, 234

Lille, 4, 115, 131–32, 153, 201; canals of, 95, 96; disinfection in, 144, 152; Pasteur Monument in, 266–69; poverty in, 96–100

Lister, Joseph, 4, 141, 173
London, 49, 243–44
Louis XIV, King of France, 106
Lyon, 130, 151, 180, 205, 214–15

MacMahon, Patrice, 58
malaria, 110–13, 134, 263, 269
malnutrition, 97, 133, 210
Marié-Davy, Hippolyte, 47, 135–37
marshes, 45, 110–13, 134
Martin, André-Justin, 144–45, 154–57
Maunoury, Gabriel, 191–93
mayors, 177–88, 204, 212, 214–19
measles, 10, 118, 122, 130, 132, 161, 177, 212–13
medical constitution, 116–20, 138
Meister, Joseph, 267
Mêlier, François, 91
mentalités, 5–6
miasmas, 1, 2, 4, 17, 19, 43–45, 91, 112–13, 122, 171; in cemeteries, 129; from crowding, 77–78, 126; disinfection of, 84, 141; from horse rendering, 68–70; and typhoid fever, 43–44, 123, 194–95; urban, 135
miasmatism, 37, 42; definition of, 45; vs. germ theory, 44–46, 95–96, 113; in Great Stink of 1880, 14, 36–49; persistence of, 194–98, 257
Michel, Arthur, 254–55
microbes. *See* germs
microbiology. *See* bacteriology
military, 50, 73; diseases in, 74, 77, 103, 115, 121, 122, 138, 166, 199, 206–8
Les Misérables (Hugo), 57
monarchists, 58, 61
Monier, Ernest, 173
Monod, Henri, 144
Montfaucon, 68–70, 72, 81–83, 94
Montpellier, 4, 210, 213
Montsouris Observatory, 41–42
morality, 86, 98; and crowding, 74–75; and disease, 3, 64, 93, 196, 212–13, 241, 265; and filth, 80, 84, 92–100, 197; and progress, 63, 68, 85; of workers, 72–73, 75, 93–94
mortality: from anthrax, 39; in children, 20–21, 60, 80, 81, 94, 117, 149, 167–68, 172, 192–93; from diarrhea, 20–21; from diphtheria, 149–50, 167–68, 192, 216, 268; and disinfection, 156–57; in Great Stink of 1880, 20–21, 31, 35; and morality, 64; from rabies, 43, 189–90, 267–68; from sweating sickness, 183; from typhoid fever, 21, 90, 268; of workers, 56–57, 64
Murard, Lion, 178–79
Murchison, Charles, 44

Nanterre, 16, 25–27, 28, 34
Napoleon I, 65
Napoleon III, 49–51
New Caledonia, 222
newspapers, 52, 60, 149, 150, 230–31, 262; vs. bureaucracy, 62; and disgust, 245–49; on disinfection, 153; exaggeration by, 32, 33; and freedom of the press, 61; in Great Stinks, 17–19, 20, 27–30, 236, 245–49
New York, 160
Nord, Philip, 61

obesity, 264, 265
odors, 12–64, 220, 229–59; asphyxiation from, 18, 69, 78, 80, 255; cataloging and measuring, 233–35; from cesspits, 23–25, 31–33, 81; from corpses, 239; and disinfection, 142, 149; exaggeration of, 248–49; from excrement, 23–25, 31–33, 52–57, 94–95, 199, 205–10, 240, 254–60; harmlessness of, 35, 234; history of, 238–40; in London, 243–44; mapping of, 233, 235; as pathogenic, 1, 12–23, 36–38, 95–96; from sewers, 24, 44, 52–58, 208; tolerance of, 240, 250, 252, 255, 257; from treatment plants, 16, 24–27, 31–36; in 20th century, 237
Ollivier, Auguste, 165, 208

Parent-Duchâtelet, Alexandre-Jean-Baptiste, 67, 68–73, 78–85, 94–95, 160
Paris: bureaucracy of, 218; City Council of, 25, 31–32, 55, 60, 61, 155; disinfection in, 144–49, 154–60, 227; growth of, 49–52, 79, 259; housing in, 14, 74, 223; in Middle Ages, 238–39; sensory environment of, 94, 232–35; sewer system of, 49–58; waste disposal in, 78–85, 208
Paris Commune (1871), 21, 58–59
Parliament (Britain), 243–44
Parliament (France), 59, 91
Pasteur, Louis, 11, 35, 47, 173, 258; as alarmist, 42–44, 48; on anthrax, 38; on disinfection, 142–44; on emanations, 96, 257; funeral of, 1–2; laboratory of, 2, 38, 41–42; legacy of, 11, 124–26, 132, 137–38, 170, 188–89, 212, 255, 262; and Lister, 4, 141; on Paris odors commission, 1, 12, 36, 38; and rabies, 42–43, 267–68; on sewers, 54–55; on spontaneous generation, 41–42; and vaccines, 38–43, 140
Pasteur Institute, 2, 11, 131–32, 193, 222, 260, 267
Pasteur Monument (Lille), 266–69
peasants, 200, 213–14; in Brittany, 88–91, 215; civilizing of, 90, 211–12, 219–28; culture of, 8, 227; housing of, 97, 211; and manure, 202–5; and republicanism, 211–12

52–57, 208; gases in, 55–56, 244; in London, 243–44; manholes and ventilation openings, 24, 27, 54, 248; modernization of, 15, 50–52; odors from, 24, 44, 52–58, 208; of Paris, 49–58; purpose of, 24–25; testing of, 129, 130; tourists in, 57–58; typhoid fever in, 54, 179; water in, 24, 231

Shapin, Steven, 6

Siegfried, Jules, 63–64

slaughterhouses, 36, 201, 216

slums. *See* housing: substandard

smallpox, 2, 20, 86, 122, 151, 177; contagiousness of, 9–10, 77, 130, 132, 170; disinfection after, 142–43; vaccine against, 10, 82, 190, 263

smoking, 67, 93, 99, 123, 174, 263, 265

"socialism of the microbe," 171

specificity: of germs, 105, 108, 125, 196–97, 199, 208–9, 223, 263–64; in Great Stink of 1895, 257–58

spontaneous generation, 41–42, 132–34

sputum, 131, 201, 221, 251, 256

Stallybrass, Peter, 250

St.-Malo, 105, 163, 164, 194–96

Straus, Isidore, 131

sulfur, 141, 149, 153, 159

swamps, 84, 86, 122, 263

sweating sickness, 182–86

syphilis, 2, 132, 220

Tableau de l'état physique et moral... (Villermé), 72–73, 75, 96

Tardieu, Ambroise, 81–82

teachers, 172, 177, 217; and contagion, 164–66; hygiene of, 175, 209; and secularism, 164, 174

Temkin, Owsei, 241

La Terre (Zola), 246

toilets, 31, 79, 99, 142, 233; and disgust, 136, 246; gas from, 171, 244; germs in, 44, 130, 151, 206; legislation on, 53; privacy in, 101–2; in schools, 175–76

Tomes, Nancy, 134, 171

tout-à-l'égout (everything into the sewers), 53–57, 229–31, 237, 252. *See also* sewers treatment plants. *See* waste treatment plants

Troisier, Emile, 138–39

tuberculosis, 9–10, 20, 124, 131, 161, 221, 264

typhoid fever, 10, 132, 151, 161, 163, 170, 180–81; caused by odors, 20, 234; contagion in, 163, 225–26; from crowding, 77, 125–26, 194–96, 198; deaths from, 21, 90, 268; decline of, 157; etiology of, 105, 108, 114–15; and food, 198–99; and germs, 38, 121, 124, 130, 195; healthy carriers of, 168; and laboratories, 132, 179; and miasmas, 43–44, 123, 194–95;

in military, 115, 121, 199; and peasants, 204, 215; in provinces, 125, 194, 204–6; and SBS, 134, 172; in schools, 198, 217; sources of, 34, 38, 43, 44, 54, 123, 171, 179, 194, 200, 202; specific microbe of, 43, 105, 115, 123, 195, 203; from water, 105, 119, 179, 186, 202–3

typhus, 77, 103, 120, 144, 152, 170, 234

Ulbach, Louis, 248–49

Universal Exposition (1900), 146

urbanization, 79, 82, 85, 94, 160, 239–40, 243; problems of, 48–52

urination, public, 79–80, 99, 100, 234, 238

urine, 6, 206, 240

vaccines: for anthrax, 2, 38, 39, 140, 189, 267; and Pasteur, 38–43, 140; for rabies, 2, 132, 138, 140, 189–90; for smallpox, 10, 82, 190, 263

Veber, Adrien, 155

venereal disease, 95

ventilation, 31, 70, 73, 74, 91, 101–2, 135–36, 141, 239

vidange. See cesspits

vidangeurs. See cesspits: cleaners of

Vigarello, Georges, 197

Villemin, Jean-Antoine, 124–25, 197

Villermé, Louis-René, 67, 85, 86, 160, 211, 262, 266; on alcohol, 99–100; on bodily separation, 101–2, 269; in Brittany, 87–91; on housing, 74, 75, 96–100; on investigation, 72–73; optimism regarding progress, 84, 200; on sexuality, 96, 99; on toilets, 101–2; on workers, 93, 96–100

von Gietl, Franz, 44

waste: from animals, 68–70, 78, 81, 199, 202–5, 212, 224, 237, 255; dumping of, 16, 35, 52–57, 229–31, 237, 252; exportation of, 16, 30, 244; history of, 238; in Paris, 78–85, 208; and population growth, 49; in public space, 78–82; in rivers, 69, 243–44; suburban vs. urban, 16. *See also* waste treatment plants

waste, human. *See* excrement

waste treatment plants, 16, 32, 34, 35, 236; animal waste in, 68–70, 237; in Great Stink of 1895, 230, 232, 237; odor from, 16, 24–27, 34; suburban, 16, 25–27, 31, 46, 236

water, 88; boiling of, 41, 153, 185, 225; in canals, 52, 95, 96; germs in, 41, 119, 130, 179, 186, 199, 202–3, 269; pollution of, 24, 69, 79, 81, 187, 188, 202, 224, 269; in sewers, 24, 52, 231; supply of, 49, 50, 52, 53, 79, 231; testing of, 110, 129, 130, 132; and typhoid fever, 105, 119, 179, 186, 202–3 weather: and disease, 2, 86, 93, 94, 110–13, 118, 138–39; in etiology, 116–17; in Great Stinks, 12, 25, 27, 33, 35, 230; and London stink, 243; and medical constitution, 118–19; and mortality, 117–18; and odor, 16–17, 237

Weber, Eugene, 196

White, Allon, 250

whooping cough, 10, 118, 162, 177, 181–82

working classes, 50, 55–57, 64, 74, 98, 178, 187, 188, 192, 215, 226, 239; and alcohol, 99–100; disgust among, 251; disinfection of, 142–43; geography of, 22–23; health of, 72–73, 83; housing for, 63, 75, 84, 96, 101–2, 196–97, 202, 225; hygiene of, 147–48; morality of, 72–73, 75, 93–94; safety of, 145–48

World's Fair (1900), 146

yellow fever, 170

Zola, Emile, 245–48

Zylberman, Patrick, 178–79